BEYOND LOVE

BEYOND LOVE

Dominique Lapierre

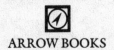

ARROW BOOKS

Arrow Books Limited
20 Vauxhall Bridge Road, London SW1V 2SA

An imprint of the Random Century Group

London Melbourne Sydney Auckland Johannesburg
and agencies throughout the world

First published in 1991 by Century
Arrow edition 1991

1 3 5 7 9 10 8 6 4 2

© 1990 by Dominique Lapierre

Printed and bound in Great Britain by
Cox & Wyman Ltd, Reading

ISBN 0 09 987370 2

To Alvin, Ananda, Bandona, Barbara, Burt, Charles, Christian, Christine, Claude, Dale, Dani, Daniel, Dannie, David, Deborah, Ellen, Flossie, Françoise, George, Gloria, Harold, Isabelle, Jack, Jacqueline, Jacques, James, Jean-Claude, Jerome, Jim, Joel, John, Josef, Joseph, Luc, Marcus, Margaret, Martha, Marty, Mary, Mathilde, Michael, Mikulas, Myron, Palma, Paul, Peng, Peter, Philippe, Prem, Randy, Richard, Robert, Ron, Samuel, Sandra, Sugar, Teresa, Terry, Willy, Zaki . . . and to all those—scientists, doctors, caring people, patients—known or unknown, who in their everyday confrontation with the disease show they are *beyond love*.

CONTENTS

CONTENTS

AUTHOR'S NOTE TO THE READER

Several protagonists of this book, among them a number of patients and their families, have asked me to respect their anonymity and to write their stories in a way that would not make them recognizable. Therefore, I felt the obligation to alter their descriptions to such an extent that they would not be identifiable from reading the book. Similarly, the characters of the sisters of Mother Teresa are actually composite portrayals. Each one is based upon several real people and real events, but because not one of these sisters is a true individual, the anonymity of all is preserved. In this way the story of these patients and of these sisters remains faithful to the spirit of their exceptional vocation and destinies.

Although this book is the result of long and careful research, it doesn't claim to depict *all* the events of the incredible human and scientific epic that took place between 1980 and 1986 on the battlefront of AIDS. It does not claim either to mention the names of all those who played a role during all those dramatic years, nor all those who continue each day to work toward finding a way to protect mankind from one of the most terrible plagues of all time.

May this book pay a tribute to all of them.

D.L.

*Only virtue gives a good karma
and the greatest of all virtues is compassion*

—BUDDHA

PART ONE

They Called It
"The Wrath of God"

1

A Frail Figure on the Banks of Immortality
Benares, India: Autumn 1980

It was there. In that setting of fire and smoke and death. Amidst
the stench of burnt flesh, the ballet of bamboo litters bearing the
deceased, and the strident crackle of flames consuming corpses. Yes,
it was there, in the putrid water some lengths from the infernal
bank, among the floating cadavers of dogs and rats, and sometimes
of men too poor or too holy to be burnt, that her frail and half-
immersed figure would show itself. With her large eyes outlined
with kohl, her ring shining in the ala of her nose, her braids tied
with ribbons, and her bright yellow blouse, which the Ganges River
glued to her skin, Ananda, the thirteen-year-old Indian girl, was
like a bouquet of flowers offered to the gods of the sacred river.
Her name meant "joy," but her nickname suggested no such idea
of happiness. She was known as "the little Ganges vulture." Her
hunting ground was the silt of that great purificatory river, near
the funeral pyres where Hindus hoped in cremation to find escape
from the cycle of rebirths, and thus attain eternal deliverance. With
the help of her two young brothers, Ananda spent her days searching
for treasure as she sifted through the pestilent mud that was thick-
ened by the ashes of the deceased. With luck she might find a ring,

a half-eroded religious pendant, a gold tooth, or simply some remnants of calcified wood.

From up on the veranda of the temple that dominated the riverbank, the girl's father squatted on a silk cushion embroidered with gold thread as if it were a throne. Amit Prakash, aged forty-one, was a small man with an air of sadness and hair that glistened with mustard oil. Like many ancestors before him, Ananda's father was director of the funeral ceremonies that prepared Hindus for immortality, the grand master in charge of the cremation of corpses. Immediately in front of him rose the symbol of his rank and power in the city, a small altar shaped like a basin in which glowed the embers of the sacrificial fire. By virtue of this trade, he and his kin belonged to the *dom* caste, the lowest and the most impure in the Hindu hierarchy. So infamous was his birth, so "untouchable" his person, that on his death his body could not be reduced to cinders on his own pyres. Instead it would be carried far afield, to a place outside the city where those considered as untouchables were burnt.

Day and night the bamboo biers brought bodies swathed in white or red for cremation on the fires laid by servants in the employ of Ananda's father. Apparently insensible to the macabre spectacle and the smell of burnt flesh, people came and went from one pyre to the next. Nearby, on steps overlooking the river, barbers carefully shaved the heads of relatives of the dead, while fat-bellied Brahmins argued the price of their priestly services. The inevitable animals participated as well. Cows and goats grazed upon the garlands from the mortuary litters, and dogs the color of ashes exhumed the scraps that had escaped incineration. Black birds awaited their share, swooping down from the sky to snap up some piece of human debris in passing.

Ananda and her family lived in a vast residence adjoining the palace of the maharaja of Jaipur. It jutted out over the Ganges. Painted black and yellow, the two stone tigers adorning its terrace balustrade looked as if they were mocking the two marble lions that decorated the neighboring palace. Legend had it that at one time the maharaja, exasperated by this irreverence, had tried to have his neighbors evicted. At the judiciary tribunal, Ananda's ancestor had retorted to the august prince: "Your Highness, are we not both kings? You are the king of life, I am the king of death." The maharaja of Jaipur had lost his suit. The cremator of corpses had won. From that day onward he would qualify for the title of "Dom raja."

As Indian tradition would have it, the family's house was also home to many of Ananda's relatives: her grandparents, uncles, and their families, in all about thirty people who lived off the proceeds of the cremations. Access was gained to the numerous rooms via a maze of staircases and inner courtyards. A distant relative had even built a family temple on a terrace within the structure, decorated with white and blue tiles and dedicated to the god Rama. But its iron gate could never be opened. The Dom raja's family were only allowed to pray outside the sanctuary: in India untouchables do not approach the gods. All they may do is ring the bell to alert them to their presence.

A billy goat lived in one of the courtyards. Once a year, for the festival of Sayr Devi, honoring one of the untouchables' goddesses, Ananda's father would enter his billy goat in a fierce contest against other billy goats. If his animal won, he would offer it as a sacrifice to the deity. The other courtyards were cluttered with piles of bamboo used to make the funeral biers, and special stocks of sandalwood destined for the cremations of the rich. Ananda's father had to be able to meet all the requirements imposed by his office. The sale of sandalwood brought in considerable revenue. Between seven and eleven *mound* of fuel, or nearly nine hundred pounds of wood, could be consumed, depending on the size of the deceased. This would cost approximately four hundred rupees, the equivalent of about twenty-four dollars. Few people had access to that sort of money. The others settled with the Dom raja on a reduced-rate cremation. The parts of the body that remained unconsumed due to insufficient fuel were thrown in the Ganges.

Ananda's father and uncles took turns relieving each other as guardians of the sacrificial fire. The family business went on day and night. They employed about thirty coolies and wardens for the pyres, the flames of which were never extinguished. The uninterrupted growth of the Indian population meant an ever-increasing afflux of old people who, sensing their impending end, came to Benares to die. The result was that funeral processions frequently caused bottlenecks in the alleyway leading to the small municipal office where relatives were required to declare the civil status of the deceased and the cause of his demise. This traffic helped build the fortunes of the numerous stall keepers along the route who specialized in the sale of shrouds, garlands, sandalwood powder, and other funerary items. Some shops offered sumptuous silk goods embroidered with gold, luxury items that only the rich could provide for their dead. From time to time, over the heads of the crowd that blocked the narrow street, a litter adorned with a dais strewn with flowers would come into view. On it a dead old man in his saffron robe would be propped up in a sitting position. The bearers sounded gongs to punctuate their mantras. This deceased was not a client for Ananda's father. He was one of the sadhus, holy men already released from the cycle of reincarnations. They were committed to the Ganges without being burnt.

*   *   *

Ananda's grandmother was a wizened woman dressed in the white cotton sari of a widow. Every morning, after her ablutions, she came to collect her thoughts in front of the portrait of her deceased husband that occupied the most prominent position on the wall of the communal room. It was hung among a collection of engravings evoking scenes from the *Ramayana*, the famous legendary epic of Hinduism. The yellowing photograph showed a splendid old man with a white beard, wearing a red turban. But for a tiny piece of material hiding his sex, he was completely naked. The exploits of this remarkable individual were often boasted of in the family. Apart from his occupation as a burner of corpses, he was renowned in Benares for his agile displays as a fakir. Sometimes he would lift enormous blocks of stone. Or he would lie for endless hours on a board studded with nails. It was in the exercise of his professional duties, however, that he had earned his principal claim to fame. Hearing on the radio on January 30, 1948, that Mahatma Gandhi, the father of the nation, had just been assassinated in New Delhi, he had leaped aboard the first train to the capital. For his only luggage he had taken with him an urn full of embers, in order that the funeral pyre of India's "Great Soul" might be lit with the sacred fire of Benares.

Ananda's mother was a frail woman whose pockmarked face bore the reminders of a smallpox attack from which she had nearly died as a small child. Her authority was undisputed for it was she who held the purse strings. Every evening her husband would passively hand over the proceeds from the cremations, which she would then put away in a padlocked chest for which, it was said, she was the only person to hold a key. It was to her that Ananda and her two brothers had to bring the fruits of their foragings in the Ganges. She was quite without equal in her capacity to evaluate the weight of a tooth or the worth of a fragment of jewel. More often than not she greeted her children with a reprimand. "Our fishing was never quite fruitful enough," Ananda would recall. "Poor mother! And yet she knew that people hardly ever left ornaments on the bodies of their dead anymore. Gold and silver had become so expensive!"

* * *

The cremator's daughter had just, that very autumn, reached the age of puberty. On the announcement of this event, her father hastened to carry out the most sacred mission that falls to any Indian father: that of finding her a husband. In fact, Ananda's parents had been thinking about her marriage ever since she was born. To prepare for it, her mother had introduced her to all the domestic duties, even the most thankless ones. For her there had been no play or school, only the care of her brothers, the drudgery of carrying water, the washing, the housework, and of course, the recovery of jewels and wood from the Ganges.

Several gentlemen soon disembarked at the Dom raja's house to engage in secret meetings with him. "My mother confirmed what I already suspected," Ananda would say. "The visitors were envoys from the family of the husband my father hàd chosen for me. They had come to discuss the financial conditions of my marriage. Here in India these negotiations are arduous and endless. I couldn't make out what was actually being said under the large-winged fan in the room into which my father and the envoys had shut themselves. But the bargaining can't have been easy because the sound of raised voices kept coming through the walls."

One day, the visitors turned up accompanied by a man in a white *dhoti* carrying some rolls of paper under his arm. He was a *joshi*, an astrologer, who had come to study the astrological charts with Ananda's father and his guests to mark the position of the planets and say whether the conjunction of the heavenly bodies at the girl's birth was compatible with that of the boy chosen for her. The test having proved positive, the *joshi* indicated the most propitious day and time for the prospective union. Ananda had neither the opportunity nor the right to express her opinion. She had not even set eyes on the man who was to become her husband.

*   *   *

Fourteen days before her wedding, just as her father was having her dowry taken to her future in-laws and workmen were already engaged in constructing a bamboo dais draped in muslin to provide shade for the ceremony, the girl noticed a slightly protruding light patch the size of a chick-pea on her cheek, just next to the gilded ring through the ala of her nose. With the tip of her finger she felt the spot and found to her astonishment that it was completely insensitive to touch. Neither the pressure of a nail nor the prick of a pin provoked the slightest sensation in that part of her face. It was as if the life had suddenly gone out of that area of her flesh.

Yet "the little Ganges vulture" was not really worried. She was used to it. In the time that she had been spending half her life in its putrid waters, the great river had hardly given her skin a moment's rest. Pimples, pustules, boils were forever swelling up at some point on her body. Her astonishing resistance had always triumphed over these onslaughts. They would disappear in two or three days.

Since this strange blemish that was insensitive to touch persisted for longer than usual, she showed it to her mother, who sent out for a *quack*, one of the backstreet healers whose concoctions and plant unctions purported to cure the most stubborn ills. The old man examined the little girl's cheek.

"There's no ointment to cure this disease," he said softly. "It's leprosy."

2

Mice and Their Executioner

Los Angeles, USA: Autumn 1980

Each of his days began with a lover's rendezvous. As soon as he got to his cramped laboratory at the University of California at Los Angeles, thirty-two-year-old Dr. Michael S. Gottlieb, a placid bear of a man with curly hair and a blond mustache, took from his attaché case the tidbits destined each morning for the companions who for years now had shared his hopes and his frustrations as a research scientist. With slow, almost religious movements he cut the potatoes into thin slices and offered them to his mice. Michael Gottlieb had more than 250 of them, all female, all brown and so fat that they could have passed for small rats. He called them his "princesses." They were members of the aristocracy of their species, the famous C3H line, the flawless products of generations of genetic selection, mice so intelligent, so cooperative, so easy to manipulate, that they inspired love and respect.

And yet every day, Michael Gottlieb martyred, mutilated, and massacred some of these endearing creatures, the objects of his tender morning attentions. With lethal rays he bombarded their spleens, their marrow, their thymus glands, and their ganglions, those organs that in mice as in men manufacture or stock the cells responsible for protecting the body against outside attack. Known

as white cells or lymphocytes, these cells are the organism's guards-.
men. As soon as a foreign agent appears, irrespective of whether it
is a microbe or a virus, they are mobilized; but they are also mobilized in the case of a graft implanted to replace a defective organ.
By inflicting such torture on his mice to destroy their immune
systems, Michael Gottlieb was seeking to discover a sure way of
neutralizing the rejection phenomena in humans that still made
organ grafting such a gamble.

*   *   *

His specialty, immunology, was the study of man's major problem: his capacity to defend himself against the artful and unseen
enemies that constantly threaten his body. Making great strides at
the beginning of the eighties, this discipline was not a totally new
science. For two centuries, thanks to Edward Jenner, discoverer of
the concept of vaccination, thanks to Louis Pasteur, to Robert
Koch, discoverer of the tuberculosis bacillus, and so many other
scientists, it had been known that the human body is endowed with
the power to protect itself. But the mechanisms ordering and con-
trolling this defense system had proved to be so sophisticated and
so complicated that it had been necessary to await the birth of
cellular immunology in the second half of the twentieth century
before their secrets could be penetrated. The instruments of this
achievement allied themselves more readily to the culinary art than
to pure science. In fact, it was in the process of finding a means of
growing cells in the laboratory, of cultivating them and keeping
them alive, that in the sixties immunologists opened up areas of
hitherto unsuspected investigation.

What prospects there were for an ambitious young doctor burning to make his contribution to the scientific community at the end
of the century! "What fascinated me about immunology was the
very nature of its field of experimentation," Michael Gottlieb would
acknowledge. "In the same way that sociology makes it possible to
explain the political and social ramifications of a culture, immunology provides the keys to a system, a system which has its logic,
its laws, its failures, its successes; a system which one can learn to
manipulate, control, modify. Not blindly like we used to, but with
all the delicacy of touch of a goldsmith, by listening to the music
of the cells, by deciphering their dialogue, by understanding the

mechanics of their relationships, with, at the very end of all this prospecting, a dream. Our dream, as doctors, of prolonging life."

* * *

The route toward this dream had revealed itself to him twelve years previously with the arrival of an unexpected guest in the family home. "What did it was a cat," Michael Gottlieb would relate, "a splendid alley tomcat called Tabby. My mother had picked it up off the street in the small New Jersey town where my father was a physical education teacher. Tabby had scarcely taken up residence and begun to purr beneath our roof before my head blew up like a pumpkin. I began to cry, blow my nose, sneeze. There was no doubt about it: I was allergic to Tabby. In her concern, my mother wanted to throw the animal back out on the streets, but I stopped her. Somewhere in my fat pumpkin head a question had just germinated. Could you overcome an allergy, stop suffering the ill effects, without removing the cause? In my case, without giving up Tabby, the cat?"

It took Michael Gottlieb three months of suffering, of blocked sinuses, sneezing attacks, swollen eye sockets, and skin rashes to get to the bottom of it. The answer was yes. "Unlike most allergies, which are aggravated by the presence of the source, in the end my system desensitized itself to contact with our cat," he would explain. "To put it another way, my body had autoimmunized itself, or even better, autovaccinated itself."

That was the future researcher's first encounter with the science of immunology. "An encounter which would decide my career," he would recall. "Why had I been the only one in my family to suffer on account of our cat's presence? Why me and not the others?" The question was so intriguing that young Michael soon found himself in the classes of the medical school at the University of Rochester.

Instead of the answer, he would find love in the somewhat unromantic setting of laboratory flasks and test tubes. With her snub nose, freckles, and mischievous air, the blond Cynthia looked a little like the actress Katharine Hepburn. She was working for a degree in hematology with a view to specializing in the field of blood transfusion.

If their shared passion had very naturally brought them together over their microscopes, it was not for the same reasons. Cynthia's interest was fixed upon the vectors of life, the red cells, those millions of tiny spherical corpuscles that provide the tissues with oxygen they collect from the lungs. "Since 1920, when the pathologist Karl Landsteiner won the Nobel Prize for his discovery of blood groups, people had known nearly everything there was to know about red cells. That's why those cells seemed so interesting to me," Cynthia would say. "With them I felt I was in control of the game. There was no danger of their letting me down, playing tricks on me, showing up the cracks in my knowledge. Red cells made good partners, not too restless and not too complicated."

Michael Gottlieb's fascination, on the other hand, focused on the other blood component, on the white cells, those prodigious chemical factories, the system's guardsmen whose deficiencies are responsible for so many fatal disorders. He tried to convince Cynthia that she should follow him and help him in his work. "That's the direction research should be moving in," he explained to her. "The study of lymphocytes is a priority. That's where the stakes for the Nobel Prizes of the future are. But all my efforts to induce Cynthia to abandon her red cells for my white ones proved abortive."

All the same, the two laboratory assistants managed to find an area of shared understanding. Having become Mrs. Michael Gottlieb, Cynthia was to obtain her degree and find a job in a blood bank. Thus the champion of the red cells made it possible for the champion of the white cells to continue his studies, become a doctor of medicine, and eventually specialize. Contrary to all expectations, he settled on medical practice, sweeping aside the thing that he had always seemed to cherish: research.

"I had suddenly become allergic to the frigid abstraction of laboratories, to their inhumanity, their assay plates, their test tubes, their centrifuges, their computers, to all the paraphernalia that seemed to belong to science fiction films. Of course it's in laboratories that our knowledge is increased, but I yearned to listen to sick people, to relieve their suffering, to cure, to save lives. I wanted to be a doctor." This ambition would take the student into cardiac surgery. "It was mind-blowing. I would build up a sympathetic relationship with a patient. Then, suddenly on the end of my scalpel, I would catch sight of his heart that had to be connected up to a machine so that the chief surgeon could repair it. For me, surgery was a school of excellence, of technical perfection, that pushed the frontiers of the impossible a little further back each day. What other branch of medicine could claim to save so many lives?"

Two years later, a research scholarship to Stanford University under Prof. Henry Kaplan, one of the world's experts in cancerous blood disorders such as Hodgkin's disease, would enable the young surgeon to return to his first love and rejoin his former accomplices, the white cells. It was there that he experienced his first scientific failure with the death of a young woman from rural Iowa, a leukemia patient whom he had given a bone marrow transplant using a technique perfected on his mice. "It was a terrible shock," he would remember, "but above all, it was a sharp warning against the temptation to use treatment that was inadequately proven. And yet, despite my frustration and sadness, I still felt a sort of pride, the pride of working at the forefront of human biology, at the crossroads of all the big problems: cancers, leukemias, unexplained cellular disorders. This awareness of being among the pioneers helped me to overcome my discouragement. It was a case of getting back to the drawing board and starting again. I still had so much to learn!"

* * *

It was precisely to keep on learning that, in June 1980, Michael Gottlieb would apply for a post as researcher and medical practitioner at UCLA, the University of California at Los Angeles, where one of the specialists in bone marrow transplants was working: the youthful Prof. Robert Gale, the man who would come to the aid of the Soviets in their attempts to save the victims of radiation from the nuclear disaster at Chernobyl. In that autumn of 1980 the UCLA researchers' work was attracting great interest. For the year 1980–81 alone some six hundred scientists there would share a number of grants amounting to some $130 million for work on the brain, the eyes, cardiovascular infections, and infantile diseases; for research into the mysteries of cancer and immunodeficiency disorders; for the perfection of diagnostic techniques; but also for a whole program of research that would enable chemistry, and nuclear medicine supported by new computer technology, to develop revolutionary medical treatments. Already that same autumn, two UCLA researchers had just carried out the first human experiment in genetic therapy by injecting human genes into patients suffering from fatal anemia. Again that same autumn, Robert Gale's team was announcing that its work on bone marrow transplants offered hope of survival in up to 60 percent of leukemia cases, which had previously been fatal in almost all adult victims.

* * *

One morning, having scattered his potato slices into their cages, Michael Gottlieb made ready to submit a batch of his mice to a new phase in the program of experiments developed by Professor Gale. This program would require their sacrifice in a test involving massive irradiation after the removal of their spleens. Asked about the cruelty to which he subjected his beloved mice, he would reply: "The conviction that their suffering would one day benefit mankind spared me too much painful soul-searching."

A knock at the door brought his mice an unexpected stay of execution. Michael Gottlieb saw the smiling face of his colleague Howard M. Schanker framed in the doorway of his tiny laboratory. Like Gottlieb, twenty-six-year-old Howard Schanker, a medical intern, came originally from the East Coast. He had obtained a scholarship to come to UCLA to take a course on the treatment of allergies. Under Michael Gottlieb's direction, this course included practical work in the university hospital's various departments for patients suffering from immunodeficiency disorders. There was no one quite like this New Yorker when it came to ferreting about in the six stories of the enormous building in the hope of unearthing some unusual disease.

"Say, Mike," he began, with the conviction of someone who really wanted to capture the attention of the person he was addressing. "I think I've just discovered an interesting case on the fifth floor. The doctors up there are all at sea. They've got a guy in his thirties on their hands. They've found an outbreak of fungoid infection in his esophagus. He's hardly got any white cells left. He appears to have lost all his immune system. It really looks like something for you. You should go and take a look. Room five sixteen."

Michael Gottlieb slipped on his white lab coat. It was about nine A.M. on Monday, October 6, 1980. The most spectacular medical adventure of modern times had just begun.

3

The Painful Metamorphosis of a Guerrilla Fighter
Latrun, Israel: Autumn 1980

That night, at three A.M., as every night, the bell of the Monastery of the Seven Agonies at Latrun, on the road from Tel Aviv to Jerusalem, summoned the community to prayer. Ever since October 31, 1890, the date on which seventeen French monks reached the biblical valley of Ayalon to found a monastery there, the inhabitants' slumbers had been regularly interrupted by this chiming nocturnal invitation. Leaving the dormitory, dressed in their white tunics, their shaven heads covered with black cowls, the monks sang as they made their way down to the choir in the church their elders had built with their bare hands. "Here we are, O Lord, we who come to glorify You," their voices repeated into the silence of the night.

Similar voices ascended each night from monasteries and convents scattered throughout the four corners of the earth, everywhere where men and women had renounced the turmoil of the world to dedicate their lives in solitude to the worship of God. It was not so much the pursuit of personal perfection and the well-being of their souls that inspired the vocation of these select Christians as the appeal of Christ to his apostles: "Pray for humanity's salvation and my Father will answer your prayer."

Few religious communities were located in so threatened a place as the Monastery of the Seven Agonies at Latrun. Over the past thirty years, the peaceful cornfields and vineyards that formed a garland of prosperity around it had seen several thousand Jewish and Arab fighters fall in the course of the three wars that had pitted the young state of Israel against its Arab neighbors. This tradition of bloodshed went back to biblical antiquity. It was here, in this very valley outside the monastery walls, that three thousand years previously, Joshua had caused the sun to stand still in order to effect his victory over the Canaanites. It was here that Samson had set fire to the crops of the Philistines and that Herod the Great's soldiers had defeated enemies of the empire. It was here that later Richard the Lionhearted's Crusaders, Saladin's mercenaries, the sultan's Turkish battalions, the Gurkhas and the Scots under the British general Allenby, would all come to perish as they forged their way to Jerusalem.

The origins of the members of the small religious community were a perfect reflection of this turbulent heritage. Besides the father abbot, a Frenchman with a worthy round face who had come from his native Burgundy more than half a century ago, there was an Italian, an Iraqi of Greek extraction, a Maltese, an Egyptian Copt who had been converted to the Roman rite, a son of an eminent Palestinian in Jerusalem, and several Lebanese Maronites. The youngest monk and the most recent arrival was a sort of archangel, twenty-five years of age, tall, delicate, and as slender as a blade.

The eldest son of a wealthy Maronite businessman who was the Ford Motor Company representative in Beirut, Brother Philippe Malouf had experienced all the luxury of a gilt-edged adolescence. After effortlessly completing his studies in economics at the American University in Beirut, he became engaged to a girl from the upper-middle business class. Until 1975, the fates had been quite generous to this spoilt young man living in a peaceful and trouble-free country. One day by accident, he came across a biography of Charles de Foucauld, a French provincial high-society profligate who, suddenly touched with grace, became an ascetic in the sands of the Sahara. More than a revelation, for Philippe Malouf the book was the awakening of a hitherto dormant religious vocation. In 1978, he left his family home on the Beirut heights for the austere dormitory of the seminary at Bkerke near Our Lady of Lebanon.

But civil war would soon snatch these pious seminarians from their study of theological mysteries and the dogma of faith. Like hundreds of their compatriots, they found themselves serving in the ranks of the Kataiebs, the Christian militia. After a few weeks of training in a camp, Philippe Malouf and his comrades had been sent to the rescue of the Christian villages on Mount Chouf threatened with extermination by their Druze neighbors. All the courage of these beardless adolescents could not, however, make up for their lack of military experience. Entire villages were wiped out, their inhabitants slaughtered, and the survivors were forced to escape to the mountains. The nightmare had lasted weeks. For the Christian camp the lesson had been so terrible that their leaders accepted without hesitation an unusual offer from the Israeli army.

So it was a few months later that one moonless night Philippe Malouf found himself on board a yacht belonging to a Lebanese millionaire businessman, sailing with all lights extinguished on the open sea off Beirut toward the Israeli gunboat that had come out to pick up him and his comrades. Three hours later the Jewish crew landed their Arab "guests" at Haifa where buses were waiting to take them to their destination: an Israeli training camp.

Located at the foot of the Judean Hills in a vast pine forest sheltered from view, the Beit Mahsir training center could accommodate some fifty recruits. It was equipped to carry out complete military training, particularly in antiterrorist operations. Arab-speaking Israeli guerrilla-warfare technicians were in charge of the instruction. Psychological tactics were also part of the program. Anxious to turn their visitors into admirers of Israel, the organizers had laced their course with films on the humanitarian activities of the Jewish state in the Arab occupied territories and in various Third World countries. Political and cultural lectures given by eminent professors from the Hebrew University in Jerusalem completed the program. The young Lebanese were not, however, permitted any movement or excursions outside the camp other than to go to Sunday worship at the nearby Christian monastery.

Philippe Malouf would long remember his first visit to the Monastery of the Seven Agonies at Latrun. "What a shock, how marvelous it was to go into that place of faith and peace, less than five kilometers away from the barracks where we were being taught how to kill and destroy," he would recall. "Inside those walls every-

thing seemed to be joy and bliss. The melody of the monks' monotonous, repetitive chanting seemed to rise to the vaulting of the
church in a never ending offering. There was so much plenitude,
so much felicity in their alleluias, that I felt as if I were being
hypnotized. I understood that it was there that Christ was calling
me, to the heart of the Palestine that nearly two thousand years
previously had been the setting for His life, His death, and His
resurrection. Yes, it was actually there that my vocation was to be
fulfilled."

*   *   *

It took Philippe Malouf several months of waiting before he was
able to return to civilian life in Israel and pass through the monastery
gate forever. Nearly a year had elapsed now since the young novice
with the tonsure and the rough homespun habit had begun to live
the austere rule of poverty, chastity, and obedience laid down in
the sixth century by Saint Benedict. It had been a year of arduous
apprenticeship, of a slow and at times painful metamorphosis from
the ex-guerrilla fighter to a man of silence and prayer turned solely
toward God and the pursuit of "higher things."

"The most difficult part was getting used to the way the monks
prayed," he would say. "For me prayer had always been a solitary
and silent activity. In the Trappist monastery it was an act undertaken together and out loud. Listening to my brothers endlessly
singing the same hymns, I came to ask myself a sacrilegious question: Wasn't there a danger of this wearisome reiteration's turning
my devotions into an insipid ritual? A bit like those prayer wheels
in Buddhist temples."

Philippe Malouf decided to confide his torment to his superior.
After listening to him, the father abbot responded with a smile of
complicity: "I'm going to let you in on a trick an elderly father told
me about when I first came to the monastery as a young novice.
At every office, during the singing of the psalms, concentrate on
one verse. It doesn't matter which one. For example: 'Hear, O Lord,
the cry of the wretched,' or 'O God, grant to Your children the joy
of hope.' Latch your thoughts onto those words while you continue
to recite the community prayer. Go over them in all directions,
project them into biblical mythology, imagine Jesus saying those
same words, then the prophets and the millions of men before you.

Try and relate them to contemporary realities. Then, you'll see, your prayer will become a meditation."

A multitude of other questions would trouble the mind of the apprentice monk on the slow path to ultimate serenity, questions such as that of the Lord's response to his monastery's incessant prayer for the salvation of mankind. "We had all consecrated our lives to prayer. We all longed to know what our dedication actually enabled God to do on this earth, we all wanted to pick up small signs of His goodness. But we never had the satisfaction of verifying the effectiveness of our efforts. It was frustrating."

Philippe's yearning would be partially answered on the day the father abbot placed him in charge of the sale of the wine and liqueurs from the abbey vineyards. "It was a marvelous opportunity to re-establish contact with the outside world, to resume communication and listen to others. Dozens of families and buses of tourists stopped off every day. At weekends or festivals crowds would form outside the abbey portals. Our products were famous all over Israel and beyond. The shop was always full. Many visitors asked to walk round the orangery to admire the sarcophaguses along the walk-ways, the frustums of Roman pillars, and the remains the monks had found as they cleared or worked the land."

$$*\quad*\quad*$$

One day Philippe Malouf received a visit from two young Americans who wanted to examine the collection of flints and carved stones kept in a storeroom that had been rearranged as a small museum. One was called Josef Stein; the other Sam Blum. With his fringe of brown beard linking up to his thick, curly hair, twenty-eight-year-old Josef Stein looked like a biblical prophet. Originally from a small industrial town in Pennsylvania where his parents ran a laundry business, in 1972 this descendant of Polish immigrants had settled in San Francisco. Working at night as a tollbooth employee on the Golden Gate Bridge, by day he had studied at the City College and then in the archaeology department of the University of San Francisco. With his degree in the bag, he had obtained a scholarship to join the American School in Jerusalem to dig the site of the Canaanite town of Gezer, some six and a half miles from the Monastery of Latrun. In the most recently excavated trenches he had met Sam Blum, an expert in biblical antiquities from Co-

lumbia University in New York City. Sam Blum, thirty-two, was
the son of a Brooklyn rabbi. With his round, metal-rimmed spectacles and his long, bony face, he looked more like an anarchist
planter of bombs than a savior of lost civilizations.

The two Americans had returned several times to the monastery
to photograph and make sketches of the most remarkable pieces in
the small museum, in particular axes, knives, and scraping tools that
dated back about a hundred thousand years. Their curiosity not
being confined to the study of prehistoric objects, Philippe Malouf
showed them the touching little cemetery surrounded by cypress
trees and asphodels.

Later, when illness confined him to a New York hospital bed,
Josef Stein would recall with intense joy the memory of that visit.
"No object found on a dig, no archaeological remains, no stone,
ever moved me quite as much as the sight of that succession of
Christian names carved on humble wooden crosses. That day I
understood what people mean by immortality."

4

"Daughter, the God Has Cursed You"
Benares, India: Autumn 1980

A tidal wave in the Ganges could not have wrought more havoc in the world of the cremator of corpses in Benares than the announcement that his daughter Ananda had leprosy. Already born into the lowest caste, the Prakashs were now afflicted by a new curse that made them doubly impure. Since the very dawn of time, India had stigmatized those infected by this repugnant disease. Centuries before Moses associated leprosy with sin, or the Middle Ages had stripped its victims of all human rights, Asia, which had probably been its birthplace, condemned lepers to the vindictiveness of the healthy. Just as Europe had once forced them to move about to the sound of a rattle, to burn their clothes, and to shut themselves away in ghettos of death, so India today still treated her lepers as pariahs. Rarely healthy Indians dared to venture into the sordid colonies in which they lived, on the outskirts of towns and villages. No leper entered the house of a nonleper. Yet there were five million of them who trailed their wounds and their stumps across the vast country.

The sacred city of Benares probably attracted the largest number of lepers. For the hundreds of thousands of pilgrims who flocked to the Ganges's liberating banks, giving alms to those they regarded as the most accursed of men was an additional opportunity to improve their karma, the credit balance of good deeds accomplished in their present life or previous existences. The lepers, who held out their bowls along the flights of steps leading down to the river, were well aware of this fact. At night, they dragged themselves to the sacred river to wash their sores and beg the gods to have them reborn into a better incarnation. It was, almost certainly, Ananda's prolonged contact with this polluted water that had overcome "the little Ganges vulture's" resistance to germs.

*　　　*　　　*

What happened next would remain forever engraved upon Ananda's memory. Driven out of his mind by the shock of the news, her father called for a cycle-rickshaw to go and present his apologies to the parents of her chosen fiancé and cancel the wedding ceremony. On his return, he summoned his daughter in the presence of the entire assembled family. Pointing to the door of the house, he announced, "Daughter, the god has cursed you. You have no place here. Go away!"

From the folds of his *longhi* he took out a few one-rupee notes and held them out to his child. His wife stepped forward with a meager bundle containing a small quantity of linen, some biscuits, and two bananas. Ananda took the parcel and remained motionless for a moment, petrified with fear and grief. Then she made her way out. Before crossing the threshold she turned around. All the members of her family were there silently watching her: uncles, aunts, cousins, her grandmother, and even her white-bearded grandfather from his picture frame upon the wall. Catching sight of her little brothers sobbing behind her father, she wanted to go back. Her mother's severe look dissuaded her. She stepped out of the door and plunged into the seething tide of the alley.

In the strict context of Hindu society this banishment amounted to a death sentence. "The little Ganges vulture" knew she could not go and knock on a single door of that vast city. The slightest physical contact with anyone was rigorously forbidden to an untouchable. All of her short life had been spent in the obsessive avoidance of any breach of this segregation. Because she was both a pariah by birth and the daughter of a cremator of corpses, she had taken care never to soil, so much as with her shadow, any Hindu of caste in the throngs of the alleys, never to buy a cone of *muri* or a stick of incense other than by throwing the money to the vendor, never to raise her dark eyes to anyone, whoever it might be. Even in the family home she had been unable to escape the oppression of her condition. Her parents had persistently imbued her with the curse of their destiny. She had been refused all tenderness, all love. To one who dared to rifle corpses, even the hope of earning rebirth into a better incarnation through merit was denied. There could not have been a karma more disastrous than hers.

Deprived of any schooling as a child, Ananda did not know how to read or write. Her father's trade, however, had familiarized her ear with all kinds of languages and dialects. In addition to Bhojpuri, the local language, she knew many words in Hindu, Urdu, Bengali, even Gujarati and Marathi, for many were the rich Hindus who came from those provinces to die in Benares, there to attain eternal peace. By contrast, since no British person had ever come to be incinerated on her father's pyres, she knew not a word of the language of the former colonizers of India.

Her particular type of work and her harsh environment had hardly spared the little girl. At thirteen, like so many Indian children, she knew all about the facts of life. She had seen and heard her parents copulating and witnessed the prostitutes, transvestites, and eunuchs plying their trade in the shameless alleys around the temples. She had seen birth, suffering, and death. Hers had been a pitiless apprenticeship that had prepared her for every possible shock, hardened her against all misfortune. At least, that was what she thought. For she could never have imagined what awaited her when she left her family home.

First there was a whole month of wandering about the streets and stairways leading down to the Ganges, of begging on temple steps, of foraging through the rubbish heaps, of furtive pilfering from the market stalls. Her already puny body became thin in the extreme. Worms inflated her stomach until it was hideously swollen. Colonies of fleas took up residence in her bush of wild, unkempt hair.

She was so hungry one day that she made up her mind to present herself at the grille of a *mahajan*, a usurer in the funeral-pyre street, in order to trade in the small gold ring still shining in the ala of her nose for a few rupees. Moved to pity by her distress, the old shylock placed a twenty-rupee note, the equivalent of a dollar and a half, on the edge of his counter instead of the fifteen the transaction was worth. With this small fortune Ananda survived for another ten days, feeding herself on bits of sugarcane and bananas.

One evening, at the very end of her resources, she slumped down onto a railway station platform and held out her hand. This time providence took the form of a smooth-tongued man wearing the reassuring white cap of a Congress Party supporter. The stranger placed an exceptionally generous donation in her hand, a crumpled ten-rupee note. Ananda did not dare look up at such a benefactor.

"Don't thank me, little one," the man was quick to insist. "I'm the one who needs you."

He squatted down on his heels and recounted that his wife had been called away to Calcutta to look after her dying father. She would not be back for two or three weeks. He was looking for someone to care for his three young children in her absence.

"I live just round the corner and you'll do nicely," he explained, in no way deterred by the somewhat defeated look and the dark skin that denoted the low birth of the girl he was addressing. "I'll give you fifteen rupees a week."

It must be the god Ganesh in person, thought the little girl, raising her head timidly. She signaled her assent with her chin, stood up, and like an animal that had found a master, fell into step with the providential stranger.

Like all the great pilgrimage centers, Benares was a favorite location for a good many profane undertakings. One of the most active and flourishing was prostitution, especially involving young girls. Here, as elsewhere, legend had it that deflowering a virgin would sustain manly virtues and cure venereal diseases. There were pleasure houses in abundance. Their residents were provided by regular suppliers who usually bought their pitiful merchandise from very poor families, notably in Nepal, or organized fictitious marriages with pretend spouses. Sometimes the victims were simply abducted.

In this holy city where all activity was fatally steeped in the sacred, some daring procurers even went so far as to use certain religious festivals to initiate their victims under a pretense of ritual. One of these festivals was Marg Purnima, the October full moon, which celebrated the glory of Vishnu, the god creator of all things. Another was Makara Sankranti, at the winter solstice, in honor of the goddess of carnal love, pleasure, and fertility. It was Ananda's bad fortune to have been discovered on the eve of one such festival.

*   *   *

"My benefactor didn't take me to his home," Ananda would recount. "He pushed me onto the backseat of a taxi and sat himself next to me. The car drove through the suburbs for a long time and ended up outside the iron gate of a temple. In the courtyard, about twenty poor creatures like me were crouched down in the custody of men with white caps on their heads. I tried to escape but two powerful hands grabbed hold of me and forced me into the court- yard. There, I was told to sit down. At that moment two older women appeared and handed us banana leaves in the hollow of which they had put a spoonful of rice and lentils. I was so hungry I swallowed it all ravenously. After a bit the men in the white caps gave us the order to get up and pushed us inside the temple.

"It was there that the nightmare began. For two days and two nights, sometimes threatening, sometimes coaxing, priests paid by the procurers expounded on how there could be no destiny more splendid for a young girl than that of being called by the gods to sate men with pleasure. These evil Brahmins were relentless in their efforts to convert us, interspersing their speeches with the sounding of gongs, resorting to all kinds of rites at the feet of the numerous divinities in the sanctuary. Eventually they turned our heads. At the end of those two days we were under their spell. Ready for anything."

What Ananda did not know was that, at that same time, identical spells were being woven in several other Indian cities. An estimated three thousand teenage girls are delivered up for prostitution each year on the occasion of Marg Purnima in the state of Karnataka alone.* Suitably bribed, the police close their eyes to what goes on.

One night, about a week later, having been transferred from one

* This figure was supplied in a survey that appeared on April 15, 1989, in the highly regarded newsmagazine *India Today*.

place to another, Ananda and her companions were penned like animals in the sordid mud houses that lined the main street of the local red light district. By a strange quirk of fate her abductors had not noticed the small patch on her cheek that was the cause of her misfortune.

5

The Enigma in Room 516
Los Angeles, USA: Autumn 1980

It had all begun with an ordinary attack of hives. When he woke up that morning, Ted Peters, thirty-one, a free-lance model working for a fashion agency in Westwood, the residential area of West Los Angeles, felt some small bumps on his tongue and the inner lining of his mouth. A mirror showed him that the whole of his mouth and tongue was covered with a strange whitish coating. Puzzled, Ted Peters rinsed his mouth with a gargle. He had often suffered from skin problems, but never before in his mouth. Like many other sexually active young men, he was prone to episodic outbreaks of herpes. He had also been the victim of several bouts of venereal disease. Appropriate treatment had always cured such irritations.

After three days the infection in his mouth still persisted, and Ted Peters was experiencing more and more difficulty in swallowing. His food remained blocked on its way to his stomach and could only be rinsed down with water. Even the passage of a mouthful of orange juice was painful. These symptoms grew worse. Soon he was unable to swallow anything at all. Worried, he decided to seek advice.

The intern in the emergency ward at the UCLA hospital deemed his condition serious enough to warrant a thorough examination.

He had him admitted. An endoscopy of his esophagus revealed that the lining was infected with *Candida*, minute fungoid growths that were extremely virulent. But it was a significant deficit in the number of his white cells that put the doctors on alert. All the evidence suggested that the patient was suffering from a serious immuno-deficiency disorder. Intensive treatment caused the infection of the mouth and esophagus to diminish rapidly, but none of the tests or analysis shed any light on why he lacked white cells. In the department of infectious diseases at the UCLA hospital, Ted Peters soon became "the enigma in room 516."

*   *   *

"If the illness of the patient in room five sixteen had broken out in some forgotten backwater in Iowa, no one would probably have taken any notice," Michael Gottlieb, the young immunologist, would say. "The doctors would quite simply have concluded: 'This guy is suffering from some mysterious disease.' He would have died and that would have been it. But in the scientific environment of a large university, that sort of enigma could hardly fail to arouse the curiosity of a whole host of brains. Which just goes to show that in research every success is based on the meeting of a problem with a fertile mind."

That morning in October 1980, the "fertile mind" of Michael Gottlieb was puzzled. "At first I thought it might be a preleukemic condition, or leukemia in its very early stages. But I'd never seen leukemia associated with a fungal *Candida* infection before. Then I considered a severe disorder of the intestinal flora, possibly caused by excessive consumption of antibiotics, something which some-times occurs in homosexuals who are hyperactive and who are there-fore particularly exposed to sexually transmitted diseases. Since the patient in room five sixteen claimed never to have gone in for any activity of that kind, I wanted to know whether the fungal infection was in any way linked to the deficiency in white cells the tests had revealed."

In an attempt to pick up some sort of scent, Michael Gottlieb had recourse to numerous medical tests. But nothing that science had invented to date by way of biological examination could provide the slightest clue. He also made a meticulous study of thousands of pages from the medical literature related to the subject. As sometimes happens in pathological investigation, the illness of the patient from Westwood "did not seem to correspond to any criteria known to date."

It was then that Michael Gottlieb had the idea of entrusting a sample of Ted Peters's blood to the biologist who occupied the laboratory almost opposite his own on the lower-basement floor of the hospital. A native of Missouri, Bob Schroff, a twenty-eight-year-old redhead, was working on a program of revolutionary experiments. The tools necessary for this pioneering work were mouse proteins that he received each week in small flasks sent by parcel post from New Jersey. Invented by a British and a German scientist, these proteins were just beginning to be manufactured. Production was still so limited, however, that only about twenty biologists in the United States could boast a few specimens destined to be tested for potential medical application.

These proteins bore the scientific name of "monoclonal antibodies." A discovery in a British laboratory had rendered them capable of interacting with all the different varieties of white cells called lymphocytes. This was remarkable because, far from being one homogeneous category, these white cells, responsible for defending the organism against external attack, are made up of several different groups and subgroups, a fact that makes identification of them singularly complicated. The most numerous type, the T lymphocytes—so named because they are dependents of the thymus gland—are divided into several subtypes, each endowed with a specific function. The T-4 lymphocytes, for instance, are in some ways the orchestral leaders of the immune system. In case of attack, they locate the foreign agent, sound the alarm, and send the system's defenses into action. They give out the signals that activate another group of white cells, the T-8 lymphocytes, which attack and kill cells infected by pathogenic agents. The T-4 lymphocytes also produce substances that stimulate the mobilization of another class of white cells, the B lymphocytes produced by the bone marrow. These B lymphocytes subject the aggressors to the sustained fire of their antibodies. As soon as the infection has been controlled, the T-8 suppressor lymphocytes restore immunologic peace by stopping the proliferation of defender B lymphocytes, thus preventing them from overreacting. But nature, ever distrustful, surrounds herself with precautionary measures. She leaves significant groups of T-4 lymphocytes patrolling the blood, ready to sound the alert again at the slightest cause for alarm.

Until the end of the seventies, there had been no microscope, no biological test capable of distinguishing between the various participants in this complex and subtle defense system contained in a drop of blood, much less of identifying any deficiency. The invention of the monoclonal antibodies filled this gap. By making them fluorescent and introducing them into a test tube containing a few ounces of blood, an immediate specific "marking" of all the varieties of lymphocytes and in particular of the famous T-4 and T-8 cells could be obtained. They could then be counted and their behavior analyzed. It was an unprecedented revolutionary step in the process of understanding the mechanics of immunity and tracking down the origins of unexplained illnesses. That October of 1980, Bob Schroff, the biologist from Missouri, was one of the few scientists in the world capable of mastering this new technology.

Three days after he had received the blood sample from the patient in room 516, his gangling form appeared in the doorway of Michael Gottlieb's small laboratory. His look of embarrassment disquieted the immunologist.

"So, it didn't work?"

"Quite the opposite," retorted Schroff. "But my results are so disturbing I'm afraid I may have made a mistake. It's such a recent technique."

"What did you find?" asked Gottlieb impatiently.

"That your number five sixteen is an extremely interesting case. I've never seen anything like it. He has hardly any T-4 lymphocytes left. But the number of his T-8s is unbelievably high."

Michael Gottlieb grimaced. Why had his patient lost the orchestral leaders of his immune system? And why, on the other hand, had his suppressor cells multiplied?

"It's such an extraordinary result that I'd like to ask you to supply me with another blood sample," added Bob Schroff. "I want to run a check."

The second test confirmed the first. In the meantime, cured of his throat infection, Ted Peters had been sent home by his doctors. A few days later he was back, this time stricken with further inexplicable clinical symptoms: extreme fatigue to a point where he had difficulty in walking from the taxi to the hospital door, and attacks of breathlessness at the least effort, rendering him incapable even of lacing up his shoes. In addition to these symptoms, he had a dry cough, a high temperature, sudden bouts of sweating, and he had lost several pounds since his previous hospitalization.

*　　*　　*

"I recognized at once the extreme gravity of these complications," Michael Gottlieb would recount. "I asked for a bronchoscopy and a bronchoalveolar washing of the lungs. The doctors on duty were amazed at my impatience. They thought it was a simple case of pneumonia, but I knew that if we didn't act urgently with the most aggressive drugs, the patient might die. The tests confirmed my fears. We were dealing not with classic pneumonia, but with *pneumocystis pneumonia*, an extremely rare parasitic disease of the lungs which only developed in subjects whose immune system was deficient. I had seen a few cases at Stanford. But there the deficiency of the immune system had always had a clinical cause, such as chemotherapy and radiotherapy against cancer, or possibly an inhibition deliberately induced to prevent the rejection of a transplanted organ.

"I rushed to the UCLA library to consult the computer linked to the central medical data bank in Washington. All the articles on pneumocystis pneumonia published in the world in the last twenty years supplied a single explanation for the failure of the immune system that had caused this illness. In every instance it was a matter of irradiation needed for an organ transplant or of a genetic deficiency as in the case of the unfortunate glass-bubble children, who are actually born without an immune system. Nobody had ever pinpointed a case of pneumocystis pneumonia with other origins.

"The mystery remained unresolved. Ted Peters's immunodeficiency did not stem from any known cause."

6

A Laboratory of Love on the Banks of the Ganges

Benares, India: Autumn 1980–Spring 1981

Everyone in Benares knew the old palace with the half-crumbled turrets overlooking the river situated at the extremity of the town. For two centuries the red-and-gold emblem of the maharajas of Nepal had fluttered from the fronton of its majestic facade now eaten away by successive monsoons. Each dawn, its wrought-iron portal had opened to an elephant covered with velvet, bearing the lord of the house under a canopy to his religious devotions on the banks of the Ganges.

The princes of the small Himalayan state had long since deserted this palace. These days a wooden notice nailed in place of their banner indicated the name and function of their successors: MISSIONARIES OF CHARITY—LEPER DISPENSARY.

Caring for lepers! This act of compassion was possibly one that best epitomized the charitable ideal of the woman who for more than twenty years had been relieving people's suffering in India and throughout the world. Mother Teresa's entire life had been haunted by the desire to bring a little peace and comfort to India's lepers. She had tended their wounds, nourished their bodies, brought peace to their souls. She had carried the dying in her arms and clasped children to her heart. Her hands had soothed away their pain and her smile had chased away their anguish. They had been her companions, her friends, the ones who had taught her the virtues of courage, sharing, and humility. They had been the source of some of her greatest joys.

Her commitment to the service of lepers shut away in their ghettos began one day in 1957 with an appeal from five workmen in a factory in Calcutta. "Mother, help us! We've just been fired from our jobs because of these marks," one of them had pleaded, pointing to some patches on the skin of his torso and those of his companions. One week later a van packed with medicines, milk powder, and sacks of rice took off for the most poverty-stricken suburbs of the big city, for the hovels where the lepers hid their distress in squalid colonies. On board were Mother Teresa and three of her sisters, three young Indian girls dressed as she was in a white sari bordered with blue. They were all ignorant of the horrors of the illness and of the often demanding and sometimes aggressive nature of its victims. The work of the foundress of the Missionaries of Charity was not, however, confined to rushing to dress the wounds of several hundred lepers. With her extraordinary talent for bringing out the best in people, she had invited the city's entire population to join with her in a massive appeal in aid of the victims of the terrible disease. As an emblem for this operation she chose the ancient symbol of the affliction, a small bell like the ones used by the condemned of former times to alert the healthy to their impure presence. Bannered in the newspapers, paraded on billboards, and postered on the sides of her van, the slogan of this appeal urged: "Touch a leper with your compassion." The outcome exceeded all hopes. Mother Teresa was soon able to launch other mobile dispensaries. Above all, on a piece of land provided by the government, nearly two hundred miles from Calcutta, she was able to found a whole town reserved for lepers, Shanti Nagar—"The City of Peace." There, hundreds of families began anew an almost normal existence and discovered peace and hope. Once started, the nun opened other leper hospitals, dispensaries, and workshops elsewhere, where weaving looms hummed and broken men and women could regain their dignity through work.

*   *   *

The center in Benares was one of her most recent creations. She had entrusted responsibility for it to one of the most remarkable workers in her community. With her almond-shaped eyes and rosy-pink cheeks, Sister Bandona looked like a Chinese statue. Her name meant "praise God." Born among the hilltops of Assam where her father cultivated a miserable plot of land, she had one day landed with her family in the abject poverty of a slum in the suburbs of Calcutta, paradoxically called "the City of Joy." To help her recently widowed mother provide for the needs of her four brothers and sisters, she had for years foraged through piles of rubbish for metal objects, which she then sold to a scrap-metal merchant. Later, she had worked in a cardboard factory, and eventually in a metal work-shop where she had made parts for trucks.

The arrival in her slum of a Polish priest who had come to serve the poor had been the catalyst for her vocation of love and charity. Hurrying about her destitute neighborhood, rescuing people day and night, she had become the life and soul of the Committee for Mutual Aid, which the priest had founded. Her memory was a card index of all ills. The quality of her expression, of her smile, of her compassion, had earned her the nickname of Anand Nagar Ka Swarga Dut—"The Angel of the City of Joy." Her encounters with Mother Teresa's sisters who came each week to tend the lepers in the slum had quite naturally induced her to choose a life in the service of others. Though brought up in the Buddhist faith, her practice of the Christian values of sharing and sacrifice had prepared her well to embrace the ideal of the Missionaries of Charity. A three-year novitiate would finally confirm her commitment. On December 8, 1975, on the Feast of the Immaculate Heart of Mary, Mother Teresa's scissors cut off her long black plait, thus making the young Buddhist forever "a bride of Christ dedicated to the service of the poorest of the poor."

*   *   *

Every morning brought the same nightmare, the same unbearable vision of a tide of living dead pressing themselves against the rail-ings. There were people with neither feet nor hands curled up like fetuses on makeshift wagons pulled by specters scarcely more able-bodied, blind men with faces eaten down to the bone, human wrecks with dressings oozing blood crawling along the ground. There were women hiding their wounds beneath the folds of *burqas* that enveloped them from head to toe like ghosts, mothers clasping their infants in arms reduced to stumps, haggard skeletons who already seemed to belong to the other world. There were also people who looked quite well but who had been cast into this encampment of the damned by a patch on their skin, a dubious lump or progressive muscular atrophy. Above all, there were little stunted bodies with stomachs swollen with worms, their bones protruding beneath their skin, their joints cracking and their limbs as thin as vine shoots. Even if most did not bear, not yet at least, the stigma of leprosy, almost all were suffering from serious illnesses: tuberculosis of the bone, chronic enteritis, and vitamin deficiencies that could make them blind.

And yet at any moment there would burst forth from all this grief some comic or marvelous spectacle that dispelled the nightmare. The buffoonery of the sick ridiculing their own infirmities or the patter of the professional storytellers invariably forced their audiences to laughter. Most surprising of all still was the children's play in the midst of all this decay, or the miraculous appearance of some woman in a sari, looking as beautiful as a temple goddess.

Most of the sick came from other parts of the country, and it was not easy for people to understand each other in this Capernaum of voices, cries, and demands. Bihar, Bengal, Orissa, the South: many had been on the road for years. They had left fragments of their skin along the way, at random ports of call on temple steps or station platforms. Most had never received treatment of any kind.

The germs that ravaged them bore the name of the Norwegian doctor who had identified them at the end of the last century. Hansen's bacilli had gravitated toward the warmth of tropical countries and settled in bodies with weakened constitutions. The extreme virulence of some made them agents of infection. It had been calculated that in a ten-minute conversation a leper could spread two hundred thousand bacilli about him. Sharing a shelter, clothes, crockery—in short, any form of cohabitation with affected individuals—was the most frequent means of contagion. A scratch, a prick, could be enough for the agents of infection to contaminate new prey. Yet these microbes were so lazy that often it took months, even years, for the first damage to be wrought on their favored targets: the skin, the nerves, the mucous membranes of the nose and mouth, the eyes, the spleen, the liver. Curiously enough, the bacillus was not directly responsible for the dreadful wounds, but rather for the fact that, in attacking the nerves, it deadened all sensibility. Thus the slightest trauma—a knock, a burn, a cut—became the cause of lesions that degenerated and eventually led to mutilation.

For centuries a shrub growing in South India had provided the only remedy capable of reducing the effects of the disease: chaulmoogra oil. Subsequently, the discovery of sulfones in the middle of the twentieth century, and then antibiotics, had revolutionized the treatment of leprosy. Except in the case of irreversible attacks, a few months of taking tablets daily generally resulted in a spectacular regression and often even in complete cure. The treatment was so inexpensive that the Frenchman Raoul Follereau, a tireless apostle of lepers, had written: "Just give me the money for a single atomic bomber, and I will cure the fifteen million lepers on this planet."

*   *   *

To cure! That was the fanciful dream of a handful of sisters in saris assailed from dawn to dusk by a terrifying reality. To try to instill some order into the macabre procession moving past their treatment table, Sister Bandona and her companions consigned the patients' names and the locations of their lesions to a rudimentary card index. Each time a patient returned they would consult his card. Then, with a few rapid but deft gestures, disregarding the smell, they would pull away the dressings, open up the wounds, disinfect them with great dabs of iodine, apply powders and ointments, and dress the wounds again with gauze and clean bandages. Sometimes they had to cut into the putrid flesh with a scalpel to free a nerve or amputate a bone consumed with gangrene. It was proper butcher's work with a few *Ave Marias* murmured under the breath as sole support and numerous resurrections from the near-dead as the only recompense. Many of those who squeezed themselves into the queue no longer had a single lesion to be seen. They were the miraculously healed of this laboratory of love set up on the banks of the Ganges.

One stifling April morning, Sister Bandona's eyes caught sight of an unexpected figure among the throng of destitute people besieging her dispensary. The daughter of the cremator of corpses in Benares had managed to escape her abductors.

7

**Five Quite Extraordinary Cases for a Chinese Magician
Los Angeles, USA: Autumn 1980–Winter 1981**

There was nothing Californian about his rosy-pink cheeks and large, balding forehead framed by curly gray locks. Like Michael Gottlieb, thirty-nine-year-old Dr. Joel D. Weisman was an expatriate of the East Coast of the United States. The son of a schoolteacher, and grandson of a launderer ruined by the advent of Laundromats, he had been born in the same maternity hospital as Michael Gottlieb, in New Brunswick, New Jersey. Life had not yet ordained that they should meet. A general practitioner, Joel Weisman shared a clinic in a pink stucco building in the Sherman Oaks neighborhood, one of the innumerable suburbs of Los Angeles. This courteous man in his sky-blue smock was unanimously appreciated for his simplicity and competence. His small waiting room, decorated with ferns and a collection of abstract engravings, was always full. It was an eclectic practice: old people, mothers with their children, teenagers in T-shirts and sneakers. On the tables in front of the black, simulated-leather wall sofas were laid out the alluring covers of the latest editions of the magazine *Being Well*. That autumn of 1980 they were offering reports on a new treatment against cholesterol, on how to stop smoking with the help of hypnosis, and a survey on pain.

"I saw a little of all life's frailties go by, both great and small," Joel Weisman would recall. "People suffering from arterial hypertension, diabetes, gout, ulcers, insignificant cases of laryngitis or colitis. It was comforting to be able to relieve and usually cure them. I hardly ever saw a patient die. I also had to treat some of the diseases which are classified today as sexually transmissible. It was the right kind of neighborhood for them: lots of gays lived there." The fact that Joel Weisman was himself gay no doubt contributed to the popularity that his clinic had found with that particular clientele. "Everyone knew that I didn't stand in judgment, that with me there were no taboos or psychological barriers, that I was there to treat them and only treat them."

*   *   *

Over the years the proportion of gays among Dr. Joel Weisman's patients had increased. The doctor saw in this increase not so much a tribute to his ability and discretion as the consequence of an upsurge in sexually transmitted diseases with a predilection for attacking this particular risk group. "From the years 1977, 1978, onwards, I began to get more and more young men with high fevers, nocturnal sweating, diarrhea, all kinds of parasitic diseases, and particularly with swollen lymph nodes the size of pigeons' eggs, in their necks, in their armpits, their groin, everywhere. The evidence suggested that these inflammations of the glands were expressions of immunodeficiency disorders. Each time, I feared the worst: cancer, leukemia. Fortunately all my biopsies came back to me marked 'benign.' True, some of the illnesses identified by analysis were not trivial. There was mononucleosis, hepatitis, lots of cases of herpes, quite a bit of venereal disease. Thank God, the viruses responsible did not kill, at least not yet. Generally, most of the symptoms disappeared after appropriate treatment. Only a few patients kept their abnormally swollen lymph nodes. They resigned themselves to living with them."

The arrival, one morning in October 1980, of a hairdresser from West Hollywood in Joel Weisman's consulting room was rudely to disrupt this relative optimism. This young gay man of twenty-five, with no known medical history, was suffering from a chronic infection of the skin, the mucous membranes, and the nails. "His epidermis is nothing but one big open wound," Joel Weisman noted on his card. Disconcerted by the extent of the infection, he picked up his telephone and dialed the number of the only person who in his view was capable of curing his patient.

*   *   *

In Los Angeles, the entire medical profession knew the man nicknamed "the doctors' doctor." His real name was Peng Thim Fan. Thirty-five years of age, he was a jovial little Chinese man with glasses who had been born in Singapore on the day in 1945 the Japanese garrison had surrendered to Mountbatten's British troops. Dr. Peng Fan had a reputation for clearing up the most bizarre cases, those that did not correspond to any previous model, that defied all logic, all analysis, all rational explanation. His thick black head of hair, always in disarray, concealed the brains of a diagnostic wizard. No one else could dissect an incomprehensible case and uncover unsuspected clues in quite the way that this inquisitive Chinese man could. A celebrated hospital in Los Angeles had once called him urgently to the rescue of a woman who had gone into a coma after a routine brain scan. The "doctor-detective" Peng Fan had saved the dying woman by finding the cause of her coma: an extremely rare and fatal allergy brought on by a substance injected to make the pictures of her skull more clearly readable.

The destiny of this rubber-tree planter's son had indeed been a strange one. Passionately interested in philosophy, he had accepted a scholarship to Oxford, but instead of flying off to Europe, in the end he left for Canada to study medicine there. Six years in Winnipeg instilled a permanent horror of the cold, so it was under the California sun that he came to take refuge at the age of twenty-five, with his brand-new MD degree. He chose a specialist field known for its legions of sufferers. Rheumatology was concerned with inflammatory ailments of the joints and blood vessels, complaints that often originated in some malfunctioning of the immune system. It was a science in its early youth, enriching itself with new discoveries every day.

Since 1975, Peng Fan had occupied a teaching post in rheumatology at Wadsworth Hospital, an important establishment linked to UCLA. Every Friday afternoon, "the doctors' doctor" held a consultation there exclusively for cases that had eluded all normal diagnosis. "One day Joel Weisman presented me with a man with acute swelling of the blood vessels in the feet and hands. His body was the color of a lobster taken out of boiling water. He was groaning like one of the damned. I ended up diagnosing erythromelalgia, an illness easily treated with aspirin but very rare."

* * *

On first examination of the hairdresser, the Chinese magician admitted he had never been confronted with quite such a riddle before. "It was a complete mystery, an enigma that would turn Alfred Hitchcock green with envy. For what reason could someone who had never suffered the slightest immune deficiency find himself suddenly in such a state of immunodepression?"

Peng Fan set himself spiritedly to work. Not a single clue, suspicion, or hypothesis escaped his investigation. He subjected the sick man to a police-style interrogation in the hope of discovering somewhere in his past some piece of information that would give him something to go on. He sifted through all the medical literature, even going as far as to dig out his old treatises in Chinese medicine. He sought the culprit amongst illnesses few people knew about, such as acrodermatitis enteropathica, the symptoms of which—infection of the mucous membranes, mycosis of the fingernails—revealed an immune deficiency of the same type. The disorders were often connected to a serious lack of zinc in the system, so he took some hair from the patient and had it analyzed. The zinc count was normal. Peng Fan then devised all sorts of treatments combining massive doses of cortisone with new substances intended to stimulate the activity of the immune system. After three week of dogged effort, the Chinese magician had to acknowledge his impotence.

An event then occurred that altered the situation dramatically: the visit in Joel Weisman's clinic of a second patient with identical symptoms. This time it was a young publicist from Hollywood, also gay and also without any previous medical history. Drs. Weisman and Peng Fan would then discover that the "pneumonia" from which their patients were suffering was in fact pneumocystis pneumonia, that extremely rare parasitic infection of the lungs that their colleague Michael Gottlieb had diagnosed in his patient in room 516.

The news of these three similar cases spread like wildfire across the medical heartland. "It was barely conceivable," Peng Fan would say. "In less than a month three young men had fallen victim in the same city to the same extremely rare illness. And for all three cases, no explanation had been found."

Peng Fan and Joel Weisman got in touch with Michael Gottlieb. "The fact that the Chinese wizard informed me that like me he was completely in the dark proved we really had something on our hands," the young immunologist would say.

The three men decided to regroup their patients in the UCLA hospital. "The appearance, at the beginning of 1981, of a fourth case of pneumocystis pneumonia, this time in a black homosexual, swiftly followed by a fifth case, suddenly made the thing look like a real epidemic," Gottlieb would explain. "I had this presentiment of a plague far worse than the Legionnaires' disease.* All the doctors in America had to be urgently alerted."

---

* In July 1976, at a convention at a Philadelphia hotel for veterans of the American Legion, 189 participants had been struck down with a mysterious form of pneumonia; 29 had died of it.

8

Millions of Orgasms in the Cause of Liberation
San Francisco–New York, USA: Autumn 1980

Neither America nor the world suspected it as yet, but the party
was over. The unidentified illness, which at the end of the year 1980
was laying out the five young Los Angeles gay men, was in the
process of tolling the death knell for the passing of an era. It had
been a thrilling, dynamic era of movements and struggles. Between
1960 and 1970, millions of blacks, women, young people, and
lesbians and gay men had fought to insure that equal rights in the
world's greatest democracy did not remain an empty formula devoid
of meaning. Of all the liberation movements conducted in the course
of those years, perhaps none had made a deeper impact on American
society than one referred to as "the sexual revolution." One day,
sociologists will most likely look into the real causes of this revolution, but there can be little doubt that the erosion of traditional
family values following the cultural shifts brought about by the
Second World War; the fall into obsolescence of monogamy; the
conquest of venereal disease thanks to the discovery of penicillin;
and above all, the widespread use of contraceptives by women were
many of the catalysts for the liberating explosion of the sixties.

No episode in this liberation process was more moving than the
coming out of the closet of many of the 17 million men and women

among America's gay and lesbian community who dared to assert their differences. The history of this minority group had been one long succession of acts of oppression and intolerance perpetrated by a puritan society that preached love between a man and a woman, marriage, and the family. The emergence of a political movement for the recognition of the right to be gay was incontestably an unprecedented historical event. For all their devotion to the rights of the individual, the founding fathers of the American Constitution could never have imagined that their laws would one day protect a minority group that based its identity not on race, religion, or language but on sexual choice.

It was on a torrid summer's night, June 29, 1969, that it all began in a cafe in New York's Greenwich Village. The "Stonewall Inn" was packed with its usual clientele of young gays and transvestites when a squad of policemen burst into the premises to turn them out. This time the representatives of public morality did not meet with the reception they had anticipated. Instead of trying, as they usually did, to make a break for it, the customers bombarded the intruders with bottles of beer and all kinds of other projectiles. When the forces of law and order beat a retreat, other gays outside tried to set fire to their vehicles. On the following evening another police raid met with the same welcome, while graffiti appeared all over the walls of Greenwich Village proclaiming the birth of a revolutionary gay movement. Two further nights of rioting put a definitive stamp on this legitimacy. The news spread like wildfire across America, to all the university campuses, bars, saunas, clubs, to the gay enclaves in the big cities, even to the offices and factories where so many men and women had hitherto lived their homosexuality in secret.

*   *   *

One of the first keynotes of policy issued by the leaders of the new movement was an invitation to all lesbians and gays to come out of the closet and openly assume their sexual identity. The call was very widely heard, especially among the young, and the opening years of the seventies witnessed a huge migratory wave from the towns and villages at the heart of America to the big outlying cities such as New York, Los Angeles, San Francisco, Chicago, Boston, Atlanta, and Houston. Of all these magnetic poles, none was more attractive than San Francisco, the shining former capital of the gold rush, planted on its crown of hills overlooking the Pacific. San Francisco had always provided a particularly open and tolerant welcome for communities more or less on the margin of accepted society. Having become the most important port on the West Coast after the wild time of the gold diggers, it had continued to attract a population of adventurers seeking to make their fortunes. The Spanish-American War and then the Second World War would turn San Francisco into an enormous transit center for naval and land operations in the Pacific. With the restoration of peace, several hundred thousand servicemen returned to civilian status in the city. A good many gay ex-soldiers and -sailors set down their roots there.

During the summer of 1968, while the Vietnam War raged on and divided America, a whole generation of young pacifists and hippies had chosen San Francisco as the place in which to affirm that only love could resolve the problems of the world. San Francisco would long remember the crowds of teenagers in jeans and sneakers who came from all over the country to camp in its parks and celebrate the cult of happiness.

If the city had always embraced a strong lesbian and gay contingent, the liberation movement of the seventies would turn San Francisco into the gay capital of the United States and doubtless also of the world. In the same way that, one century earlier, the prospect of gold had attracted thousands of Americans to its hills, so now that of liberty and tolerance propelled to San Francisco a whole generation of young men "coming out." Josef Stein, the future archaeologist at the American School in Jerusalem, was one of them. Like the majority of new immigrants he had moved into the Castro, the main homosexual area situated right in the city center, an area that would soon be nicknamed the Gay Israel by virtue of its uniform population and the fact that it was an enclave. New York, Chicago, and Los Angeles might have their areas that were predominantly homosexual, but San Francisco's Castro was the first exclusively gay colony created by the homosexual liberation movement. There, right in the heart of San Francisco, men and women bound together solely by their sexual preference undertook to build a world apart, a city within the city where they could lead a normal life out in the open, go to their offices, to the bank, to the swimming pool, to the doctor's, the laundry, the hairdresser's, eat out in a restaurant, join in political gatherings, or go to church services, without meeting anyone who was not gay. In the Castro there was even a gay synagogue, a gay Protestant church, and gay Catholic priests who celebrated gay marriage ceremonies.

To celebrate their liberation, the American gays had even gone as far as inventing gay holidays, national festivals like the renowned Gay Freedom Day, which every summer brought together more than 250,000 local residents and visitors who arrived from the four corners of the country to take part in an enormous, flamboyant carnival. On those days the whole of homosexual America, ranging from the Association of Lesbian Taxi Drivers of San Francisco to that of the Gay Cowboys of Nevada, from the transsexual organizations to the delegations of gay American Indians, from the sadomasochistic liberation front to the league of gay invalids, celebrated in the crystal-clear light of the fraternal city the right freely to proclaim its tastes and preferences.

The majority of American lesbians and gays took advantage of this right with moderation. The same was not true of a small number of young gays overtaken by an explosion of libido that translated itself, throughout the seventies, into a frenzy of revelry and experimentation such as no human society had probably known before. San Francisco's Castro became a real sexual supermarket. Day and night, thousands of young men filled its bars, restaurants, shops, and bookstores or roamed its streets in closed ranks in search of adventure. The whole neighborhood became a frenetic hunting ground. Bars and sex clubs received their clients in cubicles pierced with holes through which they could couple with other clients without even bothering to get acquainted. This opportunity to couple cost no more than three dollars. In San Francisco as elsewhere, however, the ultimate expression of liberated sex took the form of another kind of establishment. Bathhouses were clubs with, in the most luxurious instances, swimming pools, saunas, Jacuzzis, cinemas, dance floors, private cubicles, orgy rooms, and sometimes even sadomasochistic torture chambers equipped with harnesses, chains, handcuffs, and other instruments designed for violent expressions of physical love. As a bonus, New York's Continental Baths also provided a permanent variety show. As for San Francisco's legendary Hot House, with its three thousand square yards and four stories, it could take in several hundred clients at once. Over the vast bar that occupied the entire ground floor hung a giant swing. To the proprietor of this luxury bordello, it was "the symbol of all the things a child is afraid to do, especially if that child has homosexual tendencies."

Because they represented the right to get together and do anything you liked with your body, bathhouses became bastions of homosexual liberation. They increased in number. The Castro alone had at least ten, attracting thousands of tourists from all over America to their orgy chambers. A survey conducted in 1970 in the San Francisco area by two Kinsey Institute researchers, Mr. Alan P. Bell and Mr. Martin S. Weinberg, revealed that over 40 percent of the men questioned had had at least five hundred sexual partners in the back rooms of bars or the murky steam of saunas, and 28 percent had had more than a thousand. Many participants in this record rate of intercourse admitted to coupling with twenty to thirty partners in a single night. Alcohol and various chemical substances such as amyl nitrite aided such exploits.

* * *

It would not be long before the sexual excesses of the great gay liberation movement made their mark upon the country's health chart. As early as 1973, a statistic from the U.S. Department of Health indicated that two-thirds of gay men had been the victims of a venereal infection at least once, and that despite the fact that they belonged to a very small minority group, they were responsible for 50 to 60 percent of all cases of syphilis and gonorrhea. In 1978, another statistic showed that in three years the incidence of hepatitis and intestinal infections had doubled. In 1980, the San Francisco Health Department specified that 60 to 70 percent of all the city's gay men were infected with the hepatitis B virus. Heterosexuals did not come out much better. In the five years from 1971 to 1976, the number of cases of gonorrhea in the whole country had almost doubled, rising from 624,371 to 1,011,014. Of course, this figure represented only registered cases. The pattern in cases of syphilis was even more incredible: between 1960 and 1980 the number of patients had increased by 300 percent. Every year the United States was spending $50 million in psychiatric hospitals exclusively on treating the victims of neurological complications caused by the disease.

Strangely, the devastation wrought by the changing sexual mores had not seemed to worry the health authorities, the medical profession, nor even the victims. The journalist Randy Shilts would write: "Getting a dose of the clap has become a farce. Going to the dispensary is just part of the routine. You always run into plenty of friends and together you reminisce about all the reasons that have brought you there before." But according to a general practitioner named Joseph Sonnabend, with a clinic on Greenwich Village's Twelfth Street, "the flare-up of sexually transmitted diseases couldn't remain innocuous."

*   *   *

With his poorly shaven stubble, his old basketball shoes, and his shabby jeans, Joseph Sonnabend looked more like a Bowery tramp than a prince of medicine. Yet the curriculum vitae of this shy man of forty-seven totaled eight pages of distinctions and honors, and had a list of articles and scientific publications worthy of a Nobel Prize. Born in South Africa, the son of Polish Jewish émigrés, he had specialized at an early age in infectious diseases. He had treated his first patients on the decks of an Indonesian ship transporting two thousand pilgrims on their way to Mecca from Jakarta to Jedda. In 1963, the great British scientist Alec Isaacs had called Sonnabend to come and work alongside him in the laboratory where he had just discovered interferon, a powerful antiviral substance secreted by lymphocytes. Joseph Sonnabend had subsequently taught the pathology of infectious diseases in various American universities. In 1977, the health authority for New York City had entrusted him with education in its department for venereal diseases. Two years later, Joseph Sonnabend opened a private medical practice on the front line of these infections, right at the heart of New York's gay quarter.

"It was completely crazy," he would say. "A number of doctors had set themselves up in this particularly sensitive area and were treating a succession of cases of gonorrhea, syphilis, and parasitic infections. At that time antibiotics were a universal panacea. Syphilis was cured with one or two injections of penicillin. It cost only twenty-five or thirty dollars. No one was doing any detailed research, and the very idea of research was totally alien to the majority of practitioners. The most tragic part about it was their refusal to adopt an educational role with their patients. The slightest suggestion, the least warning about the dangers their lifestyle was exposing them to, could be taken as a moral judgment. It was the best way of losing your clients. In any case, irrespective of whether they were doctors in the field or representatives from the Centers for Disease Control in Atlanta and the federal Department of Health, they all thought that it was useless, indeed futile, to try and change people's behavior, that the only realistic approach was to cure them as quickly as possible. They would rather say to people: 'You keep on wrecking yourselves and we'll pick up the pieces.' "

The state of health of the first patients to come and ring his clinic doorbell literally terrified Dr. Joseph Sonnabend. Though conventional venereal disease still made up the majority of cases, the particular nature of homosexual relations had given birth to a whole new pathology of ailments that were sometimes very serious and often simultaneous. This included viral hepatitis, extensive outbreaks of genital herpes, those parasitic diseases that afflicted almost 80 percent of subjects with multiple partners, and those infections attributable to particularly aggressive viruses such as the cytomegalovirus, which attacked the lungs and digestive duct. It was above all, however, in the repeated recurrences of these attacks that Joseph Sonnabend sensed the greatest danger. Some of his patients boasted a list of ten to fifteen doses of gonorrhea, others suffered from repeated outbreaks of herpes, yet others lived with constantly inflamed lymph nodes. "It was staring us in the face: the human body could not be subjected to so many onslaughts without something fundamental beginning to give way."

The "intercity infectious diseases rounds," the meetings of specialists in infectious diseases that had been held every Monday for the last twenty years in different New York hospitals, confirmed the fears of the doctor with the ill-shaven stubble from Greenwich Village.

"Since 1978--79 we had been presented with an ever-increasing number of cases of multiple viral infections, swollen lymph nodes, hepatitis, and chronic skin eruptions. We were even presented with the case of a black man whose brain had been affected. To me, all these symptoms were indicative of the same single phenomenon: an unexplained failure of the immune defense system.

"Nobody else seemed to recognize the fact, but I, for my part, became daily more convinced of it: we were witnessing the first tremors of a cataclysm."

9

A New and Devastating Syndrome
Boston, USA: February 1981

The pressing voice of Dr. Michael Gottlieb on the telephone left no room for doubt: that morning in February 1981, he was trying to convince his listener of an impending crisis.

"The patients we've admitted are all showing the same symptoms: an unaccountable fever, abnormal weight loss, uncontrollable diarrhea. I realize that there is nothing very upsetting about that. But what is, is the fact that they are also all suffering from pneumocystis pneumonia, a form of pneumonia that is extremely rare and has such specific origins. All five are young homosexuals. And yet I don't see any correlation there because they don't know each other. But as you're well aware, if it's not recognized and treated in time, pneumocystis pneumonia causes rapid death. I have every reason to believe that we're facing a new and devastating syndrome. Other people may already have it. I'm asking your journal to let me alert my colleagues."

At the other end of the line, Dr. Arnold Relman, fifty-seven, listened in polite silence. He was used to this sort of appeal. He was the editor of the most prestigious scientific publication in the United States and possibly the world, the *New England Journal of Medicine*.

*   *   *

In its 168 years of existence the *Journal* had dealt with all, or nearly all, the major medical questions and unveiled many of the scientific discoveries relating to health. In the middle of the last century it had published a report on the first general anesthetic use of ether, then the first clinical investigation of the treatment of angina pectoris. Several decades later it had presented the first complete report on childhood leukemia. It was in 1975 that it had compiled the first series of reports proving that total removal of the breast was not necessary to check the spread of cancer. From information arising from the sites of the first nuclear explosions in Nevada, it had drawn up the most exhaustive assessment of the dangers of radiation. Coronary angiography, the treatment of pernicious anemia, the use of substances such as amygdalin against cancer, and a thousand other curative processes had found a global clinical audience through its pages.

Its eclecticism was no less complete concerning social and political issues of medicine. From the index of the various subjects dealt with in the course of the previous year, it was possible to pick out articles on equal rights to abortion, the responsibility of advertising for pharmaceutical products, the use of asbestos in the construction of schools, sanitary protection in communist China, the role of lavatory bowls in the spread of gonorrhea, patients' rights, risks run in nuclear power stations, and wrist injuries incurred through the use of skateboards.

The *Journal* did on occasion make mistakes, but everyone acknowledged the care it applied to its choice of reports and the rigor with which it checked its information. Every Thursday, 225,000 copies of it were read religiously by the majority of the 400,000 American doctors and by several thousand of their foreign colleagues. The *New England Journal of Medicine* was also read in the corridors of Congress and in offices on Wall Street. It was quoted on television and in the national press, and transmitted by satellite to publications throughout the world via press agency teleprinters. The contents for each issue could influence the treatment of millions of sick people and determine the type of care provided by hundreds of hospitals and clinics. What was said on its pages about a particular medicine had the power to set the shares of pharmaceutical laboratories into a bull rush at the stock exchange, or bring about their downfall. In short, the *Journal* was one of the undisputed bibles of the American medical world. Having his name in its columns was the highest distinction a researcher or medical practitioner could boast about apart from the Nobel Prize.

More than four thousand texts and reports of experiments landed annually on its editor's desk. Less than four hundred, not even one in ten, were used. This strict selection was evidence of a desire not to echo anything that might appear sensational or premature. The *Journal* prided itself on, among other things, extreme prudence with regard to the announcement of any new epidemic. It had waited for six months and the official alert from the Department of Health before finally rendering an account of the epidemic caused by sanitary tampons that affected thousands of women; another six months before making its point about the renowned Legionnaires' disease responsible for numerous deaths.

* * *

"Have you conducted immunological tests on your five patients?" Michael Gottlieb heard the man at the other end of the line, Dr. Arnold Relman, ask dryly.

A distinguished nephrologist from the cradle of prestigious East Coast universities, the editor of the *New England Journal of Medicine* knew the rules of the game.

"Of course," the California immunologist assured him.

"Which ones?" pressed Arnold Relman, anxious to reassure himself that he was not dealing with one of the whimsical and not very scrupulous doctors who regularly bombard the *Journal* with their pseudodiscoveries and sensationalism.

Michael Gottlieb ran through the list of tests he had carried out on his patients and even specified the techniques of investigation used, but Arnold Relman remained skeptical.

"Are you really certain that you aren't just dealing with some sort of leukemia?" he went on to ask. "Have you taken bone marrow samples?"

In vain, the young immunologist pleaded with all the strength of his conviction. The mysterious illness that had struck the five young California gay men in his hospital struck no chord of recognition in the man in charge of the world's foremost medical

magazine. Giving as his pretext the long months of delay involved
before the *Journal* was ever able to publish the briefest of texts,
Arnold Relman ended up advising his caller to address his observations to the Centers for Disease Control in Atlanta. Its weekly
bulletin would provide him with the most effective means of making
his discovery known to the medical community as swiftly as possible.
That did not mean, he concluded, that the *New England Journal of
Medicine* would not "eventually follow up the issue."

10

Rebellion in the Maharaja's Palace
Benares, India: Spring 1981

Sister Bandona had no difficulty guessing where the young girl came from. She had slipped into the throng of destitute people besieging the dispensary. The shock of tousled hair shining with mustard oil, the look of a hunted animal—everything about her betrayed the fact that she had escaped from a much tragic fate. No sooner had her procurers brought her to the main street of the Benares red light district than she had managed to run away. Ignoring the other lepers' protestations, she steered her out of the line. It took all of Sister Bandona's gentle patience to allay the timid creature's mistrust and wrest a few words out of her. In snatches she came to understand that the girl's abductors were out looking for her to force her to go back, punish her, and perhaps even stone her to death. Ananda sobbed, trying to bury her face in her hands. Suddenly, the sister spotted the mark on her cheek.

"Little sister, show me your face," she said softly.

It was a characteristic lesion. Examination of some nasal secretion under a microscope would confirm the diagnosis of leprosy. The disease was well advanced. Unless it was treated urgently there was danger of irreversible damage.

Sister Bandona stroked the young leper girl's shock of oily hair. "Don't be frightened anymore, little sister, we're going to keep you with us to look after you and cure you. No one's going to come and hurt you here."

"The little Ganges vulture" bowed her head. They were not the type of words that an untouchable was used to hearing. After a long silence she dared to look up. "I didn't really understand what was happening to me," Ananda later confessed. "It was as if my karma had been unexpectedly adorned with all the *mahajan*'s gold."

*   *   *

The young leper girl's recovery was long and hard. Despite intensive treatment with sulfone drugs, at first the disease grew worse. Ananda experienced pricking sensations, sudden attacks of itching, the feeling that vermin were running about beneath her epidermis, or that liquid was trickling over her skin. She saw small lumps with reddish, dry centers appear on her body. Her eyebrows began to fall out. These setbacks went on for several months, then stopped. Next the sick girl's skin took on the appearance of tissue paper. Little by little the skin where the two first patches had been regained its sensitivity to contact with a needle and soon to the stroking of a finger. That was the sign Sister Bandona had been waiting for: the leprosy was in retreat.

Another more subtle sickness, however, was eating away at the young Indian girl. Despite the atmosphere of love and charity into which she had found herself plunged, hers were still the reactions of a child that had been cursed. She took care never to taint others with direct contact, kept her eyes constantly lowered, and took her pittance to eat with the mangy dogs. Sister Bandona's tenderness washed over her like the monsoon rain. "The curse of my karma was too strong," she would later explain. "It had permeated every fiber of my skin with a blackness that was darker even than my color. The gods had made me a pariah. I must remain subject to their will. I had been born guilty. I had no right to be loved." To this conviction was added a visceral mistrust. She had taken too many knocks, known too many betrayals, not to look for some malevolent, hidden motive in the sisters' goodness. Had she not already cruelly been deceived by the "generosity" of a stranger on a station platform? Had she not on many occasions heard people denouncing the underhand practices of Christians trying to convert Hindus to their faith?

One day, she went to join the little workshop where several other penniless women were making up bags of powdered milk and *dhal* flour that the nuns gave out to leper mothers. It was in this room that she saw for the first time a photograph of Mother Teresa holding in her arms a child that had been abandoned at the time of the great refugee exodus from Bangladesh. This picture had made the face of the future Nobel Prize winner famous throughout the world. "Her look, so full of joy and tenderness, seemed to reach out to all the suffering of humanity. That picture needed no caption, no explanation, no commentary. You could only look at that woman, allow her look to penetrate you, and feel the sadness, the shame, the need to love, well up from the bottom of your heart."

* * *

A crucial episode would finally erase the young untouchable's suspicious reactions. It happened in the spacious vaulted room into which some thirty gravely ill lepers were crammed. It was more a place for those about to die than an infirmary. An unbearable stench of decay and ether rose from the fly-covered bodies. Sister Bandona and Ananda had just come in, carrying another stretcher on which lay an inert figure whose leg had just been amputated. In the absence of any vacant space, the nun stopped in front of one of the patients who seemed not to be in as bad a state as the others.

"Ali," she whispered, "you're going to have to give up your bed for one of your brothers who's in a much worse state than you are."

The leper propped himself up on his stumps and grumbled as he examined the body on the stretcher. It was then that the incident occurred. It happened so abruptly that the two women dropped their stretcher. Lcoming out of the shadows, from floor level, a half-naked specter with neither feet nor hands had hurled itself onto the mattress.

"This bed is for me!" he yelled, pushing the body of its occupant out of the way with his forehead. "I've been waiting for days for this character to go so I could take his place. Fuck off, you daughters of bitches!"

Turning on Sister Bandona, he dealt a blow at her knees with his head. Then, seizing a bowl between his stumps, he began to drum noisily on the ground. Another leper, a bearded fellow with a hole where his nose should have been, picked up a bowl in his turn and joined in the uproar. That was the signal. Soon, the rebellion spread to all the mattresses. A deluge of sticks, crutches, spittle, and shreds of dressing flew in the direction of the two women. Bottles shattered against the walls releasing a penetrating smell of disinfectant. A projectile disintegrated over the engraving of the crucified Christ hanging on the wall behind Ali's mattress. "We are men, not dogs!" chanted some of the voices. "We want a hospital, not a home for the dying!" shouted others.

The din of bowls, shouting, and abuse, and the bombardment with various objects, increased in volume. With her hand tightly clutching the metal crucifix on the end of her rosary, Bandona remained as motionless as a statue in the face of the unrestrained horde. Terrified, Ananda had taken refuge behind a pillar. Then she heard a voice rise above the tumult. Unbelievably calm, her eyes more serene than ever, Sister Bandona was now brandishing her rosary crucifix above the protesting heads. "O God of love, take pity on Your suffering children," she chanted. "O God of love, have pity on them."

Disconcerted, the rebels seemed to hesitate. The uproar subsided, then, all at once, stopped. The hatred that had contorted their faces gave way to an apprehensive curiosity. What punishment was the sister superior going to inflict on them? The lepers saw her advancing toward them. Passing slowly between the rows of mattresses, she asked each of their occupants to repeat after her the prayer that she was going to recite. Ananda would long recall the spectacle of "those Hindus, Muslims, and Christians racked with suffering, reciting together, one sentence at a time, in rediscovered harmony, the words of the Our Father."

The scene had thrown the young untouchable girl into confusion. Through Bandona she was discovering a God of love. Above all, she was discovering that, just like those lepers, she, too, had the right to be loved.

*   *   *

Some days later, the leader of the revolt, the legless man with the shaggy hair, lay dying. Despite his will to live, his ravaged system had been unable to resist the devasting septicemia that was consuming him. Neither Sister Bandona nor any other member of the leper hospital would ever understand how he had succeeded in installing himself in the room without anybody's noticing his presence. He had lived for weeks, ensconced behind Ali's mattress, feeding himself on insects and scraps. After the mutiny Sister Bandona had had another mattress put down for him. When gangrene set in, she took him herself in a cyclecart to the government hospital on the far side of the city. She fought like a lion to have him hospitalized and treated, but no one, no doctor or medical attendant, wanted to take on a living corpse without family or resources. Disheartened, she had been obliged to take him back to her dispensary. He died a few days later, and his body—at least what was left of it—was carried upstream to the untouchables' funeral pyre. Throughout his dying hours, Sister Bandona and her companions had taken turns to be at his bedside to spare him what Mother Teresa considers the cruelest affliction of all: loneliness.

*   *   *

It took the dauntless faith of those young Indian girls to face this confrontation with death without flinching. Above all, they needed the heartfelt conviction that death was indeed, as Mother Teresa maintained, "nothing out of the ordinary, but a person's going home to the God who has created him." No certainty of the same order helped them daily to confront that other mystery, that of life. For Sister Bandona, there was no shame at all in acknowledging that she was "sometimes overcome by the entreaties, the cries, the despair, the frenzy of the sick, to the point of admitting defeat in the face of the sacrifices inflicted on so many innocents, of giving up when confronted by so much injustice and so much misfortune." Mother Teresa prescribed only one single weapon for her sisters against rebellion and discouragement: prayer. "Pray," she urged them, "pray much and always. For without prayer there is no faith, without faith there is no love, without love there is no gift of self, without the gift of self there is no real help for people in distress." She insisted on a prayer of the heart that was continual and silent.

*   *   *

Silence! In the hubbub of Benares the very idea seemed the most fanciful of imaginings. In order to have a corner to which they could retreat, the sisters had set up a chapel in a secluded room that the architects of the palace had originally designed for quite another purpose. Apart from the distant blows of the *dhobis* beating their washing on the banks of the Ganges and the strident call of bats, not a sound disturbed the peace of the former baths of the concubines of the maharaja of Nepal. A simple table adorned with a candle served as an altar, and behind, on the mosaic wall, hung the crucified figure of Christ. Beside his head, crowned with thorns, was the inscription: "I thirst." Beneath his nail-pierced feet another inscription read: "Whatever you do to the least of my brethren, you do to me."

Every day the small community came together to hear morning Mass and receive the Eucharist from the very dark brown hands of a young priest from Kerala, a province in the South. Then Sister Bandona would recite the psalms for the day, which her companions took up in a chorus. Sometimes hymns of joy, trust, and love, sometimes cries of suffering, recrimination, and distress, each verse evoked a reality that everyone lived with difficulty here. A period of silent adoration would follow, after which the sisters would prostrate themselves with their foreheads touching the ground to say the daily invocation prescribed by Mother Teresa for her Missionaries of Charity scattered throughout the world. "O Christ Jesus, You who showed so much compassion for the distressed multitudes, You who stooped over the lepers, the blind, the sick, the crippled, the hungry, the abandoned, the prisoner. You who cared for them and spoke to them with love, who brought them hope, promised them the goodness of Your Father; O Christ Jesus, come to our aid. Help us to spread Your compassion."

One April morning Sister Bandona noticed a figure hidden in the shadows at the back of the chapel.

"Ananda!" she exclaimed in surprise.

The onetime "little Ganges vulture" took hold of the nun's hand and displayed her healed cheek.

"I've come to thank your good Lord," she said. Then, for the first time, she smiled.

* * *

The spiritual metamorphosis of the former leper girl, her outburst of gratitude to the God of her benefactresses, did not repeat itself. She would never return to the chapel. Sister Bandona did not, however, give up hope: the example of charity and love set each day in the leper hospital would undoubtedly bring the young Hindu to an eventual discovery of Christianity. As the nun herself knew from her own experience of conversion, time must be allowed to play its part. Faith cannot be given. It has to be acquired by example. For the moment, Ananda was rejecting it. The reason for this was the inherited inability of an untouchable to feel herself equal to others. In vain, the sisters had increased their demonstrations of affection and treated their protégé like one of their own. Yet the stigma of being a pariah remained indelible in Ananda. Each day, each action revealed this stigma, and it frequently became the pretext for some crisis.

It was always in connection with tasks traditionally performed by untouchables that these crises arose. The girl who had been brought up in the belief that no task was too base for her impure hands, who had spent her childhood tainting herself by her association with death, who had carried out the most repugnant of chores such as emptying the latrines near her father's funeral-pyres, was now reluctant to pick up a broom or a floorcloth to help the sisters with the housework in the leper hospital. "Her rebellion was only natural," Sister Bandona explained. "Like all pariahs suddenly snatched from their condition, Ananda imagined that when we asked her to lay out a deceased person or clean the latrines, it was because she had once more become untouchable in our eyes. Whereas a converted Brahman—many of us were high-caste Hindus —would carry out those same tasks quite spontaneously as part of our commitment to serving Christ."

* * *

It took several months to defuse Ananda's rebellion, to make her agree to wash the mortal remains of lepers, then clothe them and decorate them with flowers. The day she finally accepted, it was as if some revelation had dawned in the young Indian girl's heart. "I, too, am everybody's sister," she said to herself. "I, too, have the right to love and to be loved by everyone."

To the unflagging Bandona, this initial triumph was just one step in the grand design she was harboring: that of making Ananda understand that Christ loved her even more than His other children. She never despaired of helping her to fathom the greatest secret of them all, the secret of the love of God. There again, the surest means of achieving her objective was by example. The value of this example, however, would continue to elude the young untouchable for a long time yet.

"Why do you waste so much time shutting yourself away doing nothing in the chapel?" she asked Sister Bandona one day. "That time would be better spent on the lepers."

The nun searched for an answer likely to capture Ananda's imagination.

"Because I'm married to God," she replied. "So it's only right that I give part of my time to my husband."

Sister Bandona knew that all Indians were familiar with this idea of divine marriage. *Bhakti*, the Hindu religious philosophy, married the followers of Vishnu and Krishna to their gods, submitting them to their will "as a loving wife is subject to her lover." Consequently, the need to share one's life with one's husband was an idea that the former leper girl could readily understand.

The nun exploited the parallel adeptly. "No one would dream of accusing a man of wasting time with his wife," she further explained. Time devoted to each other was essential to the couple's harmony. People who didn't know how to take that time drew fatally apart from one another. The same was true of her and her companions at the leper clinic. Even if every one of their actions throughout the day was a witness to the love they offered up to their God-husband, it was also appropriate that they should show their love in a disinterested way and "be capable of giving up an hour or two each day for Him and with Him, without expecting anything in return."

As Sister Bandona had hoped, this image finally impressed the young Indian girl. One evening as the nun came to kneel in the chapel of the leper hospital for her hour of evening adoration, she heard the soft tread of feet on the marble. Turning round, she saw Ananda, her head covered with a white cotton veil. She motioned to her to draw nearer. Pointing to the crucifix on the wall, she said in a clear voice: "Well, Lord, here we are. We're worn out with tiredness, dying to sleep, we've had just about enough of the lepers, but we're here to be with You, just to tell You that we love You."

11

A Commando of Very Special "Supercops"
Atlanta, USA: Spring 1981

Sandy Ford put down the receiver and frowned as she carefully reread the list of medicines she had just consigned to her register. "Dear God," she thought, "another request for pentamidine!" This morning's request came from New York. That made the sixteenth. She had only registered half that number for the whole of the previous year. Pentamidine was one of the few medications that could work on the type of parasitic pneumonia that Michael Gottlieb had diagnosed in the five young gay men in Los Angeles. Until now, the illness had been so rare that the only manufacturer of pentamidine, the British pharmaceutical firm May and Baker, had not considered it worth its while to invest the funds necessary to obtain official authorization for it to be sold on the American market. Like some other drugs capable of combatting diseases, such as sleeping sickness or cholera, that were extremely rare in the West, pentamidine had become an "orphan drug." This label meant that it was only available from one place in the United States: the Parasitic Disease Drug Service where Sandy Ford worked.

The dispensary was one of the services in the most impressive organization invented by man to defend himself against sickness and death, the Centers for Disease Control, more commonly known by its initials CDC. Its headquarters, a seven-story redbrick building, took up a whole section of a suburb of Atlanta. Decorated with an imposing marble bust of Hygeia, the mythological Greek goddess of health, its entrance hall gave access to a veritable hive of hundreds of offices and laboratories. Inside, more than four thousand specialists whose sole mission was to improve and protect the health of the American people kept themselves busy. Among them the CDC had epidemiologists, microbiologists, entomologists, physicists, chemists, toxicologists, doctors, dentists, public health officers, pharmacists, veterinarians, educational advisers, statisticians, writers, social science professors, and environmental and industrial hygiene experts. Their activities covered every imaginable field.

Whether it concerned the prevention of accidents at work or of risks to the environment, family planning, the dangers certain toys represented, nutritional problems, tobacco consumption, or the international surveillance of epidemics—the competence of this army of technicians and scientists embraced practically every aspect of health. Above all, however, it was in relation to the prevention and control of infectious diseases and epidemics that the Atlanta organization had won its international reputation. The laboratory of last resort, each year the CDC received from America and the rest of the world some 170,000 blood samples or organs contaminated by diseases whose nature was still a mystery. It was the world's largest breeder of microbes and viruses, a kind of zoo of the invisible, where specimens of infectious agents were kept: some that were almost extinct such as smallpox, others freshly dated such as the hemorrhagic infections of South America, or the fevers that struck in strange places such as Lassa, Marburg, or Ebola. With its enormous bank of serums and tissues containing more than 250,000 specimens of registered illnesses, the CDC provided the collective record of all human endemic diseases. Whether it was malaria from Trinidad, strains of African cholera, encephalitis from Texas, polio, typhus fever, or influenza, every specimen was featured in an electronic index that classified the diseases into some 250 categories with different labels bearing the endorsement "available," "restricted use," or for "posterity."

*   *   *

This FBI specializing in the hunting down of microbes and viruses had been born in March 1942, three months after the Japanese attack on Pearl Harbor. Then it was called the Office of Malaria Control in War Areas. It was based in Atlanta where malaria, endemic in the South of the United States, was posing a serious threat to the numerous military training camps in the area. Gradually its scope had widened to include dengue fever, an illness spread by mosquitoes, then yellow fever and typhus. In 1945, its facilities were augmented by a laboratory mandated with ousting the tropical diseases brought back by GIs from the war zones.

The restoration of peace should have put an end to the organization's activities, but the existence of a team highly specialized in health problems seemed so seductive to the authorities in Washington that the Office was kept on and in 1946, was given the name Center for Infectious Diseases. Soon it was endowed with a whole infrastructure of laboratories equipped to study bacteria, parasites, fungoid growths, bacilli, microbes, and viruses. Its scope was broadened in 1947 to include plagues and other animal diseases liable to be transmitted to humans.

The creation, in 1951, of an operations and information branch called the Epidemiological Intelligence Service really turned the center into a research agency assigned to combatting any agent that might threaten the health of the population. Spearheading the organization was a body of about a hundred select young doctors, veterinary surgeons, and public health officers recruited for two years and put through intensive training. The detectives from the Epidemiological Intelligence Service remained available night and day, ready to catch a plane for any destination in the United States or elsewhere on the globe, to track down the culprits responsible for any new epidemic.

Christened with its current name in 1980, the Atlanta CDC constantly stepped up its interventions in all directions. "Our mission is to identify and as far as possible, eliminate unnecessary illness and death," declared its director, Bill Foege, a pioneer of the eradication of smallpox in the Third World. "That means we have to monitor the South because of the risks of equine encephalitis, dengue fever, yellow fever; monitor the borders, the arrival of planes and ships; monitor the sudden occurrence of respiratory and infectious diseases that kill hundreds of thousands of Americans every year."

A hot line responded twenty-four hours a day to requests for help. The poisoning of three New Yorkers after eating smoked salmon that had gone bad, the asphyxiation of an elderly couple in Virginia the day after the extermination of rats in their home, an epidemic of acute rheumatic fever among sailors based in San Diego, the contamination of 157 visitors to a fair in North Carolina by trimethoprim-resistant bacteria, any health problem sent the CDC into action. Its sleuths conducted more than 1,200 inquiries a year. Though nearly all of these were concerned with localized and not very significant incidents, a good hundred would warrant general intervention, such as the famous epidemic that, in July 1976 in Philadelphia, killed twenty-nine veterans of the American Legion.

In the course of its general mobilization to discover the culprits in this tragedy, the medical detectives from the CDC had sent out more than 3,500 questionnaires, interviewed hundreds of participants in the convention, the employees of the hotel where they'd stayed, the inhabitants and the frequent visitors of the neighborhood. They scrutinized the meteorological office bulletins, the room allocation plan, the program of the various events. They tested the water, ice, and food. They examined under laboratory conditions all the cooking utensils, the crockery, the air-conditioning equipment, even tracked down insects and dust. Yet they could find only one denominator common to all of the many victims: the illness itself. It became the most famous epidemic of modern times. After four months of concentrated effort, the investigators from the most prestigious medical organization in the world had not even got as far as identifying the nature of the infectious agent responsible. Was it a toxin? A fungoid growth? A bacteria? A bacillus? A virus?

Having come very close to a somewhat inglorious end, the investigation was to undergo a spectacular resurgence. Two research scientists working in their windowless laboratories finally identified in the tissue of their guinea pigs the culprit responsible for the epidemic, an ordinary bacteria that had chosen as its habitat the turbulence of the air-conditioning ducts in the hotel where the conventioneers had assembled. The discovery of *Legionella pneumophila* made it possible to put a name to numerous other cases of this fatal pneumonia of unexplained origin.

However, the history of the CDC was not blazed with victories alone. That very year of 1976 it had also been involved in a resounding fiasco. Persuaded that a fatal epidemic of porcine flu that could be transmitted to humans was on the point of breaking out, its representatives had had more than 50 million Americans vaccinated. Not only did the epidemic fail to occur, but several hundred people found themselves paralyzed as a consequence of being inoculated with the vaccine. The affair degenerated into a political scandal and resulted in the dismissal of the director of the CDC. The government, for its part, found itself condemned to handing out millions of dollars to the victims of the inopportune vaccination campaign.

*   *   *

Apart from an epidemic of fever and rashes recorded in women who used a particular make of tampon, and the sudden appearance in Ohio of cases of enteritis in consumers of marijuana, no particularly spectacular event had taxed the talents of the Atlanta detectives for a long time. As far as the placid, bespectacled Californian Dr. Harold Jaffe, a member of the Epidemiological Intelligence Service, was concerned, the only significant threat hanging over the health of the American people as the end of the century approached was "the resistance of the clap to antibiotics." It was this threat that had been the driving force behind all the activity of his colleague, thirty-seven-year-old Dr. James W. Curran, or Jim to his friends.

Jim Curran was head of the research department in the field of venereal diseases at the CDC. With his hawklike eyes, his small build, and his air of being perpetually on the alert, he was the incarnation of the perfect prototype of the organization's supersleuths. He had devoted the greater part of his career to combatting the ravages of gonorrhea, a scourge that affected nearly a million Americans every year. This infection had inspired him to write numerous scientific articles, including an astonishing comparative study of the immune system's resistance to gonococci. To make his work as incisive as possible he had no reservations about choosing his examples from two opposite extremes of society: prostitutes and nuns.

*   *   *

However, good old-fashioned clap would not remain the principal focal point of interest for the organization's experts for long. At the CDC, as in doctors' consulting rooms elsewhere, other signs were arising, during that spring of 1981, that the front line of sexually transmitted diseases was changing. Every day the hot line in Atlanta rang to report some disturbing new observation. At the beginning of April, a call from a New York dermatologist had the impact of a small bomb. Dr. Fred Siegal announced that he had treated several young gay men suffering from unusual attacks of anal herpes. The ulcerations were spreading to other parts of the body. At a loss, he wanted the CDC to tell him what course of action its experts recommended in such cases.

Two further SOS messages a few days later were enough to set Jim Curran and his team into action. The first came from Los Angeles. Having failed to convince the largest American scientific journal of his discovery of a new epidemic, Michael Gottlieb was appealing to the CDC to publish an urgent description in its bulletin of the five cases of young gay men dying of pneumocystis pneumonia in his UCLA hospital. To be sure, the Atlanta bulletin had neither the readership nor the prestige of the *New England Journal of Medicine*, but the *Morbidity and Mortality Weekly Report*—a small brochure of about twenty pages received each week by 57,000 subscribers—was an indispensable channel of information on the nation's health matters. Each issue provided a table indicating the number and the causes of deaths that had occurred in the 121 largest cities in the United States during the course of the past week. Other tables recorded all cases of infectious diseases. There were amazing things to be discovered, such as the plight of the eight Americans who, in the course of the first ten months of the year 1980, had been cursed by leprosy, the dreadful disease that had caused the little Indian girl Ananda Chowdhury to be cast out by her own family.

The *MMWR* had informants in the country's smallest towns also, and the diversity of subjects covered meant that its observations were virtually universal. There was a report from a dentist in Virginia indicating an alarming rate of tooth decay in competitive swimmers. The CDC sleuths' investigation had made it possible to establish that the water in the local swimming pool contained an acid concentration that was 100,000 times stronger than usual. Another report disclosed that after a snowstorm in Colorado, hospitals in Denver had had to deal with fourteen cases of fingers being accidentally amputated by snow-clearing machines. It would also reveal that doctors in Puerto Rico, Florida, and Texas had been surprised to record a sudden mammary growth in seventy-two male Haitians, probably due to a hormonal imbalance brought on by a sudden improvement in diet.

Half the instances of illness or death cited in the bulletin were caused specifically by poisoning occasioned by food products. There was, for instance, the outbreak of psittacosis in turkey breeders in Ohio or asthma among employees of a crab-canning factory in Alaska. It was impossible to keep track of all the cases of digestive poisoning, typhoid fever, or salmonella reported by the Atlanta journal. This eclecticism did not, however, prevent the *MMWR* from having its particular specialties. The prevention of epidemics constituted one of the absolutely prime objectives of the CDC. Barely an issue went by that did not devote at least one piece to some syndrome affecting the community at large, such as the typhus fever epidemic generated by flying squirrels, rabies in rats in East Coast areas, or viral hepatitis in a Mexican village in the Sierra Madre.

*   *   *

Duly verified by the CDC's Los Angeles representative, Dr. Michael Gottlieb's observations were an unquestionable scoop for the modest Atlanta bulletin. They appeared on June 5, 1981, under the heading "Pneumocystis Pneumonia—Los Angeles," on page 2 of Volume 30, fascicle 1, an issue that would go down in history as the first publication to mention the illness humanity would soon come to know, with terror, by the name of AIDS. Informally, history would record, however, that the editor in chief of the *MMWR* did not consider it appropriate to devote the bulletin's cover page to the subject, giving preference instead to an article about how two American tourists had contracted dengue fever, a mild form of eruptive fever, during a holiday in the Caribbean.

The five cases presented by Michael Gottlieb in his forty-six-line communication did not, in fact, supply any very startling information: they concerned five young gay men who did not know each other, who all had a substantial history of sexually transmitted diseases, who all inhaled toxic substances, and who were all suffering from this infamous parasitic pneumonia that only attacked systems deprived of immune defenses. Yet Michael Gottlieb did stipulate at the time that the infection was very serious. Two of his patients had already died of it.

*   *   *

The second SOS that spurred Jim Curran and his troops into action that spring of 1981 came from New York. A department head in the faculty of medicine at New York University, Dr. Alvin E. Friedman-Kien, revealed the existence of a sudden outbreak of another extremely rare illness. This disfiguring of the skin bore no resemblance to the symptoms that had struck in Los Angeles. Except one: it, too, attacked young gay men whose immune system had for some unexplained reason been destroyed.

12

Two Entangled Bodies Tumbling into the Abyss

Latrun, Israel: Spring 1981

"Alleluia, Alleluia," wrote Brother Philippe Malouf to his parents in Lebanon, "God has filled my cup to overflowing: He has set me at the very heart of His Creation." With these simple words, the former guerrilla fighter for the Christian militia expressed his joy at being able to fulfill his vocation in the monastery of Latrun located in the foothills of Jerusalem. He had been spending his days outside the enclosure, laboring in the monastery's vineyards and selling the wine to visitors. He had hardly gone a week without the blade of his plough wresting some prehistoric flint from the earth or scraping up the remnants of some Canaanite tablet. For Philippe Malouf, this was a continuous reminder that God had done well in choosing this place as the cradle of His Creation. With the help of Brother Anthony, a young Iraqi with a red goatee beard who came from Abraham's birthplace, Ur, Brother Philippe had moved the little museum he had found on his arrival to more spacious premises. Every evening after vespers, he would shut himself in there with his relics to mount them on small plaster stands. He would label and group them according to their periods on shelves where, for generations, bottles of Chablis and Muscadet had been stored.

The frequent visits of two American archaeologists excavating at the nearby site of the ancient city of Gezer helped Philippe Malouf to organize his objects according to their civilizations. The men occasionally exchanged information about their discoveries. On Sundays, despite their Jewish heritage, Josef Stein and Sam Blum had taken to coming to the High Mass sung by the monks beneath the ribbed vaulting of the white stone church. The monk in charge of the small monastery hostel would then invite them to have lunch in the dining room reserved for passing guests. Its pale green walls were decorated only with an olivewood crucifix. The specialties of the house—leeks vinaigrette and rabbit in mustard—were probably unique in the Middle East. These unusual monastic feasts were concluded with a cup of Turkish coffee prepared and served just as it should be, then a glass of brandy or crème de menthe distilled in the monastery caves. On feast days, Philippe Malouf would receive permission from the father abbot to accompany his two friends to Gezer "for a few fabulous hours of delving into the strata of history."

The brilliant-white hill of Gezer rose from the plain as if it were a fortress. Like a sentinel on the renowned Via Maris, the immemorial route that for thousands of years had linked the Orient to the West, the town was built upon an upper slope at the heart of one of the most ancient of man's native lands. The site of Gezer had always excited the curiosity of archaeologists. Josef Stein, Sam Blum, and their team from the American School in Jerusalem were excavating this extraordinary site to try to expose a thirtieth layer of occupation. Helped in this herculean task by a hundred Arab and Jewish laborers, they had sunk a shaft thirty yards deep. To remove the tons of debris, they had set up a whole system of winches and constructed a very daring network of scaffolding at the site of the dig.

* * *

"Christ is risen!" Never before had an Easter festival brought with it so much promise. After celebrating in his abbey's church the mystery of the resurrection of the Christ to whom he had consecrated his life, Brother Philippe Malouf was going to celebrate the resurrection of the mortal handiwork of His creatures in one of the significant places in history. To mark the young monk's Easter visit to their dig at Gezer, his archaeologist friends had kept two appropriate surprises in store for him. The first was the freshly completed excavation of a Canaanite esplanade containing ten stone blocks and a huge monolithic basin, colossal witnesses to the fact that in antiquity this city had been a prestigious religious center. The second surprise was a remarkable discovery. After digging to the thirtieth level of occupation, Josef Stein and Sam Blum had recently unearthed the entrance to a tunnel. Hollowed out of the rock and reaching a length of sixty-six yards, this tunnel led to a gigantic cavern shaped like a subterranean cathedral. It was filled in abundance with a precious substance that explained why prehistoric man had founded a city on this site in the first place, and why millions of others had lived there for thousands of years thereafter. That precious substance was water.

The visit began with a photo to record the occasion. A strange trinity they made: those three men from such different backgrounds posing together. Josef Stein, with the beard of a biblical prophet, and Sam Blum, with the metal-rimmed glasses of a militant anarchist, stood on either side of Philippe Malouf, who, with his halolike tonsure and white habit, looked like a devotional image. It was as if the Old Testament and the Revolution were providing the setting for the Messiah. With Sam Blum leading the way, the three friends set foot on the first ladder and began their descent. The entrance to the tunnel was about thirty yards down. Every now and then a piece of rock would detach itself from the shaft wall and shatter in a succession of metallic clangs against the rods of the scaffolding. "It sounded like a melody from the dawn of time," the monk would say. It was then that disaster struck.

It all happened so quickly that Josef Stein was never able to reconstruct the actual sequence of events. "I thought I saw one of Philippe's sandals get caught in the folds of his habit," he would say. "His foot had slipped. Thrown off-balance, he toppled at once into the void. He tried to get a grip on the ladder again but couldn't grab hold of the rungs. He yelled out. Realizing what was happening just above his head, Sam reached out a hand to try to stop his fall. But as he tumbled, Philippe crashed into Sam and knocked him, in turn, off-balance. I heard two screams and saw my friends disappearing together into the abyss."

13

A Viennese Doctor's Strange Violet Marks
New York, USA: Spring 1981

The New York doctor's small black eyes were suddenly agog. Dr. Alvin E. Friedman-Kien, aged thirty-six, had never seen such a proliferation of lesions before. The patient's entire face—forehead, cheeks, nose, upper lip, chin—was studded with oddly shaped purplish marks. It looked like the mask of an opera clown. Yet Alvin Friedman-Kien was used to skin disorders. The eruptions related to his particular specialty were always visual. It was, in fact, precisely this aspect of dermatology that had attracted him to a branch of medicine less prestigious than others. Shapes and colors had always fascinated him. At the age of eight he had set about painting, sculpting, and modeling objects. A visit to a marine biology laboratory a few years later had oriented this taste for visual things in a scientific direction. Astounded by the prodigious abundance of aquatic life, the young boy had become passionately interested in the study of fishes. He had begun to collect all different kinds, from the most common to the most rare. He had gazed tirelessly through the microscope at the richness and diversity of their scales, examined each square fragment of an inch of their skin, dissected the smallest of their fins. His calling to animal biology was born out of the magical scenes he saw in the aquarium. All the same, when the time came to embark upon a career, Alvin Friedman-Kien had chosen to become a doctor, abandoning aquatic fauna in favor of humankind. In the classrooms of the Yale Medical School, he met the master who would guide him into his specialist field, the famous biochemist and dermatologist Erren Learner, who had just fathomed the mystery of the formation of skin pigments.

Twenty years later, having himself become a dermatologist and a research scientist of great repute, the former fish collector occupied the dermatology and microbiology chair in the highly acclaimed faculty of medicine at New York University. Closely combining work as a medical practitioner with virological laboratory research, he had been one of the first to use interferon, the powerful antiviral substance secreted by lymphocytes, in the treatment of illnesses hitherto regarded as incurable. His experiments with acyclovir had proved the efficacy of the only medicine capable of combatting one of the afflictions born of the sexual revolution, the red blisters that Americans frequently stigmatize with a capital H, Herpes. By the spring of 1981 his work on a vaccine against that cruel infection was sufficiently advanced to make him a potential Nobel Prize winner. On that April morning, however, the professional life of Alvin Friedman-Kien was suddenly to veer in another direction.

*   *   *

The patient who had just sat down in his clinic was a young Broadway actor. Apart from his cutaneous lesions, he looked in perfect health.

"Doctor, it's horrible: I can't even manage to hide my blotches under my makeup anymore," he moaned, running his hand lightly over his face.

A single glance had been enough for the specialist to diagnose the complaint. The shape and violet color of the marks on his skin were absolutely characteristic of a well-known illness. Yet all his experience as a doctor conspired to make him reject his verdict. He knew that this illness never affected young people, and that it tended to strike only in central Africa and on the shores of the Mediterranean Sea. The Viennese dermatologist who had described it for the first time in 1872 and given it its name could never have suspected the reverberations his discovery would provoke a century later. The five cases of subsequently fatal cutaneous ulceration that Prof. Moritz Kaposi set before Austria's Royal Academy of Medicine that year would become models of a particular type of skin cancer that would one day constitute one of the characteristic conditions associated with AIDS.

Except in Africa, Kaposi's sarcoma had remained so rare that a specialist like Alvin Friedman-Kien would acknowledge having come across scarcely more than a dozen cases in his entire career. It invariably affected older men of Jewish or Latin extraction who were displayed in hospital or faculty classes as unusual specimens. Normally, the disease developed so slowly that its victims usually died of something else. And now, on this April morning, the swollen face of a young theater actor had come along to break all the established rules. That same evening a biopsy confirmed the diagnosis and threw the practitioner into a state of turmoil.

What ensued in the course of the following weeks would remain in the memory of Alvin Friedman-Kien like "a sequence of scenes from a disaster movie." One day, he received a call from a colleague in general practice. "I've got a patient with some very strange cutaneous symptoms," the latter explained. "I've never seen anything like them. Can you take a look at him?" The dermatologist would long recall the shock of that visit. "In less than a fortnight, I'd found myself confronted with two cases of an extremely rare illness. Right in the middle of New York. In two Americans in their prime."

The second victim of Kaposi's sarcoma was a young and successful Fifth Avenue decorator. The first symptoms of his illness went back some months. He had been admitted to a hospital after an abrupt weight loss accompanied by a violent fever, nocturnal sweats, and general inflammation of the lymph nodes. His spleen had doubled in size and had been removed. No tests, however, had been able to uncover the origin of these disorders. A few days later, as he was getting ready to leave the hospital, he had discovered "strange bluish patches" on his legs. The intern on duty had shrugged his shoulders. "You must have banged yourself. Those are just ordinary bruises." The young decorator had gone home. Two weeks later similar patches appeared on his torso, neck, arms, face, and even in his mouth. In a panic, he rushed to his personal physician, who, at a loss as to how to deal with such an illness, had called the dermatologist Alvin Friedman-Kien.

*   *   *

With the same zeal that Dr. Michael Gottlieb was showing in Los Angeles in relation to his mysterious pneumocystis pneumonia epidemic, the New York dermatologist set about scrutinizing some five hundred cases of Kaposi's sarcoma recorded in world medical literature since 1872. Then he subjected his two patients to a relentless interrogation. Both were very active homosexuals. They did not know each other and did not share the same partners, but both had the same medical history of syphilis, gonorrhea, amebiases, herpes, and hepatitis B. In addition, both used "poppers," the amyl-nitrite-based drug so named because the ampuls go "pop" when they are opened. They enhanced sexual activity by dilating the blood vessels, notably those in the penis and anal membrane.

For days, Alvin Friedman-Kien searched for a clue that might shed light on the source of this tragic illness. He wrote to all the gay doctors in New York known to have a sizable homosexual clientele. He asked them whether they had found violet marks on the epidermis of any of their patients. The responses were negative. Alvin Friedman-Kien was on the point of giving up when a call from a cancer specialist at his own hospital informed him that in the course of the last two years the cancer department had had to deal with several cases of various cancers with additional cutaneous symptoms similar to those of his two patients. They were all gay men under forty. They had all died. No dermatologist had been invited to examine them. "It was like some kind of aberration," Alvin Friedman-Kien would protest. "Because of the incredible insularity of departments in a large hospital, an epidemic had passed unnoticed."

Overcoming his anger, the New York doctor reached for his telephone. If it had already wrought such havoc on the gay men of his city, Kaposi's sarcoma could hardly have failed to have struck elsewhere. He called colleagues in Chicago, Los Angeles, and San Francisco. As he had expected, patients with violet marks had indeed sought consultation in several hospitals.

In San Francisco, a young cancer specialist at the General Hospital had even just discovered an eruption of similar pustules on the skin and in the mouth of a twenty-two-year-old gay male attendant operating in the saunas there. None of his medical training had prepared Dr. Paul Volberding, aged thirty-one, to tackle this kind of pathology. Born on a farm in Minnesota, an athlete over six feet tall with the build of a rugby player, he had chosen oncology after spending his childhood gazing at the glass buildings of one of the shrines of cancer treatment, the world-famous Mayo Clinic, which happened to stand on the edge of his family farm. This was his first experience with lesions of this kind. At a loss, Paul Volberding called one of the best-known dermatologists in San Francisco to the rescue.

*　*　*

Gay himself, Dr. Marcus A. Conant, aged forty-five, specialized in sexually transmitted diseases. In the sixties when thousands of "flower children" in the hippie movement had settled in Haight-Ashbury to "make love not war," Marcus Conant had generously cared for some of the victims of excesses. Now his consulting room at the University of California hospital was separated only by the crest of a hill from the steamy streets of the Castro and the gay enclave where he himself lived. The many victims of sexually transmitted diseases filled his waiting room daily. Yet he, too, had never before seen a case quite like the one with which Paul Volberding presented him.

Conant was astounded by his own diagnosis. Like any other dermatologist, he knew that Kaposi's sarcoma was extremely rare and that it only occurred in men past sixty. Marcus Conant and Paul Volberding consulted their West Coast colleagues. Down the coast, Michael Gottlieb, the immunologist at UCLA, confirmed for them that several cases of Kaposi's sarcoma involving the same type of patient had just been identified in his hospital. In Stanford, not far from San Francisco, this type of skin cancer had just killed a young member of staff for the *Advocate*, a very well-known gay publication. In New York, Alvin Friedman-Kien had no difficulty in rounding up some thirty identical cases in the space of a few days. All of them, too, involved young and very sexually active gay men.

The visible nature of their lesions made their affliction particularly difficult to accept. Most felt like lepers. Those with the means to do so went and hid themselves away in the seclusion of a room in some private clinic. Others dug themselves in at home. Yet others

tried to commit suicide. Often the tumors did not confine themselves to the skin. They also attacked the tissue of internal organs:
the pharynx, esophagus, intestines, lungs. The doctors did not know
which way to turn. No treatment produced any effective and lasting
results. Not even chemotherapy and radiotherapy. In the space of
only a few months, one of Alvin Friedman-Kien's patients was a
living corpse in his hospital bed beside the East River. One week
before his demise, just when Alvin Friedman-Kien was despairing
at his inability to relieve his patient's anguish, the dermatologist
would undergo one of the most powerful emotional experiences of
his life. Going into his patient's room, he came face-to-face with a
healthy, vigorous man, and not the dying person he had been treating for months. He thought he was the victim of a hallucination.
In fact, it was his patient's twin brother, whom the doctor had never
known existed. Ten years previously the two brothers had quarreled
and had not seen each other since that time. Alvin Friedman-Kien
had difficulty concealing his surprise. All at once, he was overcome
by a profound sense of guilt. "Dear God," he reproached himself,
"if I'd known of the existence of a twin, I could have tried a bone-
marrow transplant. It might have restored life to this poor guy's
immune system and saved him."

From that time on, the dermatologist would never fail to check
whether each new patient had a twin brother.

*   *   *

Alvin Friedman-Kien would later regret the relative slowness with
which the Centers for Disease Control of Atlanta reacted to his
appeal. Six weeks elapsed before Jim Curran arrived in New York
with a team of his medical detectives to verify his initial findings.
Strangely enough, neither Curran nor any of his colleagues made
any mention to the New York doctor of the epidemic discovered
on the other side of America by Michael Gottlieb. It would take
another several weeks for the CDC authorities to establish a link
between the two happenings. On July 4, 1981, one month after
the revelation of the pneumonia afflicting the Los Angeles gay men,
a second article in the Atlanta bulletin dropped another bombshell
on the field of international medicine. Entitled "Kaposi's sarcoma
and pneumocystis pneumonia in male homosexuals," the article
reviewed the first twenty-six cases discovered in New York and

California. It bore Friedman-Kien's signature and that of the different practitioners who had collaborated with him in his efforts. The CDC report was accompanied by a strong editorial note directed at the entire medical profession, warning it to "be alert for Kaposi's sarcoma, pneumocystis pneumonia and other opportunistic infections associated with immunosuppression in homosexual men."

At the beginning of that summer of 1981, however, in Atlanta as in New York, Los Angeles, and San Francisco, where the first victims had been identified, nobody was in a position to give any kind of answer to the only real question: Why were these gay men in a state of immunodepression?

14

An Air France Steward's Last Journey
Paris, France: Summer 1981

The celebrated bulletin issued by the antimicrobe sleuths in Atlanta, the *MMWR*—the *Morbidity and Mortality Weekly Report*—
had one faithful subscriber in France. With the unruly mop of a
merino sheep, his inseparable motorcycle helmet in his hand, and
a Gauloise cigarette permanently lodged between his lips, Dr. Willy
Rozenbaum, thirty-six, looked more like a rock singer than a prince
of the somewhat conventional medical establishment in the home-
land of Louis Pasteur. If an electric guitar or the handlebars of a
Charlie's Angels motorcycle might seem to suit him better than a
stethoscope, it remained that this enterprising little fellow, constantly on the lookout for something new, was quite a remarkable
character.

He had begun his career at the age of twenty-three in the revival
unit of a hospital that specialized in bringing the dead back to life.
The antipoison center for the Paris area, the Fernand-Widal's Hospital, took in all the main victims of accidental and suicidal poisoning. Created in the fifties to preserve the lives of victims of
respiratory problems brought on by poliomyelitis, the revival unit
represented the most exciting of horizons to a young doctor burning

with the desire to prolong life, and unconsciously, to offer a kind of immortality. "It was fantastic," Rozenbaum would say. "Just imagine: restoring life to someone who was apparently dead, to be in a position to resurrect him, to get even with death." The apprentice doctor was lucky. It was in the field of poisoning that revival techniques had made the most spectacular progress over the last few years. In 95 percent of cases, lives were saved.

His first "miracle" had worn the angelic face of a Botticelli Madonna. The whole unit had fallen in love with Véronique and made her its mascot. At sixteen, she had wanted to die. To make quite sure she did so, she had swallowed a whole box of rat poison. Since the product was no longer on sale, it had not been possible to determine its precise antidote. Hers looked like a hopeless case. The little inert body brought in by the rescue team was virtually dead: in a very deep coma, showing respiratory, circulatory, and renal collapse, and total paralysis. Six months of intensive care had finally succeeded in bringing Véronique back to life. Despite serious aftereffects—loss of hearing and a destroyed kidney—she had been able to leave the hospital. Willy Rozenbaum had seen her again. He had wanted to know what it was that drove her to suicide. In the face of her incredible appetite for life, he had given up his questioning. "Véronique was breathing in the substance of life. She was cured." All the same, one day after they attended a movie, she had asked him out of the blue to help her to commit suicide again. He had forced her to explain why. In the end she had admitted to him that even though there were plenty of beautiful things on this earth, there were just as many that dispelled her will to live. This desire to die had taught the student doctor a primary truth. "Véronique helped me to admit the idea that death is part of our destiny, that the sometimes hallucinatory fight of the doctor for an impossible immortality is a sterile struggle. As Freud says, death always has the last word."

Dr. Willy Rozenbaum would never resign himself to losing a life, but he would carry with him the message of the Fernand-Widal's Hospital's little mascot: "By improving the quality of people's existence you are doing just as much for them as by slaving to prolong it." The limitations of resuscitation did not elude him. "The wonders of toxicological revival make it possible to save bodies. People sur-

vive, but not always in the best of states in terms of the quality of
their lives. In the majority of cases the psychological suffering per-
sists."

*   *   *

To get over this problem, Willy Rozenbaum had branched out
in another direction that he immediately considered "as fantastic as
revival." Infectious diseases offered him one of the most gratifying
spheres of medicine, one of the only ones where, since the advent
of antibiotics, statistics pointed to almost 100 percent recovery.
"Diabetes, hypertension, renal deficiency, can be treated, but not
cured. Whereas after even the most serious infection, a patient can
resume a normal life."

An outstanding opportunity to make an original contribution to
this field soon presented itself. French medicine had not yet focused
on the statistical study of infectious diseases, the analysis of a health
problem not so much in individual as in collective terms. Epidemiology was not yet one of the major concerns of the descendants
of Louis Pasteur. This enormous gap was to be partially filled one
morning in February 1979, by the arrival of Dr. Willy Rozenbaum
on his Kawasaki 1,000 cm³ at the door of the Paris Claude-Bernard
Hospital. His only assets: his youthful enthusiasm, a degree in
statistics and computer science, and his ambition to give French
medicine a concern for public health.

With its forbidding appearance and its lugubrious wings that
branched out from one another like barracks in a prisoner-of-war
stalag, the hospital that took on Willy Rozenbaum did not exactly
call to mind a temple of modern medical science. Yet in the last
century, the son of the vine-grower whose name it bore had discovered one of the essential functions of the human body, the
capacity of the liver to store the energy needed by the muscles.
Apart from the strong reputation that came with this name, the
Claude-Bernard Hospital had another claim to fame. Specializing
in the treatment of infectious and tropical diseases, it was one of
the most important centers in Europe for microbic and parasitic
pathology. Generations of military men, civil servants, missionaries,
and colonial survivors of French imperial adventures had come here
for treatment of the damage done to their organisms by their service
overseas. The recent explosion in travel and tourism to distant coun-

tries had unleashed a flood of new and diverse pathologies. In short, the Claude-Bernard Hospital was an outstanding laboratory for one who dreamed of committing to its computers the individual and collective records of the diseases treated there.

Keen to take advantage of the experience and methods applied abroad, Willy Rozenbaum had naturally gone on a pilgrimage to the Mecca of world epidemiology, the Atlanta CDC. It was there that he had become a subscriber to the *Morbidity and Mortality Weekly Report*. One of the rare French readers of this astonishing little journal, he used to go through it like a prayer book. "There can be nothing more exciting than receiving every week a bulletin reporting about the collective health of a country as vast as the United States and finding out about all its important and its trivial complaints," he would say. "It gives you an appetite for research and keeps you on the alert. Every time I met with my Parisian colleagues to discuss our scientific readings, I'd be keen to pass on to them the bulletin's original reports. Sadly, I nearly always fell on my ass. At the beginning of the eighties, the French were still very wary of epidemiology."

The plague of the century was to shake them out of their apathy.

*　　*　　*

As he did every Tuesday, Dr. Willy Rozenbaum could not resist the pleasure of tearing open the brown envelope with the imprint of the U.S. Department of Health and Human Services on it. Judging by its lead article, however, the issue of the *MMWR* for June 5, 1981 promised few surprises. The fact that two American tourists had contracted type-4 dengue fever from a mosquito while on holiday in the Caribbean did not exactly constitute an event of earth-shattering importance. Willy Rozenbaum was about to stop reading when his eye was drawn to the next article, reporting that five gay men had been struck with a mysterious form of pneumocystis pneumonia in Los Angeles. That looked more like news worthy of his interest. Willy Rozenbaum was aware of the existence of this parasitic pneumonia. He knew that during the Second World War it had affected young children suffering from malnutrition in the Warsaw ghetto. He also knew that it sometimes attacked premature babies. Finally, he understood that its parasites could break out in patients whose immune system was altered or deficient. He was aware that cases of pneumocystis pneumonia had been seen in the sixties when immunodepressive treatments were used to combat cancer or to prevent rejection in organ transplants. But what could the Warsaw children, premature babies, cancer sufferers, transplant patients, and the five gay men in Los Angeles have in common?

Willy Rozenbaum was mulling this question in his mind when the nurse ushered in his first patient of the day. He was a man of about thirty, a steward for Air France by profession. He was suffering from a high fever and persistent diarrhea. He was coughing. A male friend had come with him.

"Doctor, I've just spent three weeks' holiday on the banks of the Nile," the steward announced. "I must have picked up something nasty there."

Willy Rozenbaum questioned him. His diarrhea had started in Egypt for no apparent reason and had resisted initial treatment. In the course of consultation, the doctor noted that Air France had put him on the North American route and that he made frequent runs to New York and Los Angeles.

Willy Rozenbaum had seen hundreds of similar patients with intestinal problems resulting from stays in tropical countries—dysentery, amoebic infections, typhoid, etc. They were one of the specialties of the Claude-Bernard Hospital. But such disorders in conjunction with a dry, tenacious, persistent cough were, on the other hand, something peculiar and new. He examined his patient with the greatest of care before coming back to sit down at his desk. Puzzled, he was weighing the matter silently when his eyes chanced upon the copy of the *MMWR* open before him at the second page. "It was as if something clicked in my head. The presence of the male companion at my patient's side and the mention of the frequent stopovers in Los Angeles made me link his illness to that of the young American homosexuals in the report I'd just been reading. I decided to try to get to the bottom of it at once."

Willy Rozenbaum called on the assistance of one of his colleagues, the chest specialist Charles Mayaud, and had the unfortunate steward admitted to the hospital to undergo a bronchoalveolar procedure, a washing of the lungs. This was a sophisticated technique that makes it possible to collect the microbes lodged in the pulmonary system. After several examinations came the formal result. The patient was suffering from the same affliction as the five gay men in a hospital 7,500 miles away: pneumocystis pneumonia. But the cause was not apparent.

From then on the Parisian doctor was to be confronted by the same challenge as his American colleague Michael Gottlieb, that of identifying the cause of the illness. In Paris as in Los Angeles, the assumption was the same: this type of parasitic pneumonia could only develop in a body deprived of its immune defenses for very specific reasons. Unable to explain this deficiency, the two French doctors focused their investigations on searching for possible cancer of the lymphatic system, in other words, the white cells, the organism's guardsmen, which had apparently failed.

While they were working on their tests and analysis, they recalled several previous patients with the same symptoms. All had died of unknown causes. Suddenly, a chilling thought struck them: in all probability the illness afflicting the five gay men in Los Angeles was not a new American affliction, but a worldwide epidemic that had been festering without detection.

15

Pretty Martha's Very Unusual Autopsies

Atlanta, USA: Summer 1981

Jim Curran was flying around like a bat out of hell. The unrelenting microbe hunter from the CDC was having a hard time dispelling the apathy of his enormous organization and the skepticism of a good many of his colleagues for whom "this gay business" was a "lot of hot air." To him the question was both simple and at the same time extraordinarily complex. What could be done to put an immediate stop to the spread of the epidemic? Was there, as in the case of food poisoning, some germ responsible? What did the gay men have in common that could provide some indication? The first possibility that came naturally to mind was the existence of a sexually transmitted virus as in the case of the hepatitis B epidemic. That was hardly a cheering hypothesis, because there was nothing more difficult than neutralizing a virus. Should they be looking at those famous "poppers" that many of the patients seemed to have consumed? Could they be the common denominator for all the various infections? Did the fact that the gay men met mostly in specific places such as saunas, discos, or the back rooms of certain bars imply that an environmental factor was responsible? The otherwise vigilant and efficient Atlanta organization seemed strangely ill-equipped to find the answer to so many different questions. The epidemic appeared to be eluding the CDC's usual lines of inquiry. This was not a disease that was either exclusively venereal or viral or toxicological or environmental, but probably a mixture of all four at once. Hence Jim Curran hoped to appeal to experts from several disciplines and regroup them in pursuit of a common objective.

That July morning in 1981 was the first time his endeavors had produced any results. The general staff of the CDC had assembled in its entirety in the director's conference room to decide upon the creation of a task force to combat this deceptive epidemic. Gathered there were epidemiologists, cancer experts, immunologists, experts on viruses and parasites, environmentalists, specialists in venereal and chronic disease, computer whizzes, and even sociologists.

Having appointed Jim Curran as its head, the new task force made its first decision at once. In order to act effectively, they had to know the precise parameters of the pathology they were combatting. That was a precept of epidemiology. The inventors of this young science had perfected a technique known as "case control study." This made it possible to compare a large number of victims of a given disease with a large number of healthy subjects—the control group—in order to discover the differences between the two. That was how the CDC had established, among other things, the causal relationship between tobacco consumption and cancer of the lung. A key element in this methodology was compiling a questionnaire several dozen pages long. The success of the inquiry depended on the breadth of subjects tackled and the pertinence of each question.

Now, that July morning, neither Jim Curran nor any of his colleagues felt capable of preparing a proper kind of questionnaire. "We didn't have enough data on the patients," Dr. Harold Jaffe, the quiet Californian from the Epidemiological Intelligence Service would concede. "We didn't know what line to pursue. None of us had seen this new illness from close up yet. Our first priority was to get out there and meet the victims, chat with them informally, and find out what sort of lifestyle they led."

About ten members of the task force took off from Atlanta for the first reported emergency spots where the disease seemed particularly rife: Los Angeles, San Francisco, New York, and Miami. Accompanied by a local public health officer, Harold Jaffe was able to meet several patients in San Francisco and at Stanford. What struck him first was the condition the men were in. "They were really at death's door. And yet most of them had always been concerned about their health, their diet, their weight. They had always been careful to remain athletic. They were all very young. Most enjoyed enviable jobs and came from families that were comfortably off. How had they managed to destroy all that to end up like people in the terminal stages of cancer?"

The envoy from Atlanta was also astonished to find out just how sexually active these men had been. "They had had hundreds, even thousands of partners. Their financial resources had made it possible for them to travel, and they had fulfilled their sexual fantasies in every corner of the United States." Finally, his conversations confirmed the widespread use of various toxic substances, especially poppers. "According to the people I spoke to, these poppers seemed to be endowed with all kinds of properties. Not only did they dilate the blood vessels in the penis and the anal membrane, but by lowering the arterial pressure, they induced a euphoria which prolonged orgasm." Of all his memories as an investigator none would leave a more marked impression than his venture into a San Francisco bar where several patients had informed him he could get the best poppers in town, the kind that never gave you headaches. The place was one of the sadomasochistic bars of San Francisco. It was an unusual sight with its chains and instruments of torture for decoration and its faunlike bearded men, barded with leather dungarees, boots, and studded belts. Very shy, Harold Jaffe hesitated before entering. He felt the curious looks his young executive's suit attracted. In the end he cleared himself a way to the bar. "Give me two or three vials of your best junk," he asked the barman, not without embarrassment.

The barman opened a fridge that loomed large behind him. From it he took several ampuls trademarked Burroughs Wellcome Co., the prestigious pharmaceutical laboratory that manufactured the product for patients suffering from angina. He also took out three flasks the size of miniature bottles of perfume labeled Disco Roma, the most sought after poppers. Harold Jaffe pocketed the lot, paid thirty dollars, and hurriedly left the place. "My one fear," he would say with a laugh, "was that one of those damned poppers might explode in my suitcase and release its disgusting smell of rotten bananas into the plane." Immediately on arrival in Atlanta, Harold Jaffe rushed to hand them over for analysis to the toxicology experts at the CDC.

* * *

The mass of data that Jim Curran had gone to New York to gather promised to be just as useful in the compilation of the task force questionnaire. The tireless medical detective paid systematic visits to all the persons with Kaposi's sarcoma reported by dermatologist Alvin Friedman-Kien. "I'd never seen that kind of skin cancer before," he would recount. "The violet patches were heart-rending, especially as many of the patients seemed miraculously to be otherwise in good health. The Broadway actor, in particular, was fit and athletic. As luck would have it, he and I had grown up in the same suburb of Detroit. We went to the same schools, the same church. He told me what a scandal his homosexuality had caused back there. I couldn't quite believe that all those nasty marks on his face were the direct consequence of his choosing to give expression to his difference. He forced himself to laugh as he showed me other nodules all over his body. His disease hadn't yet assumed the dreadful symptoms it would a few weeks or months later, but I knew even then that he didn't have anything to laugh about."

Back in Atlanta, Jim Curran had Sandy Ford's registers at the Parasitic Disease Drug Service examined for all requests received for pentamidine, the treatment to combat pneumocystis pneumonia. The CDC was its sole American distributor. Investigation along these lines made it possible to pick up the records of gay men who had died in 1979, 1980, and 1981. In particular, it established that they had all lived in New York, Los Angeles, San Francisco, and Miami, which supported the supposition that the epidemic had originated in those four cities. The head of the task force then undertook to have the local CDC representatives study the public health archives of America's eighteen largest cities to check for all the cases of pneumocystis pneumonia and Kaposi's sarcoma identified during the preceding three years. Finally, he had the heads of some thirty hospitals throughout the country together with a large number of private doctors questioned by telephone to make sure that not a single case of pneumocystis pneumonia or Kaposi's sarcoma escaped his organization's knowledge.

*   *   *

It was precisely five o'clock that September morning when the telephone rang in the bedroom of a young woman living on the outskirts of Atlanta. Rudely awakened, Dr. Martha Rogers picked up the receiver. A pretty, dark-haired twenty-six-year-old from Georgia, she was one of the latest doctor-sleuths to be recruited to the CDC's Epidemiological Intelligence Service. The call was from Fort Lauderdale in Florida. At the other end of the line, a man's voice directed: "Catch the next plane. He's just died."

Martha Rogers and her colleagues in the task force had been waiting for several days for this call. In fact, the CDC had been notified by the hospital in Fort Lauderdale that a thirty-five-year-old patient was about to die of generalized Kaposi's sarcoma. He had bequeathed his body to science. It was a unique opportunity. Martha Rogers had been designated to take part in the autopsy and supervise the removal of the various organs affected by the sarcoma. Analysis of the specimen tissue taken might just provide vital information as to the cause of the epidemic. Based on the sick man's medical file, the experts in Atlanta had put together an initial list of organs the young woman had been told to inspect on the spot in case other unknown lesions might come to light in the course of dissection.

Martha Rogers's adventure lasted only one day, but what a day! All through the return flight to Atlanta that evening, she did not take her eyes off the small blue simulated-leather case placed on the seat beside her. The other passengers on Delta Airlines flight 450 would have been astounded to discover that inside that ordinary piece of baggage there was an isothermic box containing two eyes, some pieces of brain, intestine, and liver, a fragment of esophagus, several shreds of epidermis, the tip of a tongue, and a tube full of blood. In short there was a variety of samples that might just harbor the key to one of the greatest enigmas of modern pathology. The aircraft's late landing prevented Martha Rogers from taking her precious parcel to the CDC laboratories. So it was that these pieces of evidence, the vital research tissues, spent their first night away from the body of their unfortunate owner wedged in her home freezer between two Dixie cups of strawberry ice cream intended for her children.

16

"What Have I Done to Deserve This Punishment, Lord?"
Jerusalem, Israel: Autumn 1981

A fly on the ceiling. Philippe Malouf's whole world was now confined to this exclusive vision of an insect's crawling about on panels punctured with little holes, a ceiling that was enough to drive one mad with its little holes. How many days had it been? How many nights? The young monk had lost all sense of time. Twenty-two days in a coma and four weeks of sleep interspersed with semiconsciousness, followed by the realization of his condition. He could no longer feel anything from the nape of his neck to the tip of his toes. His body was no longer his. He could not control his limbs or cough or swallow or sneeze or eat or speak apart from snippets of sound directed in a gasp at some visitor or doctor. For several days he had been able to pay only confused attention to what had happened to him. Then, suddenly one evening, he had recognized the large, bearded head of Josef Stein looming above him. The American archaeologist had forced a smile and even a joke. "And I thought your good Lord gave his angels wings!" It was at this point that the young monk had made the most painful discovery of all: he couldn't even laugh anymore.

Philippe Malouf had not been able to do anything to break his fall down the excavation shaft. Sam Blum, his other American friend who had preceded him on the ladder, had been luckier. Providentially, a plank projecting from the second gallery had blocked his plunge into the abyss. He had gotten away with a collarbone and two ribs broken.

Josef Stein could not forget Philippe's scream as he fell, then the dull sound of his body as it crumpled at the foot of the excavation. The cries for help, the frenzied descent into the shaft, the setting up of a winch, the arrival of an ambulance with the Star of David on it and its stretcher-bearers, bare chested and in shorts, the bracing of a stretcher to be lashed to the winch pulley, the slow ascent of the unconscious man through the millennia of rock strata, his transportation to the Hadassah hospital in Jerusalem, his disappearance into the emergency ward—all the sounds, all the images, were telescoped together in the American's memory like a surrealistic kaleidoscope. Finally, there was the sight of the surgeon, emerging from the operating room, his pale green mask dangling under his chin, his forehead beaded with perspiration, a cigarette already lit between his lips. Pale and tired, the surgeon was visibly disinclined to give anything away, mumbling simply in a neutral tone, as if to take the drama out of the unbearable:

"Fracturing of cervicals three and four, with crushing of the medullary canal. Paralysis of all four limbs."

"Permanent?"

It was as if the question had been muffled by Josef Stein's beard and by his emotion. The surgeon had taken a puff of his cigarette and slowly exhaled the smoke.

"To the best of our present knowledge, I'm afraid so."

*   *   *

Soon his inert body was overwhelmed with anguish. It was an uncontrollable anguish brought on by the thousand phenomena registering in his consciousness against the solitary background noise of the blood pounding in his temples: a sudden feeling of suffocation, a fall in blood pressure, the sensation of heat or cold, the inability to perspire, a sense of degradation or impotence at the loss of control of his bodily functions. And even more painful, he suffered the humiliation of finding himself delivered up naked, exposed, put on display to a procession of strangers.

Deeply upset by the young monk's distress, the father abbot from the monastery of Latrun looked for words that, he hoped, would bring a little comfort. Pointing his large, callused hand in the direction of the terraced roofs of Jerusalem visible from the windows, he reminded him that "it was up there, only a few hundred yards over the hill, that the One who came down to earth to redeem mankind underwent the agony of his Passion." But in his own passion, a strange obsession altogether alien to his commitment to the Christ of Golgotha, though very human, was distracting the young Trappist. In vain he turned the question over and over in his mind. Still he could not find the words to express it. It was to Josef Stein that eventually one evening he confided his torment. The two friends were listening to the distant voice of an Arab muezzin calling people to prayer from high up on a minaret.

"Tell me, Josef," the young monk asked without preamble, "do you think I'll never have an erection again?"

His anguish was succeeded by a period of rebellion, a fact that the doctors regarded as a positive sign of the paralyzed man's resistance and renewed fighting spirit. Just as Jacob had cursed his Creator for an entire night, so the young monk's imprecations were directed initially against the God of mercy to whose service he had committed himself. "What have I done to deserve this punishment, Lord? Why me?" Failing to find any satisfactory answer in his faith, the former guerrilla fighter vented his despair on those who surrounded and cared for him. Insults, cries, reproaches, threats: for some weeks the small room looking out over Jerusalem became a caldron of verbal violence that nobody dared to enter.

A complication would soon place the injured monk's life in jeopardy. Because of his immobility, parts of his skin that were in constant contact with his bed began to die. Deprived of blood and hence of oxygen because of their prolonged compression, these unirrigated areas broke out in sores, ugly, deep wounds, potential homes for irreversible infection. With urgent treatment and massage every quarter of an hour, the interns and nurses fought relentlessly to stop the tissue from mortifying and to prevent the appearance of fresh lesions. So much fervor and devotion could not fail to affect the monk's feelings of rebellion. Pondering all the events that had made up his life over the last twenty-five years, he sought desperately the strength to accept his condition. His brothers from the monastery took turns coming to help him in his attempts, bringing him the comfort of the Eucharist and the support of their prayers. It was an unexpected visit, however, that was to give Philippe the decisive shock he needed to subdue his revolt and begin to accept his condition.

*   *   *

That afternoon, he had not heard the furtive sound of two rubberized wheels gliding on the linoleum of his room. All at once, he found a girl's face next to his pillow, her forehead creased by a scarlet ribbon encircling a luxuriant shock of black, curly hair. The brightness of her expression and her smile exuded such lively strength that the monk was taken aback by it. "It was *life* that had just come into my room," he would say. "She operated a small handle with her mouth in order to control her electric wheelchair. Her hands sat motionless on the armrests, indicating that she, too, was totally tetraplegic. On her lap was a bottle. '*Shalom!*' she said cheerily. 'My name is Ruth, like the woman in the Bible. I've brought a bottle of wine for us to drink to your recovery. It comes from Mount Carmel. Just you wait and see how good it is!' Then her lips tightened on the handle again, the wheelchair did a half circle, and she left my room."

One minute later, the young Israeli girl was back, accompanied by a nurse carrying a tray with the bottle and two glasses full of the wine from Mount Carmel.

"*L'chayim*, Philippe! To life!"

The nurse poured wine in the first glass and put it between the monk's lips. He took a long sip. At once a wave of warmth flowed over him, dispelling in one shot the taste of rusty sheet metal that had been rasping at his tongue ever since the accident. Tears welled in his eyes. He tried to speak, but overwhelmed by emotion, could not manage a single word. Under the softened gaze of Ruth, who was now smiling at him, he took another mouthful.

"Thank you, little sister," he said, closing his eyes. "Your visit has been the most beautiful gift imaginable."

That evening, Philippe Malouf learned of the tragedy that had shattered Ruth's life. A member of a kibbutz located at the extreme north of Galilee, one night she had been part of a patrol along the Lebanese border when two bullets fired at close range by a fedayee had smashed her spinal column to pieces.

*   *   *

That same week, a second occurrence would contribute to the young Trappist's reemergence into the land of the living. Convinced that his cervical fractures had healed, the doctors decided to sit him up in bed for the first time. After boosting his heart with a powerful cardiotonic, a nurse set about gently raising the upper part of his body. After so many weeks of having the ceiling punctured with holes as their only vista, his eyes were suddenly lost, seeking new points of reference. "The room swiveled in all directions as if I were in an aircraft looping a series of loops," Philippe Malouf would confide. Gripped by violent nausea, he began to vomit. He had to be restored to a prostrate position. Fresh attempts were made the next day and on subsequent days, until gradually he was able to take this first step toward recovery.

17

Five Hundred Questions for a Frantic Investigation into the Mysteries of the Libido

Atlanta, USA: Autumn 1981

It was the most detailed, imaginative, daring questionnaire the brains of the young science of epidemiology could devise. Dr. Jim Curran and the members of the CDC task force had literally surpassed themselves in completing the document that, they hoped, would provide them with an answer to their riddle. All the experience acquired in their previous epidemiological inquiries into venereal disease, hepatitis A and B, and other infectious diseases had provided the basis for the structuring of this momentous questionnaire. A study, carried out four years earlier by two gay research scientists, of the sexual mores of some five hundred American homosexuals had supplied invaluable basic data. In addition, the task force had made an inventory of all the cases of pneumocystis pneumonia and Kaposi's sarcoma diagnosed in the United States at the beginning of that autumn of 1981—about forty in all—and their description in precise terms had completed the preparatory dossier.

Jim Curran had also requisitioned the services of Prof. William Darrow, the house specialist in sociological studies on groups that were sexually at risk. This work on the social dimension of sexual phenomena carried considerable weight. The forty-two-year-old scientist had devoted twenty years of his life to analyzing the practices of people who suffered recurrently from syphilis, gonorrhea, and other venereal diseases. "As far as I am concerned, there isn't a shadow of doubt about it," he affirmed. "This epidemic is passed on by sexual means." In order to clinch the case, or alternatively, to bring other factors to light, Jim Curran and his team decided it was vital to subject each patient and the healthy homosexual control group to a comprehensive interrogation made up of some five hundred questions. The list took up twenty-three pages of a document that bore the code name CDC Protocol 577.

The first part of the questionnaire was aimed at placing the respondent in a particular income and social bracket. Was he white, black, Hispanic, American Indian, a native of Alaska, indigenous to a Pacific Island, or of some other extraction? Did he earn less than ten thousand dollars or more than thirty thousand dollars a year? Was he single or married? Had he been married previously, once or more than once? For how many years had he attended school, college, university? What employment had he had in the last ten years? In the course of his professional occupation or leisure activities, had he been exposed to any industrial or agricultural chemical products, radioactive material, or defoliants? Where had he resided during the last ten years? To what countries had he traveled? Had he kept any domestic animals? For what period of time? Had the aforementioned suffered from any unusual illnesses? Had they died as a result of these illnesses? Was the subject in the habit of consuming alcoholic beverages? Occasionally? Regularly? Beer, wine, cocktails? How much a day, for how many years? Did he smoke? How many cigarettes a day, for how many years? Was there a history of cancer in his family? Had his grandparents, parents, sisters, or brothers suffered from cancer? What type of cancer? When? Along the same lines, had he in the last three years cohabited with any person, man or woman, sexual partner or not, who had suffered from cancer, or been hospitalized for any infection, or undergone an unexplained loss of weight, associated or not associated with a fever?

The questioning went on to reconstruct in minute detail the subject's medical history prior to the outbreak of his current illness. Had the subject ever suffered from syphilis, gonorrhea, nongonococcal urethritis, herpes, or genital warts? How many times? When had the last infection occurred? Where were the lesions located?

On the penis, at the entrance to or inside the rectum? The questionnaire also placed great importance upon all previous diseases that were intestinal in origin—salmonella, amebiasis, hepatitis—and on skin eruptions, inflammation of the lymph nodes, pneumonia requiring hospitalization, cancerous tumors. The nature of any medication taken during the last ten years was also a subject for detailed questioning. Had it included penicillin, and if so, in the form of injections or capsules; ampicillin in pill form, tetracycline in tablet form; particular substances for amebiasis such as Flagyl, oxyquinolines, and Humatin; cortisone; Kwell for fleas and scabies; or any other medications, which the subject was asked to remember and for which he was called upon to supply the dates and frequency of use.

Advised that his present illness could be related to drug consumption, the subject was next directed to reveal whether he had taken any such substances and if so, on what date and in what form: injections, cigarettes, inhalation, or pills consumed orally. There followed a list of possible drugs: marijuana, cocaine, heroin, amphetamines, barbiturates, LSD, Quaaludes, angel dust, etc. Poppers were naturally the object of particular interest, notably with regard to the frequency and the places where they were used: saunas, discos, bars, bookstores, cinemas, public toilets, public parks . . . and the source of their manufacture. Were they in ampuls or vials? With or without labels? Which make did the subject prefer? Bolt, Bullet, Disco Roma, Hardware, Head, Highball, Hit, Kryptonite, Locker Room, Pig Poppers, Quicksilver, Rush? If the subject had a predilection for some other sort not as yet registered in the Atlanta computers, what would this popper be called?

But "noblesse oblige": it was of course the sections relating to sexual behavior that were subjected to the CDC medical detectives' most attentive scrutiny. This part of the inquiry directly informed the subjects under question that it seemed highly likely that their illness was due to the specific nature of their sexual relations. By "sexual relations" the questionnaire specified "the introduction of your penis into a partner's mouth, vagina or anus; or the introduction of a penis into your mouth or anus." Based on this definition, the questionnaire now covered the whole gamut of homosexual and heterosexual practices down to the smallest detail. Some questions were so crude there was a chance investigators would hesitate to ask them. Dr. Martha Rogers, the young woman who had brought the first Kaposi's samples back from Florida, would admit to being reluctant to ask her interviewees whether they preferred introducing their penis or their tongues into their partner's rectum, and the percentage of times they carried out one or the other of these practices.

The CDC representatives had left nothing to chance. They had conducted "preliminary desensitization" training to prevent any eventual weaknesses on the part of their investigators. This consisted of running through the questionnaire with a specialist in sexually transmitted diseases. That was how, much to her surprise, Martha Rogers found herself confronted by Jim Curran himself, playing the role of a hypersexual gay. "I was so taken aback at finding myself face-to-face with my boss and having to ask him such intimate questions that it took a few minutes before I could utter a word," she would recall. "In the interests of my own liberation he made up the most outrageous answers I would ever be likely to hear."

The first attempt to track down the causes of the unknown disease got underway on October 1, 1981. About fifty patients—some already at death's door—and a control group of two hundred gay men who were healthy but whose behavior put them at risk would participate in Operation Protocol 577. All volunteers, they had been referred to the CDC by private doctors and the venereal disease departments at various hospitals. The inquiry was initially confined to the four cities—Los Angeles, San Francisco, New York, and Miami—where the illness had struck first. Eventually, Atlanta was added because of the unexpected discovery, in a small Georgia town, of an instance of Kaposi's sarcoma, this time in a boy of only thirteen. "That was an incomprehensible case," Jim Curran would say. "So strange it might perhaps provide us with the key to the whole enigma. With that adolescent's cancer we found ourselves like cops chasing a murderer who has killed ten prostitutes with a silk stocking and then suddenly murders the eleventh with a kitchen knife. This unexpected trail could point us in a fresh direction to the disease we were trying to identify."

* * *

For many years the impregnable ramparts of the 655 rooms in the old hotel on Manhattan's Upper East Side had safeguarded the virtue of wealthy young American girls staying in New York. The Barbizon Hotel for Women had never accepted masculine guests, and the presence in the building of any male visitor was restricted exclusively to the drawing room on the ground floor. Here, as elsewhere, however, the sexual revolution had taken its toll and eventually toppled this bastion of New York respectability. Since Valentine's Day of that same year, 1981, the Barbizon Hotel had been welcoming guests of either sex.

Jim Curran believed that its rooms, still pervaded as they were by the discreet aroma of virtue, would provide the perfect setting for the medical-sexual investigations of Operation Protocol 577. Dividing the country in two, he had entrusted the West Coast inquiry to Dr. Harold Jaffe and had assigned himself the supervision of the larger New York sector. Among his troops was the young woman he had instructed in desensitivity training. Dr. Martha Rogers would never forget her New York experience. "Every evening, after I had taken my last sample of anal secretion from my last gay visitor of the day, I would rush to the telephone to call my mother. I told her everything. Living in a very small town in the heart of Georgia, the poor woman was torn between pride at seeing her daughter belong to an institution as prestigious as the CDC and horror at the outlandish things I was having to do."

Every morning at breakfast, as he dug into his scrambled eggs, Martha Rogers's indefatigable boss went through the previous day's completed questionnaires in minute detail. "Look, Martha, you should have asked this guy how many partners he made love with last week. Dividing the total number of partners for the entire year by fifty-two doesn't necessarily give us the exact number of encounters in the course of the last week. The least little thing could be of vital importance."

*   *   *

Dr. Harold Jaffe's expense account did not entitle him to frequent the more palatial California hotels, so he and his team checked into the Best Western, a rather modest motel below Market Street in San Francisco. Mary Gynan, a young specialist in the CDC's viral diseases department, was part of his group. The constant coming and going of visitors, all young and obviously gay, eventually aroused the suspicions of the owner of the establishment. What sort of high jinks could the yuppie-type guests who claimed to be government doctors be getting into upstairs? One afternoon the proprietor got out his master key and burst into Mary Gynan's room, only to find to his amazement the young woman "bent over the rear end of a pretty blond boy, in the process of taking secretions from his backside with some cotton wool."

Their failure to take any precautions whatsoever during these proceedings would later haunt members of Operation Protocol 577. "We were oblivious to the danger," Harold Jaffe would acknowledge. "We didn't wear gloves or masks, and we used our own bedrooms as examination rooms." For a long time, Mary Gynan would recall the trauma of the blood that spurted over her when one of her healthy subjects fainted without warning while she was taking a blood sample.

The interviewers were astonished by their subjects' willingness to answer questions of even the most intimate and compromising kind, such as those relating to the use of drugs. "It was as if the people we were questioning had a presentiment of the nightmare that was to come, as if they wanted to help us stop it," Harold Jaffe would confide. Plenty of other surprises lay in store for him. One day, when he was questioning a bearded man, in black leather clothing covered with badges, and asked him where he usually indulged in his sexual revels, he found himself given the names of several of the city's top hotels. Amused by the doctor's surprised expression, the bearded man explained: "They're the only places that have spacious enough rooms for me to lay out all my gear." The man did not have to be begged to explain that he was heavily into sadomasochism. For their activities he and his partners resorted to a whole range of military uniforms and devices, the use of which did indeed require plenty of space.

When illness confined one of the subjects to his bed, the interviewers would go to his home or hospital. Martha Rogers remembers having to go out very late one evening "to the far end of Manhattan, to see a poor guy painted with the gaudy colors of Kaposi's sarcoma. He was like a Mardi Gras clown." She had walked back through the deserted streets clutching in the bottom of her pocket, as if it were treasure from the lost Ark, "a small box containing the implicating vials of blood and sperm and other secretions that were evidence of the illness that was killing him." In Los

Angeles, Harold Jaffe conducted several interviews in luxurious Hollywood homes. "It was a bit embarrassing to turn up and see people like that and asking them all those indiscreet questions beside their swimming pools," he would admit. "One day, one of my hosts, who seemed to have a particular interest in the inquiry, slipped off his trousers and began to masturbate in front of me, to provide me with a prime specimen of his sperm."

Each night, before going to bed, the envoys from the CDC would assemble in an isothermic box filled with crushed ice the tubes of blood and the other secretions that had so patiently been collected. The next morning, they would go to the nearest post office with their parcel. When asked to declare the commercial value of their shipment, the CDC representatives could only reply: "No value." How could a dollar value be established for a collection of vials that might contain the culprit of a tragedy whose magnitude was beyond calculation?

18

"Wherever People Are Suffering"
Calcutta, India: Winter 1981

54-A Lower Circular Road. The entrance to the headquarters of the mission founded by Mother Teresa was marked only by a modest wooden board. The gray, three-story edifice at the heart of Calcutta had become one of the best-known buildings in that vast city, and one of the most visited by all those Indians or foreigners who are on pilgrimage to the source of the famous nun's work. Its ever-open windows overlooked a rumbling tide of overloaded trams, lorries, cars, and rickshaws pulled by the last human horses on this earth. On the crumbling sidewalks of the avenue, a whole host of homeless people in *dhotis* that enveloped them like shrouds lived alongside dealers in scrap metal and car parts. At the hydrants, clusters of naked children splashed about in the gutters, while on every street corner vendors of tea, fritters, and puffed rice sold the poorest of the poor their daily pittance.

Entry to the building was made through a wooden door in a narrow side street constantly cluttered with crowds of beggars, lepers, and women carrying emaciated children in their arms. A simple piece of string attached to a small bell served as a doorbell. Whenever it rang, the face of a young Indian sister in a white veil with a blue border appeared. She would lead the visitor through a little courtyard adorned with a large statue of the Virgin Mary, her arms held open wide. The courtyard led to a flight of stairs. On the first floor was the chapel, a vast room furnished only with an altar but always pervaded with a vibrant atmosphere of faith and prayer. As in the chapel of the leper hospital in Benares, on the far wall, next to a wooden crucifix, an inscription proclaimed: "I thirst."

The woman who quenched the thirst of the crucified Christ in India and elsewhere came here several times a day. She would kneel on an old, patched jute sack and ask God for the strength and inspiration to continue her crusade among the most destitute, the abandoned, the lepers, the despairing, the pariahs, and the rejected of all races, castes, and creeds. It was here, in this room that also served as a dormitory and study, that Mother Teresa had prepared the thousands of girls who came from all over India and the world to take the white veil of the Missionaries of Charity and proclaim their vocation of poverty, obedience, and love. The large building at 54-A Lower Circular Road held over a hundred novices. Very early each morning, after receiving the Eucharist and singing their psalms, they would leave the convent in pairs, their rosaries in hand, to go out by tram or bus or train or most frequently, on foot to their homes for the dying, orphanages, and medical dispensaries. It was as if those frail figures carried throughout the city a wave of generosity and love. They created by their presence a resonance of hope, announcing to the wretched: "We are here, we love you. There is no longer any need to be afraid."

*   *   *

That winter of 1981, exactly twenty-nine years had elapsed since Mother Teresa had moved into this house together with a few of the pupils who had joined her from the convent school where she had previously taught geography. The owner of the building, a Muslim magistrate, had sold it to her for a song. After lengthy meditation in the neighboring mosque, the holy man of Islam had explained quite simply: "It was from God that I received this house. It is to God that I am returning it."

A few weeks later, a small procession led by Mother Teresa had emerged from the convent to make its way on foot to the Catholic cathedral of Our Lady of the Rosary. There, in the candlelit nave, in the presence of the archbishop of Calcutta and the local religious dignitaries, the first eighteen novices had taken their vows. They solemnly intoned "to seek out, in towns and villages throughout the world, the poorest of the poor, and take them temporal and spiritual care, visit them regularly, be carriers of the love of Christ for them, and so awaken in them a response to His boundless love." Out of that promise the order of the Missionaries of Charity was born, a congregation that now numbers more than three thousand sisters working in some four hundred established foundations in ninety-two countries, including Cuba, the Soviet Union, and soon China and Albania. Since that day, every December 8, on the Feast of the Immaculate Conception, an ever-increasing number of dark-skinned young Indian sisters* had passed from the mother house on Lower Circular Road to go and take their vows and renew that same promise.

Next morning, a truck transported the new Missionaries of Charity to Howrah Station or Dum Dum airport. Singing, laughter, shouts, and a few tears accompanied departures, toward all the corners of the universe everywhere people were suffering, that might well mean separation for several years. For a while, the large house on Lower Circular Road seemed deprived of life, the chapel was plunged into silence, the courtyard no longer resounded so loudly during the morning washing with the metallic clatter of buckets. It was not long, however, before the vessel found a fresh crew. Soon, postulants in white saris flew in once more from all directions. While most other religious orders suffered from a critical shortage of vocations, Mother Teresa could not take all those who flocked to the doors of her novitiate.

* * *

One morning in December 1981, a few days before Christmas, a frail Indian girl dressed in a full, red cotton skirt appeared at the wooden entrance to 54-A Lower Circular Road. The sister at the door immediately recognized the nun with the Asiatic face who was accompanying the girl. Ananda, the former leper girl from the funeral pyres of Benares had told Sister Bandona she wanted to enter the great family of the Missionaries of Charity.

*With a few rare exceptions, non-Indian postulants now complete their novitiate in San Francisco, in Washington, D.C., in Rome, in Tayuman in the Philippines, in Tabora in Tanzania, or in Zabarow in Poland.

Her application was unprecedented in a congregation where only confirmed young Christians had joined up to that point. Mother Teresa, never daunted by any challenge, saw in it an opportunity "to bring one more soul to Christ," and through Him "to the suffering people in whom He is made flesh." She relieved Sister Bandona from her duties running the Benares leper hospital for a while and put her in charge of the religious education of her protégée, a task that she had already begun. Here in Calcutta, Sister Bandona would need even more prudence and tact. She feared that the former leper girl, surrounded by women of higher birth, might at any moment be gripped again by the demons of her past. Sister Bandona knew that the stigma of a pariah was still there, lurking only skin deep, ready to reappear at the slightest provocation, either real or imagined. Even here, thirty centuries of untouchability could not be wiped out with the wave of a magic wand.

Before receiving the water and salt of baptism, Ananda had to learn English in order to communicate with her companions, who came from a wide variety of backgrounds. In Mother Teresa's communities, prayers and action were carried out in English. Paradoxically, Ananda's illiteracy stood the young postulant in good stead. Like the rickshaw pullers who know twelve thousand verses of the *Ramayana*, India's *Iliad*, by heart, she made up for her lack of education with a phenomenal auditory memory. In the space of a few weeks she knew the essential words in English.

Learning to read and write, on the other hand, was a very different matter. Her brain was not programmed for that kind of exercise. Her genetic heritage had never envisioned that the daughter of a cremator of corpses might one day need to decipher inscriptions printed on paper. To this was added her own visceral lack of interest in written things. What possible use could a book have, an inanimate object that fulfilled no practical function? Ananda was too much a stranger to this kind of concept to feel the least bit motivated by it.

Yet her tutor did not despair of awakening her pupil's curiosity by dint of patience and kindness. Two factors supported these efforts. First, there was the example of the other postulants, whose reading aloud resounded at all hours through the three stories of the convent. Then there was Ananda's discovery of the God who inspired the sisters' faith, an awareness that deepened with each passing day. Certainly, the idea of God was not strange to the young untouchable. But her religion was more of a folklore concept, a pantheon of thousands of gods and divinities with multiple incarnations, sometimes demons, sometimes spirits, in animal or human form. Hers was a fantastic mythology more inclined to arouse her imagination than to develop a personal and trusting relationship with one God. Her long stay with the sisters at the Benares leper hospital had already familiarized her with the notion of one God "who loves each one of His creatures as the dearest of His children." Nothing, Sister Bandona believed, could more surely inspire her pupil to want to learn to read than the discovery of the texts that recounted the exploits of a carpenter's son from Nazareth and relayed the message of His teaching. Ananda set to work. One by one she broke down the letters of each gospel verse, allowing their syntax to permeate her without even trying, for the moment, to understand their meaning. It was a long trial and a unique experience in the annals of the community.

Soon, among the chorus of youthful recitations, Mother Teresa could make out a new sound: the timid, awkward voice of the little refugee from the funeral pyres of Benares, as she sounded out the parables.

19

They Called It "The Wrath of God"

Atlanta, USA: Autumn 1981

The field activities of Operation Protocol 577 carried out by the CDC came to an end on December 1, 1981. The Atlanta sleuths then began sifting through the harvest of information gleaned from the respondents. The piles of documents spewed out by the computers, programmed to analyze the thousands of answers, soon submerged the offices of Dr. Jim Curran and all his task force members in a sea of paper. "What struck us at once when we examined the initial results," Dr. Harold Jaffe would confide, "was the way in which the affected subjects had been much more sexually active than the healthy ones. Although they had also consumed more poppers, ultimately that seemed secondary to us by comparison with the margin in the number of sexual encounters. We were very swiftly faced with the virtual certainty that everything was pointing to an epidemic that was sexually transmitted."

But what was being transmitted? A virus seemed the most probable hypothesis, a virus that destroyed the immune system and left its victims weakened against opportunistic infections that take advantage of the body's impaired defenses. A number of these illnesses were known, such as the pneumocystis pneumonia of the first patients diagnosed in Los Angeles, and the New York actor's Kaposi's sarcoma.

Not since the Legionnaire's disease effort had the world's capital of epidemiology engaged as many resources as it did now in its attempt to identify the mysterious virus. The CDC staffers used every possible experiment that their genius and imagination could conceive to force the cells to reveal the presence of the offending agents. Every biological specimen, every secretion, every drop of blood, sperm, and urine that arrived via the investigators' parcel post was passed through a mesh of microscopes, chemical reagents, centrifuges, and computers.

Much to the relief of her family, Martha Rogers had returned to Atlanta at the end of October to organize and coordinate the distribution of the material gathered on location to the numerous units of the CDC. The various laboratories that tracked down the multifarious herpes viruses set to work at once. One of them specialized in the detection and study of herpes simplex, a variety of virus that attacks primarily the mucous membranes of the genital area and sometimes ulcerates into lesions so devastating that its victims die. This virus also assails the lungs, the digestive tract, and even the brain and the nerve fibers. Another laboratory devoted itself exclusively to the study of the notorious cytomegalovirus, a long-established herpes-related virus widely found in homosexuals. Although more often than not benign, this virus had been shown to have disturbing links with Kaposi's sarcoma. Fearing that some inexplicable mutation of the cytomegalovirus might be responsible for this sudden virulence, the researchers were quick to make up a substantial culture from the specimens provided by Martha Rogers. They hoped that a study comparing these cultivated viruses with the old strains of the same virus stored in the CDC's freezers would provide them with some clue. Another laboratory specialized in the Epstein-Barr virus, named after the two British scientists who had discovered it and known as the cause of "yuppie flu." This virus was responsible for infectious mononucleosis and was connected with certain cancers of the lymph nodes, nose, and throat. A fourth laboratory, specializing in the chicken pox virus, benign in children but capable of giving adults terrible shingles that even affected the eyes, also joined the fray. As could be expected, the department of parasitic diseases threw itself into a systematic examination of the microorganisms that transmit pneumocystis pneumonia. The department also conducted research into the numerous parasitic diseases such as toxoplasmosis, aspergillosis, and cryptococcosis, responsible for the dreadful affliction of the central nervous system found in several victims. Other teams working on amoebic diseases and hepatitis concerned themselves with the microbes and bacteria found in the pathology of the patients questioned.

For more than eight weeks this titanic effort went on. It would prove to be abortive. Although the presence of innumerable infectious agents was identified many times over, no single one of them on its own could be found responsible for instigating the extraordinary disease. Unable to find a culprit, the Atlanta medical detectives devised a name for it, GRID, the four initials of a somewhat brutal periphrasis: "gay-related immuno-deficiency."

Many doctors and nurses who came face-to-face with this particularly horrible illness, that autumn of 1981, preferred a more unfortunate name. They called it "the wrath of God."

20

Indifference to a "Weird Gay Epidemic"
Bethesda, USA: Autumn 1981

Nearly a thousand of them are known to man. They are the most assiduous enemies of God's creation. Since the beginning of the world, viruses, those minute particles of death, have wiped out more people, more animals and vegetables, than all the natural disasters and historical conflicts put together. The mummified skin of Rameses II, studded with smallpox scars, bears witness to their onslaughts in antiquity. Humanity would have to wait for the twentieth century and the mastery of cellular research techniques to unveil these infinitely small corpuscles. Incapable of reproducing by themselves, in order to survive they need the complicity of the cells they attack. Everything that lives attracts them, and no cell is safe from their covetousness. Since 1952, when two American biologists discovered that the genetic material of these killer agents is made up of nucleic acids analogous to those of healthy cells, the study of viruses—virology—has brought about a giant leap forward in molecular biology, a young science trying to fathom the mysteries of life.

The forms and targets of viruses are as manifold as the families to which they belong. More than 60 percent of infectious illnesses are attributed to them. They attack nearly all organs and all func-

tions. Among the most devastating, there is, for example, the grace-
ful papillomavirus, shaped like a cut diamond, responsible not only
for hideous cancerous tumors but also for ordinary warts; there is
the adenovirus with its six little antennae, which causes respiratory
infections; the dread herpes virus in the shape of a notched wheel;
the variola poxvirus enclosed in a crenellated case; the rabies rhab-
dovirus, as hairy as a caterpillar; and like a microscopic sun, the
influenza and mumps myxovirus. There is also an exceptionally small
lozenge-shaped virus, the polio virus, responsible for poliomyelitis,
the last great epidemic to terrorize America and much of the world.

*   *   *

Dr. Jim Curran and his medical detectives from the CDC were
too young to have been involved personally in the struggle against
poliomyelitis, but they knew all about the different phases of the
nightmare that had preceded ultimate victory. At a time when SOS
calls relating to a new scourge were coming in by the dozen, the
specter of the terrible American summer of 1953 lingered in their
minds as one of the most distressing precedents. For that had been
a summer of panic. The polio virus attacked its victims through the
intestinal or respiratory canals. It multiplied there before going on
to invade, in the most serious cases, the central nervous system,
destroying the motor neurons of the spinal cord and the brain in
the process. Whole strands of muscle visibly dissolved or disappeared. An adolescent weighing some 130 pounds could lose half
that weight in less than a week. The first symptoms of the disease
took the form of a stiffness in the lower back and neck. Next came
general fatigue accompanied by nausea, buzzing in the ears, and
motor problems in the limbs. Then violent pains occurred all over
the body, with a high fever. These last signs confirmed the dread
diagnosis.

Every week the statistics had appeared in the papers. In six months
the polio virus had struck down nearly five thousand Americans.
Soon, official records would show some sixty thousand victims. Yet
it was not just the numbers that were so distressing, but the fact
that no one could tell where or when it was going to strike next.
All that scientists knew was that it had a predilection for children.
Known as infantile paralysis, polio drove parents mad with anxiety.
That summer, America's hospitals were full of thousands of inert

little bodies before whom medical science was compelled to acknowledge itself tragically impotent. The only treatment to diminish the effects of the illness was the injection of gamma globulin, a blood extract containing antibodies. Stocks were so limited, however, that it had been necessary to restrict the administration of the injections to pregnant women and people under thirty who were likely to have been infected. In New York, parents laid siege to the Department of Health for twenty-seven hours to obtain ampuls of gamma globulin for their children. To prevent abuse and the creation of a black market, distribution had been entrusted to the incorruptible members of the Office of Defense Mobilization. But the hope vested in this precious substance was to founder in June 1953 with the publication of a scientific article demonstrating its ineffectiveness.

Though it had been possible to cure some victims of poliomyelitis, how many others had died of it? This did not include those who had been left paralyzed in all four limbs or only able to move one arm, the fingers of one hand, or their eyes. America had seen newspaper pictures of tortured children hobbling on two crutches with their dead legs supported with metal splints, or slumped between the arms of a wheelchair, their complexions pale, their features drawn, their expressions helpless, and their inert bodies partly concealed beneath a blanket. Other pictures had shown an incredulous nation the coffin-shaped containers in which victims of the polio virus fought against death with an iron lung.

It had been a time of weeping, wailing, and revolt, and then one of resignation. Suddenly in the middle of that cruel summer an unknown doctor had brought an unexpected burst of hope to the country. Dr. Jonas E. Salk, a thirty-nine-year-old New Yorker and the son of an employee in the garment trade, revealed that he had managed to produce antibodies in his laboratory effective against three strains of the poliomyelitis virus. He had followed up this result with the development of a vaccine, which he had tried first on himself, his wife, and their three sons, before inoculating 161 children. Overnight the portrait of this half-bald man with protruding ears had appeared on the front pages of all the national newspapers. Jonas Salk had become one of the most famous people in the United States, a benefactor acclaimed by a nation beside itself with gratitude. Though other scientists would subsequently invent new and more effective vaccines against the polio virus, Jonas Salk would still go down in history as the man who had put an end to the nightmare.

* * *

On a September morning in 1981, the indefatigable scientist driving through Maryland's luxuriant autumn foliage at the steering wheel of a rented car had no doubt about it: twenty-eight years after the polio crisis, another, equally tragic plague was bearing down upon an unsuspecting contemporary America. The attaché case beside him was crammed with all the evidence Dr. Jim Curran and his Atlanta team had collected: analysis reports, microphotographs, slides, the comparative results of Operation Protocol 577's two hundred and fifty questionnaires completed on the sick and the healthy gay men. "As an epidemiologist, my urgent primary concern was to convince scientists and laboratories that we were actually dealing with a new epidemic," he would say, "and that in order to find the culprit as quickly as possible, we had to channel all our energies in a realistic direction."

Jim Curran was a pragmatist who liked to take the bull by the horns. He preferred the philosophy of the outlaw Willy Sutton to the so-called dogma of medical research. "Are you familiar with Sutton's theory?" he liked to inquire. To those who were not, he would explain with a sly smile: "When Willy Sutton was asked why he robbed banks, he would answer: 'Because that's where the money is.'" For the chief of the Atlanta medical sleuths, he wanted to go where the action was, in the sperm and blood of American gay men.

That autumn of 1981, the logic of his line of reasoning had not yet struck any chord of recognition in the world of research scientists, nor among the Washington officials responsible for allocating their funds to medical research. The editors of the *New England Journal of Medicine* had not yet even judged it expedient to relay the various alarms sounded by the first witnesses to the epidemic in the CDC's modest weekly report. For their part, the national press and the other media, usually so fond of medical scoops, showed a surprising discretion, as if the disease were a shameful punishment confined to a guilty minority. In any case, why be alarmed? Were not important scientific figures predicting that if subjects at risk stopped using their infamous poppers and curbed their sexual activity this epidemic had every chance of disappearing just as quickly as it had come?

It was because he disagreed fundamentally with this prognosis that Dr. Jim Curran was heading, that autumn morning of 1981, for the largest medical/scientific complex in the world.

* * *

In the small town of Bethesda, less than half an hour from the capital of the United States, there was a campus of three hundred acres. There, in a rural setting of lawns, hundred-year-old trees, and clusters of flowers, were located the thirteen national institutes responsible for safeguarding the health of the American people. All together, ranging from the cancer institute to the heart-and-lung institute, from the eye institute to those of gerontology, diabetes, arthritis, and skin diseases, the National Institutes of Health comprise four departments, eleven research centers, 1,420 ultramodern laboratories, a hospital with up to 540 beds, and the most important medical library in the world, endowed with several million volumes, more than 2,500 international periodicals, and an electronic bank of scientific data available for consultation day or night by any one of the 470,000 American doctors. Some 14,000 people work fulltime on this campus, of whom 2,300 are holders of degrees in advanced studies and several thousand others are medical doctors. This was possibly the world's most impressive concentration of gray matter.

This prodigious institution had at its disposal for the year 1981 six billion dollars, a budget almost four times larger than that of the United Nations. A quarter of that incredible sum went to the organization exclusively responsible for officially combatting America's "dread disease," cancer. Ever since President Richard Nixon had, in 1971, introduced a law pledged to the total eradication of an affliction that was killing nearly one million Americans a year, the National Cancer Institute had constituted the spearhead of that unprecedented initiative.

Both on its own premises and in associated laboratories elsewhere, the NCI was conducting a formidable research program geared to discovering the causes of the disease and defining its prevention, diagnosis, and treatment. Thanks to the NCI's inexhaustible financial resources, it provided universities, hospitals, independent research centers, and all kinds of public and private bodies with the means to carry out specific research. It also offered individual doctors and innumerable scientists, from both America and abroad, private scholarships and grants. It collaborated with a whole host of professional organizations, associations, and industries engaged in educational activities. The resources distributed by the NCI for cancer research amounted to several hundred million dollars each year, making the American institute the world's leading promoter of the battle against the disease. With its data bank that gathered, classified, stocked, and distributed all the results obtained daily from all over the world, the NCI played a pivotal role in the circulation of information enabling scientists and doctors from every country to keep themselves constantly informed of the slightest progress.

True, all was not exclusively sweetness and light on the Bethesda campus that autumn of 1981. Power struggles, personal rivalries, and political interference paralyzed many an initiative and discouraged or buried many an ambition. Promises of imminent and decisive victory regularly made by those in control had scarcely been fulfilled, and the aim set down in 1971 by President Nixon's plan still seemed, ten years later, a distant objective. The "dread disease" continued inexorably to fill the cemeteries.

Nevertheless, enormous progress had been made as far as knowledge of the mechanics of the disease and the manner of treating it were concerned, to a point where the National Cancer Institute had proudly been able to give one of its brochures the heading: "1971–1981—A decade of discoveries." The brochure cited two "heartening" trends—improvements in treatment for children and women with breast cancer.

But the crop of cancerous pustules appearing on the skin of a growing number of young gay men had come to cast a rude shadow over the end of that decade. Since the middle of 1981, appeals from doctors had been coming through to the treatment department of the NCI, indicating an abnormal increase in cases of Kaposi's sarcoma and calling urgently for new methods of treatment. It had not been long before the suppliant voices of numerous patients had joined in the chorus. After some hesitation, eventually in September the Bethesda authorities contacted the Centers for Disease Control in Atlanta. The CDC suggested a meeting of all doctors currently treating patients with Kaposi's sarcoma or infectious pneumocystis pneumonia, the two diseases that had just brought the strange epidemic to light.

That morning, in the middle of September, Dr. Jim Curran turned up at the meeting that was to assemble the early witnesses to what the world would soon know by the name of AIDS. Although used to his colleagues' lack of experience when it came to epidemiology, he was left by this confrontation with a somewhat bitter memory. "My aim was to show them that the epidemic of infectious pneumocystis pneumonia and that of skin cancer were the results of one and the same disease," he would recount. "No one would believe me, for the simple reason that cancer experts had no experience with infectious diseases, and specialists in infectious diseases didn't have any with cancer. One lot didn't recognize the other. It was almost unbelievable: entrenched in their own particular specialist field, they refused to acknowledge that such different manifestations could originate from the same single source."

*   *   *

That first encounter in the citadel of American cancer research was not all negative as it sounded the alarm for the scientific community. All the same, Jim Curran harbored no illusions. The NCI might have timidly half-opened its doors, but it remained a cumbersome machine subject to the goodwill of numerous committees that determined the direction of its scientific and medical undertakings. For the time being, no one on the Bethesda campus thought it should "get mixed up in this pitiable little epidemic" while it had other more immediate and important subjects for study such as cancer of the breast and lungs. Other more subtle considerations also had a role to play. Wasn't there a rumor circulating in certain laboratories that someone high up in Bethesda, himself a homosexual, was leading an active campaign to prevent the prestigious institution from getting mixed up in the affair at any price?

But Jim Curran was not a man to be easily disheartened. He knew that inside the concrete blocks of the science complex scattered among the dogwood groves and the azalea bushes there were brains capable of solving his mystery. One such building bore the number 37. There, on the sixth floor, at the heart of a whole network of experimental laboratories, in office 6A09, worked a supremely gifted biologist of Italian extraction with the profile of a Roman emperor.

Robert Gallo was one of the most ambitious scientists in American medical research. He was only thirty-five when he had been, in 1972, appointed chief of the Laboratory of Tumor Cell Biology of the National Cancer Institute. He was today at the zenith of his glory. By identifying the first virus of a new family of viruses, called retroviruses—this one associated with a malignant human tumor —Robert Gallo had indeed opened up an entirely new sphere in man's knowledge of the behavior of the microscopic agents that threatened the life of humanity. His revolutionary discovery was probably as significant for the future of mankind as Pasteur's isolation of the rabies virus or Koch's finding of the tuberculosis bacillus had been in their time.

But how, Jim Curran asked himself, was he to persuade so accomplished a scientist to put his reputation and hence perhaps his career on the line for a venture that so many authorities persisted in regarding as "a weird gay epidemic"?

21

A Genius in the Guise of a Faun
Bethesda, USA: Winter 1982

People may envy him, even hate him, but in the end they always fall prey to his charm. With his irresistible smile, his predatory jaw, his shock of barely graying hair, shapeless trousers, and carelessly knotted tie, the forty-five-year-old Dr. Robert C. Gallo looks more like the eternal student than a prince of science. The son of Italian immigrants, he is one of the most fascinating characters on the Bethesda campus, possibly even of the entire American scientific community. Behind the thick lenses of his unframed spectacles, his expression is by turns roguish, jocular, or suddenly capable of a severity that can hypnotize even the least susceptible. Most striking of all, Gallo gives the impression of always following several trains of thought at once. Feared and adulated by the small set of international scientists that cluster about him, he had turned his experimental unit doing research on tumors into one of the brightest beacons of American and world virological science. Those fortunate enough to belong to this unit cosigned more articles in important scientific magazines than most other laboratory teams. To work with Robert Gallo was an opportunity to find oneself at the very source of discovery, to bask in an uninterrupted flux of original ideas, to plunge into a seething tide of hypotheses and intuitions that attracted some of the earth's best brains.

This scientific genius had the strength and originality to leave his doors ever open to the world, to know hundreds of other scientists on a personal basis, and to welcome visitors and frequently the most productive deserters from other laboratories to the microscopes and centrifuges of his workrooms. His taste for publicity allied to his unequaled ability to make himself accessible to even the most un-tutored of journalists had made him a darling of the media. His Hollywood-style ease in front of television cameras, his gift for popularizing the most complex biological phenomena with dem-onstrations a child could understand, and his consummate skill in obtaining the applause of scientific publications, all combined to place him in a league of his own. Yet all these talents would not have been enough to single him out to such a degree had not Gallo also contributed to the wealth of medical and scientific knowledge of the end of this century with the fundamental discovery that would earn him that November of 1982 the prestigious Lasker Award.

*   *   *

His career had been born from a tragedy. Illness had snatched his much loved younger sister from him when she was just thirteen.

"I didn't know she was ill," he would later relate. "Nobody had told me. Her illness had broken out during a summer holiday at the seashore. It took the form of shivering, fever, terrible fatigue. My parents thought it was straightforward flu. One evening when I got home from school, I went rushing into her bedroom. Judith had gone. My parents had taken her to the university hospital in Boston where they were trying out some new medicines at the time. The following Sunday they took me to see her. I'd never been in a hospital before. A crowd of doctors were lining up at her bedside, examining her as if she were a guinea pig. They dripped blood transfusions into her. They also administered endless IVs of the chemical substances whose curative powers they were testing. They made her feel so sick she couldn't swallow anything anymore. Her face became more hollow by the day. The most moving thing was the way her skin turned yellow. She ended up looking like some lugubrious theatrical mask. Still, her condition improved and the

doctors authorized my parents to take her home. We all went together to fetch her on the following Sunday. Then she had a relapse.

"One day when I went into her room, she tried to sit up and
hold out her arms to me. In her exhaustion, she fell straight back
onto her pillow. She tried to speak to me. A gush of blood issued
from her mouth. The chemical treatment had destroyed her blood
platelets and she suffered one hemorrhage after another. Later I
discovered that she was only the third or fourth patient in the world
to be treated with chemotherapy. Well, at that time they didn't have
blood platelets in concentrated form at their disposal to rectify the
damage the new therapy did. She died a few weeks later. It was
only on the day she died, when we were all crying over her body,
that I heard the dreadful name of the illness that had taken her from
us. My little sister Judith had died of leukemia. That was the first
shock of my life and the end of my youth."

The tragedy plunged the Gallo family into such despair that Robert's father nearly went out of his mind. Leaving his metal factory,
he went and camped for weeks on end beside his daughter's grave.
Back home, he wandered about from room to room all night,
embracing the pictures of Judith he had plastered everywhere. Overwhelmed with guilt, he tried to transfer to his son all the affection
that he had not had time to give his daughter. Thus, he had spoiled
the young Gallo beyond all reason.

Nothing could appease the teenager's grief, nor his sense of anger.
"I had seen my sister die with all those doctors bending over her,
all those learned men who emerged from their laboratories to examine her like some object for their experiments. I had seen them
inject bottles full of blood and their famous medication into her.
For all their knowledge, they hadn't been able to cure her. *They
didn't know enough.*"

*   *   *

Aware of this frustration, a close friend of the family would steer
the young Gallo into a life he would never otherwise have contemplated. Dr. Marcus Cox was the anatomopathologist at the Virgin
Mary's hospital in the town of Waterbury, Connecticut, where the
Gallo parents had settled when they first arrived from Italy. He was
the one who had originally diagnosed the implacable illness that

had killed Judith. With a mind that was ever alert, he was as curious about the latest scientific discoveries as he was mistrustful of them. He questioned everything constantly. A man of percussive cynicism, he spared no one his criticism. In short, he was the ideal master for a boy who was gifted but cruelly disappointed by his first contact with the medical world.

Robert Gallo spent his high school holidays following Dr. Cox religiously about his daily work at the Virgin Mary's hospital. The doctor was in an exceptionally good position to appraise his colleagues' competence: he was the one who examined their pathological samples and performed their autopsies. "That Sherlock Holmes with a scalpel and microscope didn't miss a thing," Robert Gallo would recall. "He could tell instantly whether or not a particular doctor had treated a patient correctly. My vocation developed in the course of that apprenticeship. Well before I set foot in a university, I had decided to be a doctor. All the same, Cox's harsh judgment of the profession put me off treating people. The anger against those who had been unable to save my sister was still smoldering in me. What I wanted to do was research, to know more, ever more, and help science to avenge Judith."

The avenging of Judith was a stirring ambition from which the young Robert Gallo would nevertheless deviate once he began his medical studies. "I was still too shocked by my sister's death to be directly interested in the world of cells. The very word 'leukemia' gave me goose pimples." It was to a discipline devoid of all emotional associations, therefore, that he turned initially, to that of metabolic disorders. A meeting with one of the greatest biologists of the time, the Danish-born Allan Preslav, would soon, however, return him to his prime objective. Allan Preslav ran the department of cellular biology at the University of Philadelphia. Recognizing the abilities of a brilliant student, he took him on his team.

* * *

Robert Gallo would grow attached to his new master, who "seemed so very un-Scandinavian, with his volcanic, seething, passionate personality." One summer, the scientist entrusted an experiment on bone marrow cells to him. It was a fiasco. The cells died without warning. Young Robert brought disgrace on himself. But the first step had been taken. He had entered the world of centrifuges and test tubes for good. To redeem himself, he suggested he could look into the reasons why patients with chronic lung complaints did not produce enough red cells. This original piece of research earned him the satisfaction of seeing his signature at the bottom of a scientific article for the first time. Convinced that his disciple had what it took to succeed, Allan Preslav urged him to do his internship at the University of Chicago, a center renowned for its instruction in cellular biology and a bastion of Nobel Prize winners. The university hospital drew the most unusual and hopeless cases from all over America, a fact that made it possible for the young intern to make friends with personalities as diverse as the black athlete Jesse Owens and Mahalia Jackson, the remarkable gospel singer; and to meet the widow of Enrico Fermi, one of the pioneers of the atomic bomb. In the evenings and on Sundays, Robert Gallo would abandon his young wife, Mary Jane, and their baby, Marcus (so named in honor of his mentor Dr. Marcus Cox), to shut himself away in a laboratory and carry on with his research into blood cells. His tenacity would soon earn him a transfer to an important research post at the Bethesda National Cancer Institute near Washington. He had just turned twenty-eight.

In the absence of any immediate vacancy in a biology laboratory, Robert Gallo was assigned to a place where he had once promised himself he would never again set foot: the children's leukemia ward attached to the research institute. Sixteen years had elapsed since his sister's death, sixteen years during which numerous treatments devised on the same Bethesda campus had been able to slow down the onslaught of cancer of the blood. By a strange stroke of luck, one of the architects of this progress was a woman who had formerly treated Judith. She had in her laboratory archives a surprise for the newcomer. One day, she showed him a series of slides that depicted the infected white cells of his little sister struck down by leukemia.

It was a shock and a revelation. After years of intimate contact with red cells, Robert Gallo decided to set about fathoming the secrets of white cells, the lifeguards whose breakdowns condemned people to death.

* * *

This choice coincided with the advent of a new era in medical research. Two factors were at that time providing research scientists with new means of conquest. On the one hand, there were the huge allocations of funds made available for the fight against cancer since the eradication of infectious diseases by antibiotics. On the other, there was the revolution that had recently come about in the practice of cellular biology. Since the end of the fifties, science had known nearly all the secrets of cell life. Scientists knew how to make cells grow, how to cultivate them, how to reproduce them under laboratory conditions. Above all, the mastery of a very ordinary substance, plastic, had enabled researchers to equip themselves with instruments made to specification and so increase their experimentation and extend the field of their knowledge beyond all previous limits. The marriage of plastic implements to cellular biology had given birth to the industrialization of research equipment, thus providing a larger number of technicians and laboratories with new opportunities to study cell life.

The year Robert Gallo spent among the children with leukemia at the National Cancer Institute was a decisive experience. "At the faculty in Chicago I had only worked on cells that were physiologically normal. Now, there I was, suddenly confronted with cells that were completely crazy, cells in a state of total delirium, cells that were suicidal." As soon as he was appointed to a laboratory, he set to work. "I was lucky enough to find myself in a pool of brains engaged in frenetic competition. I was quick to take advantage of this fact to build up a whole network of professional contacts. A tennis match against a Chinese research scientist was to open up new horizons. The scientist had previously collaborated with a Nobel Prize winner in molecular biology. 'Listen, Bob,' he advised me one day between sets, 'the best way to study cancerous human cells is to use animal tumors caused by viruses as models.' "

Viruses! The tennis partner had uttered the magic word that obsessed so many oncologists. But Robert Gallo merely shrugged his shoulders. "I'd never had an ounce of interest in virology," he would confide candidly. "I'd never worked with any virologists. I hadn't the faintest idea about the blasted little creatures and thought those who had ventured to specialize in them were quite naive."

Yet what hope had been inspired by the hypothesis of a viral cause at the roots of numerous cancers! Ever since the day in 1910 when an American by the name of Francis Peyton Rous had announced his ability to infect chickens with cancerous tumors, scientists' imaginations had been inflamed by the idea of the virus as an agent for cancer. Forty years later, the discovery of a virus causing leukemia in mice had proved the viral origins in the case of certain cancers. It was a hypothesis backed by the highest authorities. In 1962, the head of the department for infectious diseases at the National Institutes of Health had not hesitated to affirm that "human cancers could also be caused by viruses," and that they should in that case be "regarded as ordinary infectious diseases." The conviction had given birth to a special research program financed with considerable resources. From then on, a whole generation of scientists would try to identify those microscopic killer agents in order to be able to combat them with appropriate vaccines. The example of Jonas Salk, the man who had conquered poliomyelitis, was there to encourage such aspirations. Heated competition developed between the different research centers, giving rise throughout the sixties to a shower of purported discoveries relating to the role of viruses in human cancers. These pseudotriumphs were just flashes in the pan. At the very most it had been possible to show that some viruses had a limited role as cofactors in the development of certain tumors. For example, the virus responsible for infectious mononucleosis described by the English doctors Michael A. Epstein and Y. Barr would prove to be involved in the formation of lymphomas or cancer of the rhinopharynx. Also implicated were the papillomavirus in tumors of the cervix and uterus, and the hepatitis B virus in cancer of the liver.

On the other hand, no one had ever been able to show the direct culpability of one particular virus family—that of the retroviruses —that had consistently intrigued scientists since the discovery in 1910 of the first retrovirus in cancerous tumors found in chickens. In fact, the parasites' behavior violated all the laws of biology. These laws that govern the mechanics of the reproduction of life follow a well-known and immutable process. At the heart of each cell nucleus is a nucleic acid called DNA,* which transmits the genetic information it carries to another nucleic acid called RNA,† which

---

* A double strand of deoxyribonucleic acid rolled up in the form of a helical ladder. In 1962, the American biochemist James Dewey Watson and his British colleagues Maurice H.F. Wilkins and Francis H.C. Crick received the Nobel Prize for medicine and physiology for their discovery of the molecular structure of DNA in the form of a "double helix."

† A ribonucleic acid.

converts this information into specific proteins that the cells need in order to live and function. Conventional viruses being endowed with a similar biological system, their DNA will mix with the DNA of the cells they attack. When they multiply, the host cells will automatically reproduce the viruses they are harboring. Not having any DNA but only RNA, retroviruses are obliged to resort to an outside intermediary in order to have themselves accepted by the DNA of the cells they want to invade in order to be reproduced by them.

This intermediary* had not been discovered until 1970. The enzyme in question was known as "reverse transcriptase" because it enabled retroviruses to carry out a procedure that was the reverse of the usual method of viral reproduction. It converted their RNA into the DNA they lacked and without which they could not reproduce. This enzyme was the "signature" of the presence of a retrovirus in an organism. Its discovery was to provide an incomparably useful research tool. The detection of its presence alone was enough to prove that one was dealing not with an ordinary virus but with a retrovirus.

Robert Gallo saw in this biological "signature" the means he needed to pursue his intuition and send him rushing toward a new objective: that of proving that retroviruses did not exist only in animals but that they also attacked human beings. This approach would provoke widespread skepticism on the Bethesda campus, where no one believed in the existence of human retroviruses. One of the objections raised by his incredulous colleagues begged an answer: the most powerful electronic microscopes had revealed no trace of them in diseased human cells. This finding was all the more disturbing for the fact that whenever it occurred in animals, this type of virus was extremely prolific. Hence the official line: if retroviruses also attacked man, their existence would have been detected long ago.

* * *

Robert Gallo's genius lay in considering the reverse hypothesis. Why was the idea so inconceivable of retroviruses so artful and

---

* A discovery made by three young American scientists, David Baltimore, Renato Dulbecco, and Howard Temin. It earned them the 1975 Nobel Prize for medicine.

discreet that no microscope had yet been able to pick them out? Oblivious to all the skeptics, the impetuous researcher set to work. He began by studying all the reports, articles, and documents in which veterinarians and virologists, famous ones and anonymous ones, dealt with unexplained illnesses, primarily forms of leukemia occurring in cats, monkeys, cows, squirrels, and even kangaroos. Gallo's search convinced him of the existence of a number of other, as yet unregistered, retroviruses in the animal world. Their activity was often carried out so secretly that it was virtually impossible to detect them. Even the "signature" of their reverse transcriptase enzyme proved to be illegible.

The sarcasm and the mockery redoubled where Robert Gallo was concerned. He was a man "fishing in the Dead Sea." His colleagues would not let go of the idea that there were no retroviruses other than those the existence of which had scientifically been proved in chickens, mice, and cats. "If ever they give me a Nobel Prize," the scientist would later say as he recalled all these fluctuations of fortune, "it will be for all the knocks I've taken. Not a meeting, discussion, or scientific conference went by without my being put ferociously in the pillory."

One of the major obstacles he encountered in trying to demonstrate the existence of retroviruses in man was his persistent inability to find their famous "signature" in cancerous cells. In vain he made cultures of the cells, coddled them, treated them with every conceivable care. They refused to divide and reproduce in sufficient numbers to disclose a viral presence in their nuclei.

Discouraged, Robert Gallo was on the point of giving up when serendipity, in the form of an ostensibly insignificant scientific article, came to his aid. A laboratory at the University of Pennsylvania had just extracted from a plant a protein called phytohemagglutinin, which had surprising effects on certain white cells. On contact with it, lymphocytes grew suddenly, became incredibly active, and divided. Robert Gallo established that this vegetable protein stimulated the T lymphocytes in particular, those cells responsible for mobilizing the organism's defenses against outside attack. Above all, he noticed that in the presence of this protein, the lymphocytes began to secrete a sort of cell food that was particularly potent. He called this growth factor, which was unique to T lymphocytes, interleukin-2. Was this the miraculous nutrient he needed to induce cancerous human cells to reproduce en masse and force them to reveal in the process the possible signature of a retroviral presence?

In 1980, five years after the rest of the scientific community at Bethesda had abandoned all research into the possible viral origins of certain cancers, little Judith's brother announced that two scientists in his laboratory, Bernard Poiesz and Frank Ruscetti, had found evidence of a first human retrovirus. The cells that had made this momentous conclusion possible had come from a group of patients with a rare form of leukemia that produced an anarchic proliferation of their lymphocytes. The first of these patients, a former basketball player, lived on a farm in Alabama; the second, a New Yorker who was also black, was of Caribbean origin; the third, an Irish sailor, had retired to Boston. Robert Gallo discovered that this sailor had spent a good part of his life sailing on the Sea of Japan and used to frequent the brothels of Kyushu. This information excited him all the more for the fact that a Japanese scientist by the name of Kiyoshi Takatsuki had, in 1977, alerted the scientific world to the existence of several cases of an identical leukemia in the southern islands of Japan. According to the Japanese scientist, this leukemia was transmitted through the blood, through sex, and by congenital means from mother to child. This triple mode of transmission suggested the presence of an infectious agent. The same leukemia would soon manifest itself in Africa also. All the evidence suggested that this agent was already infecting a certain number of individuals in the world.

Robert Gallo invented a name for it: the HTLV (H for human, T for T lymphocyte, L for leukemia, and V for virus).* The advent of this abbreviation marked the beginning of a new era in the understanding of the development process of certain human cancers and of other unexplained infections that were decimating humanity. The "Dead Sea fisherman" could once again hold his head up high and savor the "avalanche of scientific awards that began to rain down upon me and my team in place of all the kicks in the ass we had been receiving up till then." He was specially to receive, on November 19, 1982, the Lasker Award, the most prestigious medical honor in the U.S. This award was named after a publicity baron

---

*"Human T-cell leukemia virus" or "human T lymphotropic virus." In 1982, Robert Gallo would discover a second human retrovirus belonging to the same family as the first. The two viruses would then bear the respective names of HTLV-I and HTLV-II.

of the twenties who had launched Lucky Strike cigarettes and persuaded the whole of America to smoke them. In the twilight of his life, millionaire Albert Lasker had given up both cigarettes and publicity to devote himself to a passionate struggle against cancer.

A few years later, the work of Robert Gallo would win this exceptional scientist the unprecedented honor of receiving the Lasker Award for a second time.

22

"For Heaven's Sake, Don't Just Rest on Your Laurels!"
Bethesda, USA: Winter–Spring 1982

Was it a forecast of doom? A front of Siberian cold had descended upon the Bethesda campus. Yet that day in February 1982, Dr. Jim Curran would have braved the arctic ice to come and have his say in front of a committee from the National Cancer Institute responsible for allocating research resources. He not only hoped to convince the suppliers of funds that the need was critical, but he particularly wanted to impress one of the NCI superstars who would be present. Robert Gallo had also been invited to address the assembled company on the subject of his revolutionary discovery of the first human retrovirus.

The file of the CDC task force had gained dramatically in weight since his last attempt to rally the Bethesda research scientists to his crusade. The CDC's records currently indicated 202 Americans had contracted the immune-deficiency syndrome. In the course of a few months the mortality rate had reached 40 percent. The leaders of the medical press, headed by the *New England Journal of Medicine* and the London *Lancet*, had at last broken their silence. Five articles signed by five separate groups of scientists had just revealed that points of startling similarity existed between the epidemic's various manifestations.

The first patient identified in October 1980 in Los Angeles by Dr. Michael Gottlieb, the one nicknamed "the enigma in room 516," had died in the following May. The four other first cases described in the CDC bulletin had likewise succumbed as a result of the failure of their immune systems. The young Broadway actor had been unable to hide for long beneath his makeup the ravages of the skin cancer that had finally killed him. At Bethesda itself, a man had died at the beginning of the spring of 1981 in the care of Dr. Samuel Broder, the young, mustached director of the clinical oncology program at the National Cancer Institute. Broder's unit only accepted exceptional cases likely to be of use to medical research. He would recall with horror the memory of "the thirty-year-old living corpse suffering from infections such as we'd never seen before." After his death, the doctor and his assistants simply hoped they would "never have to live through that kind of tragedy again." After eight months of agony, the Air France steward at the Claude-Bernard Hospital in Paris had also perished of a final viral attack, this one in the brain. "We would hardly get through one infection," his doctor, Willy Rozenbaum, would say, "before another even more serious one would put everything on the line again." Every day brought confirmation of this sad fact. "There was definitely a yawning gulf between our usual practice and this totally new situation. We clearly had an epidemic on our hands."

After six months on the trail, there was no longer any doubt in Jim Curran's mind. Only a virus—probably one not yet discovered—could be responsible. That was the thesis he was coming to defend before the members of the National Cancer Institute that day. He had made the journey in the hope of inducing them urgently to initiate a national research program. To support his theory he was counting on one shocking piece of evidence: the statistical picture conveyed by a slide made up in Atlanta. More eloquent than any discourse, it showed that the principal difference between the sick gay men and the healthy ones questioned by his CDC colleagues was the number of their respective sexual partners over an identical period. In the diseased group this figure was ten to twelve times higher. For Jim Curran and his team this was sufficient evidence of a sexually transmitted infectious agent, probably the mysterious virus that their high-powered microscopes had been unable to detect. "I knew what hostility I was going to provoke by advocating the viral hypothesis," Jim Curran would later acknowledge. "Because as far as research scientists and doctors are concerned, there is no more complex scientific venture than that of having to deal with a virus."

The reception he received from the Bethesda brass seemed as chilly to him as the snow that covered the Maryland countryside that day. Even Robert Gallo's usual Mediterranean enthusiasm seemed cooled by an attitude of glacial skepticism. Turning spiritedly to the prestigious scientist, Jim Curran tried to warm him to the cause. "For heaven's sake, don't just rest on your laurels," he urged, raising his hand in the direction of an imaginary point beyond the walls of the room. "I swear to you that there's a mortal virus roaming freely at large out there."

*   *   *

"Of course it was a peculiar business, but isn't all research made up of peculiar things?" Robert Gallo would say later in justification of his deafness to the CDC envoy's appeal. "Actually it was the sensationalist aspect of it, with all its disturbing and slightly distasteful implications, that put me resolutely off the venture. The CDC had done a superb piece of detective work, but for a laboratory like mine already engaged in all kinds of long-term work, it was unthinkable to stop everything and throw in our lot with some story of homosexuals with multiple partners."

The medical detectives from the Atlanta CDC were soon to discover that this was also the attitude adopted by most of the large research centers. Furthermore, apart from this general standpoint there were other considerations of a practical nature. Robert Gallo and the majority of his colleagues shared the conviction that they were facing something so complicated that there was little chance of their being able to find it. "Patients seemed to be suffering from so many different infections that it looked as if it would be impossible to find the precise cause of their illness," Gallo would say. "So what was the point in wearing yourself out banging your head against a wall?" The scientists' evasiveness during those initial months of the epidemic derived finally from a third, possibly more pressing, motive: fear, the fear of introducing a mysterious killer agent into their laboratories. The Nobel Prize winner David Baltimore, codiscoverer of the reverse transcriptase enzyme that had enabled Robert Gallo to identify the first human retrovirus, decided he would not have any tissue or blood samples taken from AIDS patients in his laboratory at the Massachusetts Institute of Technology in Boston. He has not to this day reversed his decision.

Most American molecular biology centers displayed the same lack of courage. Robert Gallo would later defend their attitude by underlining the very real danger of introducing an infectious agent with totally unknown properties into a workplace. "How were we to know that a virus that had already shown itself to be so devastating wasn't going to jump out in our faces at the very first experiment, that it wasn't passed on in conversation or simply by shaking hands?" On top of that, there were all the other microorganisms that caused the multiple infections from which the victims of this very particular epidemic were suffering. "These are agents that would not perhaps have affected healthy subjects like you and me. But did we have the right to take that risk?" In his defense, Gallo would recall that several Bethesda scientists had previously perished, mysteriously infected by unknown viruses within their ultraprotected laboratories.

* * *

In June, around three months after this unproductive reaction on the part of the Bethesda establishment, Jim Curran received a note written by the person in charge of the CDC pharmacy informing him of a new fact capable of reversing even the scientific community's attitude to the epidemic. A doctor in Denver, Colorado, was asking for the urgent dispatch of doses of pentamidine for one of his patients who was suffering from chronic pneumocystis pneumonia. Unlike earlier requests received over the past year by the CDC, the exclusive distributor of this drug in the United States, this one was different. The medication was not sought for a subject deprived of his immune defenses as a consequence of an organ transplant or for a homosexual victim of the new epidemic. The patient in Denver suffering from this rare type of pneumonia did not comply with any of the usual criteria. He was not a frequenter of bathhouses nor a drug addict nor did he snort poppers. He was the fifty-nine-year-old father of a large family, a quiet man who had always lived in the same respectable neighborhood in deepest America. He had never undergone any immunosuppressive treatment of any kind. In short, there was nothing about him that should have opened the doors of his organism to the fatal parasitic invasion now afflicting him, nothing except an anomaly in his genetic heritage that made him susceptible to a special risk of infection. He was a hemophiliac.

That morning in June 1982 this piece of information stirred up powerful emotions in the Atlanta headquarters. Jim Curran grasped the implications immediately. The patient in Denver belonged to the small group of Americans—about twenty thousand—who, as a result of their blood's inability to clot, were periodically given transfusions of coagulation factors to protect them from hemorrhages. In order to prevent risk of rejection and comply with American health regulations, these blood products, which had been produced on a commercial basis since the beginning of the sixties, were created from a group of at least a thousand different donors. In fact, most batches were made up of the blood of between ten and twenty thousand donors scattered throughout the United States. With an average of ten transfusions a year, each hemophiliac could thus be receiving blood from some two hundred thousand donors annually. The rigorous filtering processes that these products underwent had eliminated all risk of contamination by infectious agents such as bacteria or microbes. The only living elements small enough to penetrate such barriers were viruses.

*   *   *

"The hemophiliac patient in Denver enabled us to put a decisive stage behind us," Jim Curran would relate. "He brought us peremptory proof of the viral origins of the AIDS epidemic. From then on no research scientist could play the ostrich role with regard to our claims and the validity of our hypothesis. The hemophiliacs were a particularly interesting category of subjects for study. Due to the continuous, diversified sources of the blood batches injected into them, they were to ordinary blood transfusions what homosexuals with multiple partners were to gays having normal sexual relations."

Scarcely three hours after the alert from Denver, a CDC medical investigator caught a plane to Colorado. For ten days Dr. Dale Lawrence subjected the patient, members of his family, and his doctors to a barrage of verifications. He checked in minute detail the patient's medical history. The doctor had new pulmonary biopsies carried out, reviewed all samples of blood concentrates received by the patient in the previous five years with a fine-tooth comb. His painstaking study served to confirm that this family man was indeed suffering from the same illness that was attacking gay men. Clearly, the virus had been transmitted through blood transfusion.

Less than a week later, the Centers for Disease Control in Atlanta learned of the existence of a second similar case. This patient was a twenty-seven-year-old hemophiliac who had been born in a small town in northeast Ohio and never left it. Once more, Dr. Dale Lawrence boarded a plane. With all the relentlessness of an FBI agent, he questioned every one of the young man's past and present acquaintances. He met his parents, brothers, sisters, his old school friends, his athletic and work contacts, and his girlfriends, in an attempt to discover whether he had a secret life. Dr. Lawrence rummaged through the tiniest details of his past. Knowing that hemophiliacs sometimes resort to drugs to ease the pain in their joints, he asked the patient endless questions on that particular point. Here again, however, the case was transparently clear. Only the transfusions of blood concentrates could be at the root of his illness.

Dale Lawrence had just returned to Atlanta when a third case threw the CDC into a state of fresh turmoil. A doctor from Westchester County, a residential suburb of New York, let it be known that a biopsy carried out on the lungs of one of his patients, a retired man of sixty-two, had revealed a widespread infection of *Pneumocystis carinii*, the usual agents of pneumocystis pneumonia. Like the two earlier cases, this patient, too, was a hemophiliac and had been receiving regular injections of blood-clotting factors.

*　　*　　*

Medical history would not preserve the names of those three victims. Yet, as Jim Curran would confide, "their sacrifice completely altered the rules of the game." Despite the terrifying implications, the head of the Atlanta task force was triumphant. The scientific community that had so disdained his "seedy gay epidemic" was at last going to have to step down from its Olympian heights and enter the arena. Apart from the twenty thousand hemophiliacs, some three and a half million other Americans underwent blood transfusions every year. Curran believed that identifying the infectious agent would become a matter of national priority. Along with that challenge came an assortment of urgent tasks: a detection test would have to be devised, all blood products and composites would have to be made subject to draconian control, antiviral substances and treatment would have to be invented. Finally, a vaccine must be developed. It was a phenomenal task that would take mountains of dollars and the mobilization of masses of scientists.

The men in charge of the Centers for Disease Control decided to launch this next decisive stage by giving the epidemic a new name. Sensitive to the legitimate indignation in gay circles toward a disease then known as Gay Related Immune Deficiency (GRID), they rechristened the epidemic AIDS,* four letters that would soon resound like the curse of this millennium's end.

* Acquired immunodeficiency syndrome.

PART TWO

The Victory of the Magicians of the Unseeable

23

Links to Form a Chain of Love Around the World

Antwerp, Belgium: Winter 1982

She had been a beautiful, rich young woman, destined to receive all the blessings of a golden future. The daughter of prominent members of the upper-middle class in the Belgian port of Antwerp, she had grown up in the velveted opulence of one of those homes that Rubens had so loved to paint. Her height and sporting appearance contrasted with the fineness of a face lit up by two huge eyes of periwinkle blue. At eighteen, Jacqueline de Decker was one of the most attractive marriage prospects in the kingdom of Belgium. Her beauty and position turned many a head. At an age, however, when all the other young ladies of her circle dreamed of dancing the night away on the arm of some Prince Charming or of escaping to the golden beaches of the French Riviera, she preferred to shut herself away in a chapel for long hours each day to listen to the inner voice that was calling her to quite another vocation. Persuaded that God was asking her to enter a religious order, to go to India and care for the poor and the lepers, she packed her suitcase one day in 1939 and knocked on the door of the local convent of the Missionary Sisters of Mary. Delighted to welcome a young woman from such a good family, the nuns wanted to give her a royal banquet. But the tin of salmon opened in her honor was tainted. Jacqueline nearly died in the night. Taking her food poisoning to be a sign, at daybreak she dragged herself to the mother superior's office to tell her that she was going home. "I was determined to dedicate myself to God and to go to India to care for the poor of the Gospels," she would say, "but as a lay worker."

A Belgian Jesuit friend of the Indian bishop of Madras was just then seeking volunteers to set up a medical social center in an impoverished area of Tamil Nadu, a province in southern India. Seven young women from Antwerp had already formed the nucleus of a team. Jacqueline de Decker enthusiastically joined them. The invasion of Europe by Hitler's tanks, however, was to rudely shatter her beautiful dream. As Belgium fell prey to poverty and suffering, Jacqueline and her companions quickly earned their nursing diplomas and joined the Red Cross. Four years of bombing and overcrowded hospitals provided the young heiress with a harsh preparation for her ideal of charity. By the time Liberation came, her unfaltering dedication had earned her recognition as a heroine. Several eminent people were already interceding with her parents on behalf of their sons seeking the hand of this angel dressed in white and decorated with medals. Jacqueline had no thoughts of marriage. War had disrupted the plans of the group of friends with whom she had originally wanted to go and serve in India. Several had been killed in the bombing, one had gone into a convent, the others had married. Only Jacqueline was still ready to embark on the great adventure. On December 31, 1946, she boarded a ship leaving for Madras.

On her arrival, she discovered that the Belgian Jesuit who had inspired her coming to India had died the very day she left Antwerp. She found herself completely isolated. For two years, dressed like the village women in a cotton sari, she lived among the poor in an improvised dispensary set up in a village not far from Madras. She provided for her daily sustenance with a bowl of rice seasoned with chili beans and some cups of tea, sleeping on the bare earth in a wooden hovel infested with rats and cockroaches. The only European for miles around, she shared the life of suffering and deprivation of landless peasants, among people who could find no work, among tuberculosis sufferers and lepers. It was a tough apprenticeship. Her steadfast faith was challenged by the emotional and spiritual isolation, particularly as the presence of this white foreigner in a place crying out for miracles sometimes gave rise to hostile reactions.

One day, in a state of profound discouragement, Jacqueline de Decker made the journey to Madras on foot along the irrigation dikes that ran across the rice fields to seek the spiritual consolation of a priest. There, another missionary told her about a European nun who had just left her convent in Calcutta to found a new religious order whose vocation was, like Jacqueline's, to live in the slums among the most disinherited, to care for the sick and the dying, to educate the street children, take care of the beggars, give shelter to the abandoned. Two days later, the young Belgian nurse stepped out of a third-class carriage in the great metropolis of Bengal. After several days of searching, she finally found the woman she was seeking, temporarily living with some American medical missionaries in Patna, in the neighboring state of Bihar. Prior to immersing herself in the poverty and suffering of the slums, the future Mother Teresa had gone there to learn the rudiments of first aid and medical care.

At thirty-eight, this tiny slip of a woman with a luminous smile had already been living in India for nineteen years. Born in Skopje, then part of Albania, the daughter of a prosperous merchant, Agnes Bojaxhiu had been called to the religious life at a very early age. At eighteen, taking the name Teresa as a tribute to the humility of the "little flower" of Lisieux to whom she was fervently devoted, she had entered the Irish order of Loreto. On January 6, 1929, she had disembarked from a steamship onto the quay in Calcutta, then the largest metropolis in the British Empire after London. For sixteen years, wearing the black veil of the nuns of her congregation, she had taught geography to the daughters of relatively well-to-do Bengali families. It was in 1946, on a train taking her for her annual retreat to Darjeeling in the foothills of the Himalayas, that another call from God turned her life upside down. A voice resounded in her heart. "It was an order. I was to leave the comfort of my convent and give up everything to follow him, Jesus Christ, into the slums to serve Him in the distressing disguise of the poorest of the poor."

Her mother superior, the archbishop of Calcutta, the whole hierarchy, had joined forces to try to make her give up the project. They argued that this new "call" was probably no more than a hallucination brought on by the fatigue of an overpowering climate and the tension prevailing in a country on the brink of independence. But she had shown herself to be unwavering: she had written to Rome and after two years of waiting, obtained the Holy Father's permission. On August 8, 1948 she had stepped out of her convent and exchanged her habit for the cheapest sari she could find in the bazaar. At the American nursing sisters' dispensary, her first confrontation with disease and suffering had been far from glorious. At the sight of blood, she fainted. Gradually, however, her indomitable will and her faith would inure her to the most painful tasks. In the evening, exhausted, she would recover her strength through prayer and contemplation in front of the crucifix in the mission chapel.

It was there that Jacqueline de Decker met Teresa for the first time in an encounter that neither of them would forget. They had so much to say to each other, so many feelings to share. The two trying years that the young Belgian woman had spent alone, relieving the wretchedness of the peasants in Madras, offered Teresa the invaluable fruits of firsthand experience. For her part, Teresa brought Jacqueline a long-term project: the creation of a religious congregation uniquely dedicated to the poorest of the poor. She hoped to draw to her other generous souls wanting to share her ideal of poverty. A few of her former pupils had already given her to understand that they would join her. While she waited, she had to compile the rules of this new community, submit them to Rome, and pray that a papal bull would authorize her to found the Order of the Missionaries of Charity, which, in addition to the usual vows of poverty, chastity, and obedience, would also respect a fourth, that of "wholehearted free service to the poorest of the poor."

Filled with enthusiasm at the prospect of living her own ideal as part of a team, Jacqueline de Decker immediately committed herself to Teresa's project. She would be her first companion. Destiny, however, would ordain otherwise.

While she was making ready to follow her new friend into the slums of Calcutta, Jacqueline found herself suddenly crippled with unbearable pain in the spinal column. An injury she had experienced at the age of fifteen when diving into a swimming pool was possibly the root cause of her illness. Despite intensive care, her condition worsened to the point where it seemed her life was in danger. Soon she had to resign herself to being repatriated to Belgium.

Jacqueline de Decker promised Teresa she would rejoin her as soon as she was better. On the ship that took her back to Antwerp, such a sense of failure came over her that several times she thought of throwing herself overboard. "Now that I was useless, I had only one thought: of killing myself. God had called me to India and I had betrayed His call. I never stopped praying to Him, but I could no longer feel His presence. If I still had a role to play in this world, the Lord would have to give me a sign."

She would wait for this sign all through her months of suffering in the hospitals of her native city where surgeons carried out several operations and fifteen grafts to try to save her from total paralysis. She went through agony. There were months of unbearable pain. Finally she found herself imprisoned from the nape of her neck to the base of her hips in a plaster corset. On realizing that she would never be able to return to India to work with her friend, she wrote Teresa a heartrending letter, the desperate farewell of a woman who saw her dream and the meaning of her life slipping away from her.

Sometime later, she received a blue aerogram bearing the postmark of the central post office in Calcutta. In the space of a few lines Mother Teresa outlined for her a unique project: the creation of an association that would weave across land and ocean, the links of a mystical communion between those who suffer in their bodies and need to be active and those who are active and need the prayers of others in order to be so. "Today I am going to propose something to you that will fill you with joy," Teresa wrote to her Belgian friend that October 8, 1952. "Will you become my twin Sister and a true Missionary of Charity, being in body in Belgium but in soul in India? By becoming spiritually linked to our efforts, through the offering of your suffering and your prayers you will share in our work in the slums. The work here is tremendous and needs workers but I also need souls like you to pray and suffer for the success of our undertaking. Will you accept to offer your suffering for your Sisters here in order that they may have the strength each day to carry out their works of mercy?"

Wasn't this the sign she had been waiting for? To her fervent acceptance Jacqueline de Decker added her readiness to enlist other handicapped people able to share this same ideal, an ideal that would manage to combine two great mysteries of the Christian faith, that of the redemptive power of suffering and that of the "communion of saints," which claims to unite all souls of goodwill. Thus was born the Link for the Sick and Suffering Coworkers of Mother Teresa, affiliated to the Missionaries of Charity, a "chain of love which would encircle the world like a rosary." The first links were formed by twenty-seven severely handicapped and incurable people, all of whom wanted to offer the suffering of their bodies for the success of the work of the first twenty-seven sisters—twenty-five Indians and two Europeans—who had followed Mother Teresa into the Calcutta slums. Thirty-five years later, there would be thousands of sick and incurable people linked, through prayer and the offering of their suffering, to Mother Teresa's sisters working away in the leper clinics, the dispensaries, the orphanages, and the homes for the dying all over the world. Despite her age and her straitjacket of pain, Jacqueline de Decker now coordinated this worldwide communion of souls from her apartment in the suburbs of Antwerp, gathering up each morning the piles of envelopes that the postman had just delivered, bearing stamps from every part of the planet.

*   *   *

One morning in the winter of 1982, she found herself moved by a letter posted in Jerusalem. Unable to write himself, Brother Philippe Malouf had dictated it to one of his friends.

Dear Jacqueline, my sister,

They say that for a rose to be beautiful, sometimes some of the branches of the rose bush must be sacrificed. Since the accident that deprived me of the use of my limbs, I have been unable to feel the sap of that rose rising in me. On the contrary, I have allowed myself to succumb to angry shouting, sobbing, and rebellion. Even with the affection of all those around me, I have not been able to rise above my handicap, to find in God the strength to accept all that humanly speaking I have lost.

And yet after a young Israeli girl who was paralyzed like me and in a wheelchair visited me in my hospital room, I was filled with hope. That girl invited me to drink a toast "to life." She shook me out of my bitterness, swept away my rage. I

*realized that I had to stop giving in, that I must at last come
to grips with my misfortune and find fulfillment in some other
way. But when I went back to the monastery, the world knocked
me back again, the demons of revolt began once more to turn
the screws on me: revolt against the God who created life, revolt
against the healthy people around me. My handicap was turning me against everything alive. It was making me egoistical,
centering me on myself, wiping out everything else. Yet I
wanted to fight this fall.*

*How often did I try to muster all my faith to think of Christ
on his cross? Then a voice would say: "Don't waste your suffering. You can't move, you can no longer take part in the
works of men, but you have God and with Him you can save
the world. . . ."*

Philippe Malouf went on to explain how an American archaeologist friend had, one day, brought him an issue of *Life* magazine
devoted to Mother Teresa of Calcutta that mentioned particularly
the Link for the Sick and Suffering that united the Missionaries of
Charity with thousands of volunteers throughout the world. He
had written at once to the nun, who had replied in her round, neatly
formed script. She had interspersed her words of practical advice
with a spiritual message: "You can do much more on your bed of
pain than I can with my legs." Then she had firmly reminded the
young monk that suffering was a school for heroism and holiness.
She had urged him to transcend his trial, to offer it with his prayers
for one of her sisters. "We need you to have the strength to carry
out our active work in the service of God's poor." Mother Teresa
had concluded by suggesting that her correspondent write to Antwerp, to the person who "married" each sister to her spiritual support.

Jacqueline de Decker reread the letter from the invalid monk
several times before placing it on top of her pile of current correspondence. Then she took out of a file a sheet of paper on which
the sister in charge at the mother house of the Missionaries of
Charity in Calcutta had written the names of the most recent en-
trants to the congregation. At the top was that of a girl from Benares

who had just been assigned to one of the most trying places founded by Mother Teresa, the home for the dying in Calcutta. This was the last resting place on this earth for the dying picked up off the streets of that inhuman city. Due to her painful past, this novice would definitely have need of staunch spiritual support. Jacqueline de Decker wrote Brother Philippe Malouf's name opposite that of the former "little Ganges vulture." Rather than change her name to that of one of the Christian saints, Mother Teresa had suggested that she keep in her religious life the name her parents had given her at birth. Thus the daughter of the cremator of corpses in Benares was now known as Sister Ananda—Sister Joy.

24

The Musicians in Block 37

Bethesda, USA: Summer 1982

The tall young man with the unruly locks who arrived at the Bethesda campus direct from Paris on that stifling July morning had no mandate from any French scientific authority, body of research scientists, or doctors' association. Intuition alone had impelled him to jump on a plane and cross the Atlantic to try to persuade the discoverer of the first human retrovirus to throw himself body and soul into the fight against AIDS. Thirty-three-year-old Dr. Jacques Leibowitch, the son of a renowned Parisian dentist, who had also been cabaret singer and actor when the mood struck him, had started life brandishing a conductor's baton. His paltry musical gifts had very swiftly convinced him to switch from the orchestral stand to the benches of the faculty of medicine in Paris. At twenty, just as he was finishing his second year of studies, an American biologist friend of his family had invited him to the United States for his summer vacation. There, in addition to the New World, he had discovered the world of medical research. Not one of the pretty American girls he courted each evening on the terrace of Greenwich Village's Café Figaro would ever have suspected that their charming companion had just spent his day slaughtering rats to extract from their livers the cells needed for work being carried out by the team of one of New York University's laboratories. "It was," he would say, "a revealing experience."

As Robert Gallo had so cruelly discovered on the death of his sister, Jacques Leibowitch would come back convinced that "in order to be able to treat people effectively, you had first to learn how things work. Above all, you had to know the mysteries of life." The key was there: in the form of cellular biology, a discipline almost as young as he was. Having become a doctor of medicine in Paris, he would go back to the United States to pursue that additional study at Harvard. There followed two years of relentless servitude, cultivating, cooking, and manipulating cells to the point of nausea. Back in France, Leibowitch chose to teach immunology at the Raymond-Poincaré University's hospital center in Garches.

News of the strange epidemic among American gay men immediately fired the imagination of one so habitually curious and reminded him that, a few years previously, he had come across several similar cases, in particular that of a Portuguese immigrant worker. Felix Pereira, a thirty-two-year-old truck driver, had originally come from Lisbon. In August 1977, three and a half years before the first patient was identified in Los Angeles by Dr. Michael Gottlieb, he had presented his Paris doctors with the same surprising sequence of clinical signs: fungal *Candida albicans* infection in the mouth and the esophagus lining, cutaneous eruptions on various parts of the body, a dry cough, persistent, inexplicable. These disorders had at first led Jacques Leibowitch and his colleagues to diagnose *Pneumocystis carinii* parasitic pneumonia. The condition was aggravated by abscesses on the brain with serious neurological complications. These different symptoms had been accompanied by a general deficiency in white T-4 cells, revealing the breakdown of the immune system. Eventually Felix Pereira returned to his home country where, after a year of agony, he died on March 10, 1980.

An ominous light had just been shed on this case, which went unnoticed at the time. There was no doubt in Jacques Leibowitch's mind. "That man had died of AIDS." Unlike the cases recorded on the other side of the Atlantic, the Portuguese was neither gay nor a drug addict nor a hemophiliac. So how had he managed to catch the disease? The young Parisian immunologist set off in search of a trail. He reconstructed the sick man's route. Before emigrating to France, for five years Felix Pereira had been a taxi driver in Maputo, the capital of Mozambique, and Luanda, capital of Angola, both Portuguese colonies at the time. After much prospecting, Jacques Leibowitch came across two more cases, those of two women who had died in Paris at about the same time, both of similar infections. At last he was on the track he had been looking for. Although those two women had nothing in common with the American gay men, they had at least one thing in common with the Portuguese taxi driver: both had lived for a long time in Zaire, an African country. Angola? Mozambique? Zaire? . . . Could it be that three years before the epidemic broke out in the New World, the African continent had provided a cradle for it?

At about the same time, Jacques Leibowitch learned that researchers had established in Africans the presence of the HTLV, the first human retrovirus discovered by Robert Gallo. From there it was only a short step to seeing this agent as also responsible for AIDS, albeit possibly in a slightly different form. "It wasn't a farfetched idea at all," he would later say. "If the HTLV retrovirus produced certain rare leukemias by causing the anarchic multiplication of white cells, it was easy to imagine that a very subtle genetic modification in the virus might conversely bring about, as in AIDS cases, the death of those same infected lymphocytes. It was a seductive piece of deduction."

His hypothesis seemed to him all the more convincing when he discovered the case of a young French geologist who had died in 1979 on a Caribbean island that had close links with Africa. Surprising as it might seem, at twenty-four, Claude Chardon had come to his marriage a virgin and just like in a fairy tale, had been so much in love with his wife that he had never so much as looked at another woman. Posted to Haiti to do his national service in the French Peace Corps, he devoted his weekends to exploring the wonders of the West Indies with his wife. One day, on a winding road, their driver suddenly lost control of his vehicle and crashed into a tree. Seriously injured, the geologist was taken to the French hospital in Port-au-Prince where he underwent a blood transfusion. He was given eight units provided by eight different indigenous donors. Thirteen months later he was dead.

Dr. Jacques Leibowitch saw this new case as substantial confirmation of his intuition. He decided on the spot to place a transatlantic call to Bethesda. Robert Gallo was out, he was informed, but Louise Burkhardt, his secretary, was willing to take down a message, a cryptic message in the form of an equation: "Africa–Haiti–Heterosexuals–Transfusions–HTLV = AIDS." Jacques Leibowitch had then given his telephone number "in case Professor Gallo should wish to contact me."

The message hit home. Despite his initial reluctance to involve his laboratory in the AIDS question, Robert Gallo called the French immunologist back to suggest that he come to see him at Bethesda.

*   *   *

The isothermic box Jacques Leibowitch deposited on the illustrious American scientist's desk, that summer's day of 1982, contained none of the gastronomic delicacies of which Robert Gallo was so fond: no Normandy Camembert, no Périgord pâté, much less rillettes from Le Mans, but rather a gift of inestimable value for the head of a research laboratory. Meticulously packed and filled with crushed ice, there was ranged inside a whole collection of tubes and flasks containing a real treasure. Before taking off for America, Jacques Leibowitch had raided the freezers of the Parisian hospitals to bring away with him blood samples from all patients suspected of being AIDS victims.

The evidence was there, in that suitcase brought to the celebrated virologist by the most anonymous of his colleagues. "The explosive arrival of an individual with such infectious enthusiasm together with his precious samples seriously undermined my reticence," Robert Gallo would confide. " 'Bob, Bob,' he said to me. 'We've got to move fast! Very fast! You're going to have to plunge in, give it everything you've got, and find that damned virus!' "

*   *   *

Give it everything he'd got! How could anyone reasonably imagine that the ever prudent Robert Gallo would hurl himself headlong in pursuit of such an elusive, hypothetical virus? Nevertheless, the spread of the epidemic beyond the gay community and the clinical specimens brought by Jacques Leibowitch would, in the end, dispel his hesitation. The very next time his laboratory assembled, he would suggest that one of his assistants try to decipher the AIDS mystery.

The auditorium was jammed that day beneath the neon lighting at the very center of the protected universe of freezers, centrifuges, and microscopes of block 37 on the Bethesda campus. It was a sheltered world in which the notions of illness, agony, and death remained as abstract as paintings by Mondrian, where it was possible to spend a whole lifetime handling killer viruses without ever actually seeing the monstrous spectacle of their assaults; a world a thousand leagues away from the field of battle, but a world inhabited by a handful of magicians endowed with the power to save more lives than all the earth's doctors put together.

The master took up his usual position in front of the blackboard and surveyed the team of assorted people he had gathered about him over the years, men and women of all ages and backgrounds who had come to him because of his prestige, bound together by the same mad passion for the invisible particles that make up the mysterious thread of life. They looked more like a band of students or kibbutzniks than a gathering of elite brains, but he was proud of them. Curiously enough, his team included only a very small number of his fellow countrymen. "Young Americans today prefer the big dollars that private laboratories and biotechnological organizations have to offer, to the mystique of fundamental research," he would often lament. His best performers were nearly all foreigners: Germans, Japanese, Pakistanis, Indians, French, Chinese, Swedes, Finns, etc. All of them were crack scientists in their specialist field. For example, no one was better at dissecting a viral culture and making its genes talk than a delightful thirty-five-year-old Chinese woman by the name of Flossie Wong-Staal. A doctor of molecular biology and a very top-level research scientist, in ten years she had become the master's alter ego. Similarly, there was Syed Zaki Salahuddin, a jovial Pakistani, lacking in degrees but such a sorcerer in the art of growing and cultivating cells that he was said to be able to make pebbles reproduce. Then there was another artist of the invisible life, the Czech Mikulas Popovic, a scientist who had come in from the cold, a genius so obsessed with secrecy and espionage that he had turned his experimental laboratory into a bunker. In short, there was no lack of talented people on the sixth floor of block 37. They were so numerous, in fact, that their master would have no difficulty in taking one off other assignments to put him onto the AIDS mystery.

Robert Gallo waited until all the other subjects on the day's agenda had been dealt with before revealing his intentions. He sketched a succinct picture of what was known about the AIDS epidemic and pleaded the case for possible viral transmission. "The fact that the AIDS agent attacks the same lymphocytes as our HTLV retrovirus allows us to suppose that we are dealing with a retrovirus belonging to the same family," he declared. Other discoveries reinforced the idea that this hypothesis was well-founded. Recent work on the Gallo retrovirus, which produced rare leukemias in humans, had confirmed that it, too, was transmitted by sexual means and by contamination of the blood, and furthermore that it was rife in the African countries where the AIDS cases had been discovered. There was also corroboration in the work of an eminent research scientist at Harvard University, the veterinarian and retrovirologist Myron R. Essex. A specialist in leukemia in cats, Essex had established that the infectious agent for this disease in animals was almost identical to the retrovirus that caused the same illness in humans. The only difference lay in a slight disparity when it came to its envelope, the outer coat. "Regardless of how many retroviruses exist in nature, it is logical to imagine that they all belong to related families and that the AIDS one is a lesser variety of the one we have already identified," Robert Gallo concluded.

It was without much lightness of heart that the eminent scientist contemplated his first timid steps in the direction of the epidemic. That summer, the wildest rumors were spreading as to the dangers involved in handling such a mysterious virus. Gallo knew that research centers had seen their staff melt away like snow in the sun as soon as the first samples of contaminated blood arrived within their confines. Even in his own laboratory, when the word spread that his team would almost certainly be going to work on AIDS, vacancies for certain technician's posts had remained without applicants. He also knew that the safety conditions provided in his facilities did not meet with the maximum requirements, but then few American laboratories had the very costly maximum-confinement "P4" equipment reserved for the handling of large concentrates of viruses reputed to be highly contaminant. While they waited for improvements, he and his team would therefore have to make do with the old laboratory hoods with their sterile air fluxes. All the same, Robert Gallo did take one precaution. He gave the order that no one was to use syringes or instruments of any kind made out of glass. Since one prick of a needle, one tiny cut, could cause fatal contamination, only plastic would be used.

But for some reason, which he would later attribute to the "persistent lack of real motivation" that paralyzed him that summer, Robert Gallo entrusted the AIDS operation to a timid fifty-two-year-old biochemist of Indian origins whose expertise lay more in the direction of administrative work. Launched by his leader upon a trail that would prove to be false, incapable of sensing the evil genius of the adversary he was assigned to track down, and left almost totally to his own devices, the unfortunate Prem Sarin would steer the celebrated laboratory for American virology into the most humiliating of fiascos.

25

A Fashion Designer Comes to the Aid of Men of Science

Paris, France: Autumn 1982–Winter 1983

It was no good, thought the energetic doctor dashing fiendishly about with his unruly mop of hair. French scientists were displaying the same indifference with regard to the "weird gay epidemic" as their American colleagues. Yet Dr. Willy Rozenbaum was leading a vigorous crusade aimed at mobilizing the attention of the health officials in the land of Louis Pasteur. In June of 1981, he had no sooner been confronted with the tragedy of the Air France steward—the first official case of AIDS in France—than he had taken the initiative of setting up a rudimentary monitoring center in his building at the Claude-Bernard Hospital, which looked like a German stalag barracks. He began by alerting all the specialists in infectious diseases he knew: pneumologists, dermatologists, and immunologists. Then he turned his attention to the association of gay doctors in Paris. This move would leave him with a somewhat bitter memory. "The homosexual practitioners gave me a suspicious reception. They were afraid of possible political exploitation of the AIDS phenomenon. There was a chance that moralists would once more join forces against homosexuality. How could it be explained to them that we couldn't play the ostrich for much longer, that we were faced with a fatal disease and that information must be circulated at all costs? Fortunately, in the end my pleading did win the active support of those who were very often the first to witness the ravages of this new epidemic."

To the same end, the imaginative Willy Rozenbaum set up a sort of anti-AIDS brain trust with a small group of specialists, among them several cancer experts. One of the most dynamic figures in this team turned out to be Jacques Leibowitch, the young immunologist who had gone to the United States to entice Robert Gallo into the quest. Having become an intimate associate of the illustrious American virologist, Jacques Leibowitch provided his Parisian colleagues with a valuable link to U.S. medical research. This was critical if the French were to avail themselves of the best human and material resources capable of broaching so complex a problem. In France the number of sizable laboratories specializing in human retroviruses could be counted on the fingers of one hand. Willy Rozenbaum and Jacques Leibowitch contacted them one after the other. Using the pretext of other work already in progress, they declined with one voice.*

However, the first French AIDS doctor did not succumb to despair. Strictly speaking, the invitation to come and talk about the epidemic in front of some forty medical practitioners, virologists, and immunologists from the Pasteur Institute was not the product of a sudden upsurge of interest in the disease on the part of the prestigious research center. The meeting had been arranged by an old friend from his intern days who was sympathetic to the cause. Willy Rozenbaum seized upon this opportunity to arouse the French scientists' sympathies. With all the ardor of youth, he painted the somber realities of the mysterious disease and stressed the dangers of its spreading. Holding back until the end the information that he was counting on to rally his audience, he set out in detail the reasons that made it possible to point a finger with virtual certainty at a particular culprit. In this illustrious place where for nearly a century so many battles against microbes and their misdeeds had been instigated, he thought it would be enough for him merely to utter the word *retrovirus* to produce the desired effect.

"Is there a retrovirologist in the room?" he inquired, surveying

---

* Including Prof. Dominique Stehelin of the Pasteur Institute in Lille, one of the fathers of the discovery of oncogenes, the genes that allow the transformation of normal cells into abnormal, cancerous cells.

the assembled group. Not a single hand went up. The three principal specialists who could have responded to his appeal had not been given notice of Dr. Rozenbaum's talk.

*   *   *

With his baby face, rosy cheeks, and slow, measured voice, one of those absent specialists might more readily have been taken for a provincial lawyer than a scientist inflamed with a passion for research. Prof. Luc Montagnier, aged fifty, head of the viral oncology unit at the Pasteur Institute, was the living antithesis of the American Robert Gallo. The two scientists had but one conviction in common: like Gallo, Montagnier was persuaded that retroviruses were responsible for numerous human ailments, particularly in the field of cancer.

As early as 1975, he had set up a research laboratory in his unit devoted to the study of human retroviruses. With two research scientists, two technicians, and some modest equipment, the enterprise was a modest operation in comparison to Robert Gallo's center at Bethesda. Starting with the retroviruses implicated in leukemia and other cancers found in mice, the small team had looked for identical pathogenic agents in humans, notably in breast cancer. Thus far, its work had not produced any spectacular discoveries.

The outbreak of AIDS on the world's virological scene did not immediately attract the attention of this handful of French research scientists. Faces disfigured with the violet pustules of Kaposi's sarcoma, lungs consumed with *Pneumocystis carinii*, brains destroyed by toxoplasma—all the horrors that haunted Willy Rozenbaum and his practitioner colleagues were only vague and distant abstractions to the laboratory's personnel.

Toward the middle of November 1982, two telephone calls swept Luc Montagnier and his collaborators into the very center of the tragedy. The first was an SOS from Paul Prunet, the scientific director of Pasteur Institute Productions. As the senior man in charge of the manufacture and sale of vaccines and serums produced by the celebrated research center, he was alarmed at the possibility of the AIDS agent's contaminating its products. The vaccine against hepatitis B recently produced by the institute was indeed manufactured from large quantities of blood plasma bought in the United States and Africa, two areas where the killer virus was now being spotted with increasing frequency. The implications did not escape Montagnier. He promised to give some thought to the problem.

He did not have to think for long before he received a second call, this time from a pretty young woman who had once been one of his students. Françoise Brun-Vézinet, aged thirty-four and the daughter of a general practitioner, was in charge of work at the Claude-Bernard Hospital's virology laboratory. Her job meant that in the course of the year most of the viruses causing the infectious diseases in which the establishment specialized passed through her hands. For eighteen months now, one of her most active suppliers of blood samples and infected tissue happened to have been her hospital neighbor, Dr. Willy Rozenbaum. Not one patient with AIDS symptoms left Rozenbaum's consulting room without a little of his blood, his skin, or his lymph nodes being dispatched at once to Françoise Brun-Vézinet's laboratory. Throughout that year of 1982, they had both sought obstinately to discover the role of different viruses in the instigation of the disease. But their results were so meager that the young woman had finally suggested to her colleague that they appeal to Luc Montagnier, under whom she had studied retroviruses at the Pasteur Institute. She thought it judicious to establish a link between practitioners in immediate contact with the disease and a research laboratory working on retroviruses.

So the die was cast on the eve of Christmas, 1982: eight weeks after the American Robert Gallo, France made its cautious entry into the race to discover the agent responsible for AIDS.

* * *

The news from across the Atlantic at the end of 1982 was hardly designed to fill the French researchers with optimism. The quest was not progressing. The medical detectives from the Atlanta CDC had not been able to incriminate any known virus. As for the Indian virologist in Bethesda's block 37, he had still not found anything to confirm the culpability of the HTLV his boss had discovered. Yet the team at the Pasteur Institute believed that a retrovirus might provide the answer. However, unlike the Indian researcher who, on Gallo's orders, had charged headlong into the complex procedures of such research, the French decided to proceed with caution. First, they wanted to get to know their adversary better, an aspiration that was to sow the seed of an original idea with incalculable consequences. The French researchers had noted that the particular characteristic of the incriminated virus was its ability to introduce itself into the white-cell lymphocytes to reproduce inside them before destroying them and perishing with them in the same holocaust. It would therefore be better to look for this virus right at the beginning of an infection rather than at the bitter end of the illness; in other words, at a stage when it had every chance of being well and truly alive and active and thus more easily identifiable. They would need to study patients in the early stages of the illness.

A few days before Christmas, a fair-haired young man dressed in leather trousers and jacket turned up at the consulting room of Dr. Willy Rozenbaum. By virtue of his profession, the fashion designer Frédéric Brugère had made numerous trips to New York. He readily acknowledged both his homosexuality and his relations with a significant number of sexual partners; he had suffered from frequent bouts of venereal disease. But it was only when he undid his silk scarf that the doctor understood the real reason for his visit. Frédéric Brugère was afraid that he had AIDS. At the base of his neck he had a swollen lymph node the size of a pigeon's egg. Further examination would reveal other swollen nodes in other parts of his body. It looked as if the patient's fears were justified. "A biopsy on this nodule would be advisable," the doctor announced as he probed his neck. "And the sooner the better."

Even as he uttered these words, it dawned on Willy Rozenbaum that this reservoir of freshly infected cells probably contained the ideal research cultures for Luc Montagnier and his team at the Pasteur Institute. Perhaps this was the material that might just make it possible for them to achieve what Robert Gallo and his superlaboratory had so far failed to do: isolate the agent responsible for the fatal epidemic.

26

A Waiting Room for the Father's House

Calcutta, India: Autumn 1982–Winter 1983

No virus either known or unknown, no new epidemic, could account for the presence of the 170 men and women who lay dying in the transparent light of the old building with the round towers. The cold that followed hard upon the tropical heat of summer and the monsoon deluge brought a constant succession of people at the point of death, victims of the most ancient plague: poverty. There were three hundred thousand people in Calcutta living in the streets, without any kind of shelter, feeding on refuse from the rubbish heaps. For those who no longer had any family, Mother Teresa's home for the dying represented one last hope of not leaving this world like an animal, of being cared for, of hearing a few words of compassion.

The "saint of Calcutta" had created a unique institution right in the middle of a militant Hindu quarter, a few steps away from the temple dedicated to Kali, the goddess with the bloodthirsty image who is the city's patron deity. Called the Place of the Immaculate Heart, it was the first creation of her crusade in the service of the poor. That morning in November 1982, the nun was preparing to celebrate its thirtieth anniversary. For three days in her little white Renault driven by her old Muslim chauffeur, Aslan, himself a survivor of a long journey to the farthest reaches of horror, Mother Teresa had been making the rounds of everyone she knew in the locality, inviting them to join in the celebrations. An endless round of Mercedes were depositing at the home's narrow door baskets overflowing with vegetables, fruit, fish, meat, and pastries, along with parcels of linen and clothes. Often the wealthy lady donors in their festive saris accompanied the piles of presents. Other gifts came from organizations, clubs, shops, and industrial organizations.

Inside, the hospice had been transformed into a carnival of festivity. The smell of disinfectant and the haunting spectacle of the rows of skeletal bodies huddled on straw mattresses were almost lost among the perfume and the joyous color of garlands of Indian marigolds, bouquets of jasmine, and rose petals strewn in patterns on the floor. In the hallway that linked the men's and women's dormitories, an improvised altar had been erected where Mass would be celebrated. The cloth that covered it was the handiwork of the lepers from another refuge. Today, a place usually beset with calmness and serenity had become a hive of activity. The four novices assigned to the home for the dying were busy attending to the inhabitants' morning toilet. The translucent skin of some of their faces was stretched so tautly over their cheekbones that it looked as if it would tear. Bodies lay helpless in a state of rigidity that foreshadowed death, their eyes turned back in their sockets seemingly already focused on the next world. Wide-open mouths remained fixed in strange grins. Some of the hands reached out feebly as the sisters passed, seeking a gentle touch or an appreciative greeting.

These waifs had been collected from station platforms, temple steps, from the edge of some sidewalk, or even from the carriageway itself. No hospital would have taken them. Most of them were poor peasants suddenly catapulted into this seductive city by one of the climatic catastrophes so frequent in the region. The shock had been terrible. Their resistance was broken down by the air pollution, the lack of a roof over their heads, the hazardous camping on a patch of sidewalk among the vermin and the rats, the unsanitary condition of the water, the difference in temperature between day and night, or simply from being forced to become beasts of burden and pull inhuman loads to earn barely enough to survive for one more day. One day they had collapsed, never to get up again. Deprived of all immune defenses because of nutritional deficiencies, they had been unable to resist the onslaughts of tuberculosis, dysentery, typhoid, and cholera. No longer supported by their muscles, their skin cracked, eventually broke up into shreds, and became infected through its many sores. As long as the energy requirements of the brain were satisfied, these disintegrating tatters of human beings could still talk, groan, or beg. But soon a state of somnolence, interspersed with convulsions, would overtake them. Defeated at last, these living dead would then sink into a coma. Ten to fifteen thousand poverty-stricken people of Calcutta—thirty or forty times the number of AIDS victims recorded in the West for that year of 1982—would perish like that annually amid almost general indifference.

Those figures would have been worse had not Mother Teresa wrested thousands of the dying from the oblivion of the city's sidewalks. On that anniversary morning, an entry in the admissions book for her home for the dying spoke eloquently of the magnitude of her rescue operation. At dawn a truck from the municipal council refuse dump had brought in the 52,410th poverty-stricken person to be picked up since 1952.

* * *

That autumn, the nursing team had been augmented with a new recruit. Ananda, the former "Ganges vulture," had just begun the second year of her novitiate. With goodwill and courage that had won her the admiration of all her companions, she had overcome her handicaps one by one. Now she could speak, read, and write enough English to be able to take a full part in the life of the community. She had yielded to the implacable discipline of the Missionaries of Charity and to the austerity of their existence. She had learned to get up at half past four in the morning to read her prayer book and sing the verses of the psalmists while she was still reeling with sleep.

It was in the spiritual domain that the metamorphosis of the young untouchable was particularly remarkable. With patience and tenderness, Sister Bandona, her benefactress from Benares, had relentlessly worked to help her discover the values of the religious life, to help her to an understanding of the greatness of the God of love whose "bride" she would soon become. Persuading a young

Indian girl to deny the fatality of a condemnatory karma, helping her to cast off the carapace of disdain and defilement in which she felt herself imprisoned, convincing her that the God of the Gospels loved her as much as and even more than all His other creatures, and that she should not be afraid but rather surrender herself to His mercy—none of this had been easy. To complete her education, one morning Bandona took her protégée on foot to the far side of the city to the door of the home for the dying, the Place of the Immaculate Heart.

Ananda's Story

When I went into that large room full of dying people, I was gripped by a sudden feeling of revulsion. I wanted to turn on my heels and run away. Bandona kept hold of my hand. "Don't be frightened," she said to me, "all these men are our brothers. You are their sister. You have a duty to touch them, serve them, relieve their suffering. Jesus loves each one of them with the same love that he has for you." But I could already tell from some of their eyes that they had recognized me. They were Brahmans and they had inevitably seen that I was a pariah. They would reject me, strike me, spit in my face. I was sure they would. There were sisters and voluntary helpers there cleaning the excrement off mattresses. Others were washing a corpse in a corner. I had obviously been brought there to do that sort of dirty work. What a shock it was! Suddenly all my past as an untouchable came flooding back to me. I wanted to get out of there. Bandona tried to reason with me. She pointed to a poor skeleton, all curled up like a fetus. He was a Hindu. He was hardly breathing. And she said to me, "Look at that man and tell yourself that it's Christ you're seeing."

Then Sister Paul, the sister in charge of this home for the dying, arrived. Bandona said something to her in Bengali and Sister Paul smiled at me. She took me by the hand and asked me to go with her to the women's dormitory. She exuded such quiet, reassuring strength that I found myself wanting to follow her. I said good-bye to Bandona. From then on the home for the dying, the Place of the Immaculate Heart, became my new home.

Sister Paul had been working there for fourteen years. She was a stout woman from the South who liked to laugh and sing. From time to time she would pause between two outstretched people, take hold of her rosary, and recite a dozen *Hail Marys*. She had an incomparable gift for making you forget that most of those people were there to die. She seemed to know each one personally and never went past any of them without touching their hands and saying a few words. That didn't involve much effort on her part because as soon as she appeared countless hands would reach out to her spontaneously. The dying called her *Ma* or Mother. Sister Paul maintained that this physical contact was more important than any medical treatment, that as a way of showing our love for unfortunate people who had perhaps never had any in their lives, it was more effective than any injection. She was right. I often had occasion to see for myself the miraculous effect of the mere touch of a hand, the sound of a soothing voice. There were times when it didn't work. Some of the dying would shut themselves off in total silence and preferred to keep their eyes closed, as if, having lost all taste for living, they didn't want to see any more of life. It was a dreadful notion.

Most of the time, we didn't know anything about these people, about their past, what dialect they spoke, what their religion was, how old they were. Someone had just brought them to us and that was all there was to it.

One day, a lady brought one of these poor unfortunates to us by taxi. She had found him near the large railway station at Howrah. He was covered in machine oil. His skin was peeling off in strips to reveal large white patches. He couldn't have been more than thirty and the only word he uttered was "Pakistan." Ten days later he died without ever having said anything else. Sister Paul knew instinctively how to figure out where an unknown dying person came from. The smallest thing was enough: a facial feature, someone's general appearance, the way he behaved. For example, the way a person exercised his natural functions could be revealing. It made it possible to identify those who had lived in huts or houses. Sister Paul called the latter "house persons." The others, those who had only ever known the sidewalks, were "street persons." The first group would always ask to be taken to the toilet or for a bucket. The others soiled themselves without restraint.

Because she knew smatterings of a whole host of languages and dialects, Sister Paul nearly always managed to reawaken some memory or elicit some answer to her questions. Apart from the Bengalis, a number of our residents came from other, sometimes distant, regions such as Karnataka, Kerala, or Nepal. Working out what religion they were was difficult. In the absence of any exterior indication, such as a goatee beard for a Muslim, how were we to know whether an individual brought in in a coma was Hindu, Muslim, Buddhist, or possibly even Christian? Yet this became a rather crucial question at the moment of death because the funeral rites and the destination of the bodies were not the same. With the men, there was always one way to distinguish Muslims: in case of doubt Sister Paul would examine the deceased to see whether they had been circumcised.

Many people arrived in such a state of exhaustion they couldn't take the smallest mouthful of food. In such cases a sugar-water drip had to be inserted into a vein. There was a risk otherwise of their dehydrating completely and dying within a matter of hours. Sister Paul never gave up hope. "*Babu, babu*, little father, you've got to try and live," she would say very softly to those who had given up the struggle. "Only God has the right to withdraw your life, not you. And as long as God has decided not to open the gates of His paradise to you, you must stay with us." Sometimes she would have to make three or four attempts before getting any reaction. But it was rare for her to fail altogether. The first sign that her words had struck home was a natural gesture of survival: the mouth would open to take in a little food. Only later would the eyes open. A victory like that was a moment of great rejoicing for us. We would rush off to look for clean clothes to put on the man or woman who had finally opted to live. We would wash them, cut their nails, shave them, tidy their hair, in short, we would titivate them in every possible way.

These "resurrections" were the occasion for some very special treats. Either one of the sisters or one of the voluntary helpers would rush off to the neighboring bazaar to buy *rasa gula*, the delicious sweetmeats made out of highly sweetened milk, or a tumbler of *doi*, the local yogurt. Sometimes, too, Sister Paul would send out for a packet of *bidis*.* She would light the cigarette herself and then place it between her protégé's lips. I was always amazed at the beneficial effect of a cigarette. It was as if in some way it enabled the person who, a few moments previously, had wanted to die to step over the threshold of his return to life.

The occupants of the home for the dying were not all at death's door. Many had walked in under their own steam in the hope of finding shelter and recuperating for a few days, especially during the monsoon. It wasn't always easy to tell which ones really needed to be admitted as a matter of priority. We had to keep our wits about us: in a city of several million inhabitants where there was so much anguish, shelter for one hundred and sixty or seventy people was really only a drop in the ocean. But as Mother Teresa always says: "Without that drop the ocean would be that bit smaller." Sister Paul had found an infallible way of spotting gate-crashers. She would examine their hair. In India, men and women rub mustard oil into their hair, and you have to be absolutely poverty-stricken before you give up that practice. All those with traces of oil in their hair had to relinquish their place for those poorer than themselves.

Although the home for the dying was not so much a clinic as a haven of rest and peace where people could wait for death, we did give medicines to the most ill and to those who were in unbearable pain. One small metal cupboard housed our dispensary, and the foreign doctors who came to help us were always astonished at the small amount of medication we had. They tell me there are about eighteen thousand patent medicines in a country like France alone, whereas we, in Calcutta, only use a dozen kinds of medicine together with a few vitamin, iron, and mineral tablets for the most serious anemia cases.

We had a logbook in which the prescriptions to be administered to the patients were noted together with their reference number. In the home of the dying each person was known by the number of his mattress. "Number fifty-seven has pulled out his drip," we would say, or, "Twenty-four has died." The lids from used tins of tuna fish sent by a charitable organization in Italy served as containers in which each patient's tablets were distributed. Their manufacturer† would

* Indian hand-rolled cigarettes.

† Maruzella, Genova, Italy.

no doubt have been very surprised to discover the use they were being put to. It was the unpaid Indian doctor attached to the home for the dying who wrote out his prescriptions in the logbook himself. He came twice a week as a rule. Some foreign volunteer doctors came at intervals, too. Their visits were vital to us because none of the novices assigned to work there had had any medical instruction. It wasn't part of the training that Mother had ordained for her sisters, and I know that people sometimes reproached her for that. Luckily, we had the good fortune to be taught by Sister Paul, who had learned everything there was to know in the course of so many years of contact with thousands of poor people. No one else could position a catheter in the vein of an arm as thin as a matchstick at a single go in quite the way she could. With people reduced to skeletons, that was really quite an achievement. She tried in vain to teach me the secrets of her technique. I never managed to match her deftness. I used to prefer using veins in the foot: they burst less easily than those in the arm. But it seems it is dangerous for the patients because it can cause blood clots and embolisms.

Mealtimes were the only times when the home seemed to emerge from its extraordinary calm. On most of the mattresses you could see prostrate bodies recovering on the arrival of the cooking pots full of steaming rice that smelt so sweetly of saffron. For the foreign volunteers passing through, this was always a source of astonishment. They rediscovered the importance of that vital element which they took for granted because, for them, it was not a daily source of anxiety: food.

Paradox would have it that at the end of their poor lives, there were many who no longer even showed any desire to eat, as if their stomachs had given up on them once and for all. That meant we had to take an infinite number of precautions: the first mouthfuls could cause nausea, sharp drops in blood pressure, diarrhea, vomiting. Only very small quantities of easily digestible food—a little rice, a mashed potato—taken in several installments over the day would get their engines going again. Even these precautions were sometimes not enough. After so many years of deprivation the shock was sometimes too great and people died swiftly after the very first mouthfuls.

Despite such accidents, meals for us novices and for the voluntary helpers were rewarding opportunities to deepen our relationship with the men and women we were serving. Most of the residents no longer had the strength to feed themselves. We had to help them eat very slowly with a spoon. Expressions overflowing with gratitude rewarded us for our patience. They always made me think that what we were doing might well be just as important as the food itself.

Strangely, I was to discover that the men were much more sensitive to our demonstrations of affection than the women; they were more appreciative of our pampering them, enveloping them with kindness, with the result that they were also more demanding, more difficult. They wanted more attention, more looking after. Whereas the women seemed less touched by our compassion. They were also tougher, better able to rise above their suffering. Sister Paul explained this phenomenon by pointing out that in our country, from childhood onward, women are used to doing the most arduous work and that they are brought up with the idea of total submission to masculine whims and fancies. That kind of education, she said, strengthens their character, whereas having things too easy makes men soft.

Days were long in the home for the dying, often exhausting, but nearly always enriching. What a joy it was to see someone who had been on the brink of death recover after so much care, as if resurrected from the dead; to see him smile, then one day salute us with a bow, and walk away unaided. Especially when it was an adolescent who had arrived several weeks or months previously in a state of apparently fatal malnutrition. Yet Sister Paul was careful to see that these everyday miracles did not deflect us from our primary task, the one that Mother had assigned to us: that of helping those in our care to enter the Father's House peacefully.

The foreign friends who passed through the home for the dying never ceased to be surprised at this. Death was so natural there that it seemed just like the continuation of life. There was no weeping or wailing or rebellion, only the serene acceptance of a passage into the beyond. What struck them in particular was the absence of any apparent anguish. They said that where they came from people didn't experience death in this way, that they never dared look it in the face, that it was always an occasion for revolt, that it came in the guise of a hideous skeleton carrying a scythe, that it was just an injustice, a terrible punishment, ultimate defeat.

Sister Paul explained that in the West people were afraid of death because they didn't know where it is going to take them. She added that when you'd been fortunate enough to have a good life on this earth and you didn't believe in the kingdom of heaven, it was only natural that death should frighten you. Conversely, here in India, people are convinced that they will be happier in the life hereafter, especially the poor to whom God can only grant a better life. In any case, whatever their religion, Indians have such faith that they accept the divine will.

For all that, the agony of the dying was no less a trial for all those who worked in the home for the dying, even for Sister Paul. She knew instinctively when a person's hour had come. He would then be carried into a kind of alcove between the men's and women's dormitories, in the privacy of the passageway. We would wash and dress him in a new *longhi*. Sister Paul would send for a garland of golden marigolds from the bazaar, which would be put round his neck as on festival days. Then we would take turns at his bedside to hold his hand, mop his brow, comfort him, and pray. Sister Paul had a special way of talking to the dying. She would go into raptures about how lucky they were to be "going home" and describe the marvelous life that lay ahead for them in paradise, starting with the abundance of things they would find to eat there. If the dying remained conscious, I can bear witness to the fact that those talks helped them to pass away in peace. Their fingers would grip our hands with unusual vigor then relax suddenly. It was all over.

It took only a few minutes to lay them out. We would wrap the body in a white cotton sheet. If it was a Hindu, Sister Paul would ask someone to go and tell one of the Brahman priests in the neighboring temple dedicated to the goddess Kali. An undertaker belonging to the Dom caste, my family's caste, would then come with a litter to fetch the dead person and take him to a funeral pyre on the banks of the Hooghly. In the case of a Muslim, Sister Paul would telephone an Islamic organization that looked after deceased persons without families. A few hours later a van would come to take delivery of the corpse and drive it to the paupers' grave at the Muslim cemetery in Gobra. As for the rare Christians, our ambulance would take them to the burial vault in Tollygunge cemetery, to the south of the city.

It's true that in the Place of the Immaculate-Heart, death was just a formality. My childhood years amongst the smoke and the smell of the funeral pyres had no doubt prepared me better than most to accept it as such. Yet it didn't stop a kind of anger from welling over me sometimes at the cruelty of certain deaths. I shall never forget that of a young twenty-year-old Muslim who was reduced to a skeleton with his body covered with sores. He had been found in the toilet on a train from Madras. Contrary to usual practice, which precluded all desperate attempts at medical treatment, I really fought to try and save him. I don't know how many bottles of serum I managed to pour into his veins, nor how many bottles of antibiotics, vitamins, and iron I made him swallow. With his protruding ears and his frizzy hair, he looked a bit like my little brother, the one with whom I used to go dipping in the Ganges, looking for teeth and jewelry in gold from the cremated bodies of the rich. His name was Abdul. But he had gone through too much: he hadn't the strength to get his engine going again. We spent hours together. He didn't want to let go of my hands. He called me *didi*—"big sister."

Every evening when the time came for us to go back to our convent on the other side of the city, Abdul would sink into a state of despair. He would cling to my sari with a strength you would never have expected of so weakened a body. "Don't leave me, big sister," he would plead. One evening when his groans had particularly upset me, I gave him the greatest token of love that I could offer him. I unpinned from my shoulder the small metal crucifix that Mother Teresa had given me when I entered my novitiate.

"Take this, little brother," I said, placing it in the hollow of his hand, "it's the thing I prize most in all the world. It's as if your 'big sister' were staying with you."

His face at once became more peaceful. "*Didi*, you can go now," he murmured.

Next day, when I returned to the home for the dying, Abdul was dead, the small crucifix pressed between his hands folded across his chest. I fell to my knees and sobbed.

I was still crying when I felt Sister Paul's hand on my shoulder.

She was holding an envelope covered in foreign stamps with my name typed on it. A young Lebanese monk had written to me from Israel. He wanted to offer his prayers and his suffering as a paralytic to help me "to be strong and courageous in my work in the service of God's poor."

27

A Snug Night for the Harborers of an Assassin
Paris, France: Winter 1983

Frédéric Brugère, the young gay fashion designer, was stretched out on the operating table, sleeping peacefully. As soon as the surgeon had completed the removal of his lymph node, Dr. Françoise Brun-Vézinet, the attractive head of the virology laboratory at the Claude-Bernard Hospital, took charge of it to divide it up into several pieces. Collecting biopsies was part of her work: night or day, over the weekend, from any of the hospitals in the vast conglomerate of Paris. She was involved wherever a small piece of flesh taken under emergency conditions from a sick or dead person might facilitate the immediate diagnosis of a tumor, the study of brain cells while they were still warm, or the discovery of a virus responsible for some unexplained illness.

The young virologist placed each of the fragments in the bottom of different flasks. The first two she would send to the hospital's pathology and bacteriology laboratories, and the third she would keep for her own personal virological tests. As for the fourth, the largest, that was the present she and Dr. Willy Rozenbaum wanted to give Luc Montagnier, the professor under whom she had studied retroviruses, and his team at the Pasteur Institute. To make quite sure that this precious sample of an infected gland would come to no harm in transit, she had immersed it in a sterile solution. One last fragment remained. That one was not destined for any particular experiment or treatment. Instead, it would constitute the memorial to a lymph node removed that evening from the Parisian stylist. Preserved in the depths of a freezer, it would become one of the capital assets of a cell bank. In a year, ten years, or possibly a century's time, scientists endowed with fresh knowledge would be able to wake it from its icy slumbers and induce it to reveal some piece of information that today's techniques could not yet persuade it to disclose.

Twenty minutes later Françoise Brun-Vézinet was lining up her red Alfa Romeo under the hundred-year-old chestnut trees outside the Pasteur Institute in Paris. If there was one place in the world where men had succeeded in fathoming the mysteries of infection, it was here in this hall of discovery, at the very heart of the French capital. It was here, within these walls, that widespread outbreaks of diphtheria, smallpox, cholera, typhus, plague, tetanus, yellow fever, tuberculosis, and poliomyelitis had been conquered. It was here that the first anti-infective medicines and sulfonamides had been developed; here that the first malaria parasite responsible for the death of a million children a year had been discovered; here that the involvement of protozoans in the incidence of parasitoses had been proved; here that the principles of cellular immunity, the role of antibodies in the body's defense against attack, and of antihistamines in the treatment of allergies, had been revealed. It was here that the behavior of genes and the manner in which they expressed themselves in living organisms had been codified.

It was barely one P.M. by the time the young woman reached her former professor's laboratory in the building adjoining the one where Louis Pasteur had spent the last years of his life and where he rested now in a marble tomb. As it happened, Luc Montagnier's virology course was starting that day. He would not be able to make a culture of the cells from the lymph node of the designer with the precursory signs of AIDS until that evening.

*   *   *

Ever since he had first dabbled in chemistry at the age of twelve in the cellar of his family's home in Châtellerault, right in the heart of France, Luc Montagnier had consistently been possessed by the demon of experimentation. He liked to spend his Sundays distilling perfumes or making Bengal fireworks. The provincial son of a father from Auvergne and a mother from Berri, he went up to Paris to study medicine and take a science degree. Having put his degrees behind him, he had opted for the researcher's microscope rather than the practitioner's stethoscope. It was a vocation that would take him, at twenty-three, into one of the Curie Foundation laboratories where he was to discover the fascinating world of cell biology, which was currently undergoing a revival. New techniques of culturing cells and viruses devised in America were in the process of opening up revolutionary research opportunities. Filled with wonder, the young scientist decided to devote himself to the study of lymphocytes, the white cells that would one day have such a crucial role to play in his life.

One of the most virulent assailants of these white cells, the foot-and-mouth-disease virus, every cattle breeder's nightmare, provided Luc Montagnier with the subject for his doctoral thesis in medicine. This work would orient his career in the direction of virology. A scholarship enabled him to enter one of the great scientific shrines of the day, the British Institute in Carshalton. There, side by side with Kingsley Sanders, an English Francophile and smoker of Gitane cigarettes, he would witness the first halting utterances of a new discipline that bore the promise of a fantastic future, a science that transcended the mere study of cell life to concern itself with the actual nature of cells' genetic inheritance: molecular biology. Because they were relatively simple biological systems, viruses were ideal subjects for study and enabled the pioneers of molecular biology to make rapid headway. The young man from Auvergne was able to make his personal contribution to his masters' efforts by shedding light on certain reproductive mechanisms in a virus that killed mice in under forty-eight hours. This timorous flash of brilliance would give him the legitimate satisfaction of seeing his name inscribed at the bottom of an article published by the celebrated British scientific magazine *Nature*.

After Carshalton, it was on to Glasgow. This long stay on the other side of the Channel would bring the young French scientist into contact with the greatest brains of the period and give him a mastery of English, thenceforth the indispensable vehicle for all scientific communication. Luc Montagnier spent the next eight years in various Parisian laboratories developing the evidence for the involvement of viruses in the incidence of certain cancers. His persistent efforts earned him the honor of admission to the Pasteur Institute in Paris at the age of forty.

To become a "Pasteurian" is to belong to an order that has its own soul, style, and unity; and its clans, too. Many Pasteurians had no desire to see the name of their prestigious institute mixed up with that of an epidemic with connotations they considered distasteful. And yet, as Luc Montagnier would later point out, "if any research was in line with Louis Pasteur's calling, it was research into AIDS. There was no doubt in my mind that if he'd still been alive he would have been the first to put all his energies into the venture." One hundred years later, fortune ordained that Luc Montagnier's laboratory should be the one to continue that vocation.

* * *

It was no mean task. Of all the hardships with which nature challenged virologists, the identification of a human retrovirus was possibly the most arduous. In fact, after nearly a century of unflagging effort, only one of these "superviruses" with their complex mode of functioning had been unmasked in man, the HTLV responsible for certain rare forms of leukemia, which Robert Gallo had discovered in 1977. Luc Montagnier had already cultivated billions of cells suspected of harboring such viruses. He knew their tastes, their whims, their favorite foods. One of his refrigerators was stocked with vials full of the dishes and sauces of which they were especially fond, particularly a cunning mixture of mineral salts, calcium, magnesium, and the serum of a fetal calf. This serum was the ultimate dish in cell gastronomy. Like all great wines it had its vintage years and its pedigrees. The best, it was said, came from New Zealand. The scientist also had at his disposal a powerful stimulant extracted from a bean that increased their strength tenfold in much the same way that spinach did Popeye's. This substance settled on the wall of the cells and imitated the signal that mobilized them in the event of attack.

* * *

Eager to start without delay on a piece of research he recognized to be important, the little man with the air of a provincial lawyer shut himself in his laboratory as soon as he had finished his instruction, to make a culture of the cells from the infected lymph node Françoise Brun-Vézinet had brought him. He knew that handling an unknown virus was always a dangerous exercise. He put his white jacket back on, slipped on rubber gloves, protected his face with a gauze mask, and placed the flask entrusted to him by his former pupil under the only safety hood currently available to him. To prevent any contamination in either direction, this apparatus emitted a current of sterile air that formed a screen between the handler and the subjects of his experiments. Montagnier had performed the procedures he was about to go through hundreds of times. Culturing cells, to keep them alive and enable them to reproduce, is a routine operation in a virology unit. It is also a subtle art not unlike music, because of the harmony it requires, or like haute cuisine, because of the necessary judicious choice of nutritional ingredients. And finally it requires a juggler's dexterity to handle the diverse elements.

The scientist cut up the piece of lymph node, pulverized it, teased it to extract the white cells, centrifuged it, purified it, and reduced it to a liquid, which he then divided between five small cone-shaped flasks. Into each one he poured a few drops of his elixir-of-life factors together with a little carbon gas and some nitrogen to keep the preparation breathing easily. He sealed each flask hermetically and put them into water at 98.6° F. Then Montagnier took off his mask, jacket, and gloves and committed the procedures he had just followed to the notebook in which he recorded his experiments. One by one he turned out the lights, bolted the doors, then slipped on his heavy winter coat and made his way slowly down to the courtyard where his gray Lancia awaited him. In half an hour he would be back in his villa in Robinson having dinner with his family.

Well fed, warm, and snug, the designer Frédéric Brugère's infected cells would have a good night. Tomorrow the team at the retrovirology laboratory would be able to start looking for the mysterious AIDS virus they were suspected of harboring in their nuclei.

It was 9:15 P.M. on Monday, January 3, 1983.

28

"How Many Deaths Will You Need?"
Atlanta, USA: Winter 1983

The head of the anti-AIDS task force at the Centers for Disease Control could be proud. Dr. Jim Curran had once again surpassed himself. Despite the fact that he had only decided upon and organized it at the last minute, his conference was a success. That morning of January 4, 1983, more participants were packing themselves into auditorium A at his headquarters than even his most optimistic projections had envisioned. The 150 visitors had arrived the previous day and throughout the night from all four corners of the United States. They were all concerned with one of the country's ultrasensitive undertakings, the industry that collected, stocked, and sold the substance that was undoubtedly the most precious of all the nation's riches, the irreplaceable liquid that safeguarded the health and life of three and a half million Americans a year. This was the blood used for transfusions. It was such a flourishing business that its annual sales of $2.5 billion would have placed it high within the Fortune 500 listing. The American Red Cross alone distributed some six million liters of blood, enough to transfuse one million individuals from their first to their last drop. The industry's particular source of pride, however, was the esteem and renown it enjoyed. Indeed, no other enterprise could boast such care and attention to the handling and sale of its products. The whole world imported them.

Jim Curran was aware that the news he was about to break could deal a fatal blow to this noble empire; but there was so much at stake that it was his duty to reveal the truth. His call of alarm could hardly fail to have immediate repercussions. In his mind's eye he could already see his guests leaping out of their chairs and making for the telephones to dictate the emergency measures to be taken in their respective areas of responsibility. They were, after all, dealing with one of the most tragic problems America had ever had to face. Jim Curran himself had difficulty believing such a catastrophe was possible: the United States blood stocks had been contaminated by the AIDS virus.

*   *   *

The proof collected by the CDC was irrefutable. After the first three hemophiliacs had died the previous autumn as a result of infection by an injection of blood products, nine other hemophiliacs had recently succumbed in their turn. And now an astonishing case discovered just before Christmas was necessitating this extraordinary mobilization at the beginning of 1983. This time the disease had abandoned its known targets to strike in a completely new direction and manner.

A San Francisco pediatrician had just diagnosed AIDS in a twenty-month-old baby. Initial investigation had been unable to pinpoint the precise origins of the illness. Unlike the rare instances of children infected with AIDS because of parental contamination, this baby had not been born of a mother who was a drug addict, prostitute, or Haitian who could have transmitted the virus to her child in the course of pregnancy. On further investigation, Jim Curran's medical team had eventually discovered that the child had come into the world under difficult conditions. A cesarean delivery had been necessary. Suffering from a rare blood abnormality, the baby was given several transfusions. In the first four weeks of its life, nineteen units of blood had been injected in this way. Although AIDS had not yet been linked to the transfusion of fresh blood, the investigators sought out the nineteen donors. They could all be eliminated as possible carriers, except the last.

He was an unmarried businessman in San Francisco, aged forty-eight, who had died eight months previously. Like millions of other Americans who regularly undertake this same act of charity, he had given his blood on a voluntary basis. On March 10, 1981, when he had presented himself at the counter for the local Memorial Blood Bank, he had seemed in excellent health. Nothing about him had prompted the supposition that he belonged to a high-risk group. Six months later he had complained of extreme fatigue and loss of appetite. His doctor had noticed the inflammation of a lymph node under his right armpit. Suspicious patches appeared on the retina of his left eye, and the following month, he had been admitted to the hospital with infective pneumonia. Tests then revealed a severe decline of his immune system. His protective lymphocytes had almost totally disappeared. There could be no doubt about the nature of his illness. Three weeks later, the unfortunate blood donor died of AIDS.

The discovery of this tragedy reduced the Atlanta investigators to a state of terror. "It was reasonable to suppose that thousands of pints of blood stocked in the country's hospitals and blood banks had been contaminated by the virus," Jim Curran would recount. "That meant thousands of Americans destined to have transfusions were in danger of contracting AIDS and possibly dying. There was only one way to avert this catastrophe and prevent any future ones, and that was to subject immediately all existing stocks to control checks. What was more, we had to do something without delay to keep all donors at risk away from the banks."

*　　*　　*

To induce his listeners—known as "the American red gold barons"—to accept this strategy, Jim Curran had his assistant Harold Jaffe paint them a graphic picture of the situation. AIDS had struck 880 Americans to date. Some 317 were already dead. The death rate was higher than that of the most devastating epidemics of the Middle Ages. Even the survivors were only on reprieve. Patients with Kaposi's sarcoma died within sixteen months, those with infective pneumonia within nine months. As for the number of cases, it doubled every six months. At this rate, one hundred thousand Americans would be affected in less than five years.

The doctors from the Atlanta CDC had foreseen everything except the incredible reaction of their audience. "They quite simply refused to believe us," Harold Jaffe would remember. "They claimed our figures weren't conclusive and that they involved too few cases for blood transfusions to be definitely incriminated, that checks would be astronomically expensive and out of all proportion to the reality of the risk, that to stop homosexuals from giving blood would be considered an infringement of the rights of the individual."

That January 4 would remain one of the blackest days in the Atlanta team's crusade against the galloping AIDS epidemic. No protective measures, no decision to control what was happening, could be wrested from the incredulous audience. Before the end of the meeting, one of the organization's young research scientists, Dr. Donald Francis, summed up his colleagues' disappointment and the fear that haunted them.

"So, how many deaths will you need," he inquired of the assembled company, "before you finally decide to act?"*

*   *   *

To make up for this, another piece of news came as a much appreciated gift. After the failure they had just experienced with the blood bankers, Jim Curran and his medical detectives welcomed with special gratitude the French entry into the competition to find a virus. They could see at once the many advantages of the Pasteur Institute's involvement. Their fellow countryman Robert Gallo was now going to have to take up the challenge, muster his troops, give them more resources; in short, make their success inevitable. His reputation as the world's leading retrovirologist required it of him. The whole body of American medical research, one that had been so fertile in recent years, would also have to move into action.

The team from the Atlanta CDC was wrong. Robert Gallo had no desire to change one iota of his program. He did not consider he had anything to fear from those French "beginners" who, in his mind, had no international standing when it came to retrovirology. Could people who ate frogs' legs be seriously considered competitors? At most he considered them killjoys. If the AIDS agent was really a retrovirus, it was he, Robert Gallo, and he alone, who would identify it. Wasn't he the one who had discovered the first human

---

* More than a year would elapse before the leaders of the blood industry in the United States began seriously to respond to this question. During that period more than one and a half million units of blood would be collected, stocked, and distributed by American blood banks and hospitals without any anti-AIDS control checks.

retrovirus? The one who had perfected specific techniques for this kind of research? It was only natural therefore that he should continue to show so little enthusiasm for committing himself fully to the fray. "I was so convinced that Prem Sarin, my researcher, would eventually come up with something," he would admit, "that it didn't seem necessary for me to stand over him like a schoolmaster. In any case I wouldn't have dared to: he was older than I. That was my mistake."

In fact, the eminent scientist's real mistake lay elsewhere. It derived from an excess of confidence. The man who had discovered the only human retrovirus to date refused to let go of the idea that if other human retroviruses existed in nature, they must necessarily belong to the same family. The AIDS carrier must be a close relative of the specimen he had found. On the strength of this assumption he had failed to advise his associate to follow standard virus research procedure. There was no point in observing cell cultures day after day in the hope of seeing a virus emerge from them when it was already known that its model only showed itself after about thirty days. It would be enough to wait for this period to elapse, then demonstrate and confirm by means of genetic comparison the ineluctable family link with the HTLV that Gallo had discovered, and that would be it.

His Indian associate had therefore arranged his research program in terms of this calendar. It was only after the thirtieth day that he began to examine the cultures in his test tubes. Like the disciplined technician he was, he then consigned his observations to the notebook in which he recorded his experiments. And curiously, the consistency of their negative results never seemed to surprise him. Yet such results were astonishing. Instead of the anarchic proliferation of white cells habitually found after thirty days in the case of cultures infected with Robert Gallo's first HTLV retrovirus, he found only a graveyard of dead lymphocytes at the bottom of his test tubes, without any trace of a virus. It would be months before the prestigious American laboratory registered any alarm at this extraordinary phenomenon.

29

"Let the Illustrious Old Lady Raise the Flag of Rebellion!"
Calcutta, India: Winter 1983

Two by two, frail white sails on a hostile ocean, they set off across the teeming city in the direction of some leper hospital, orphanage, dispensary, school, or home for the dying. Every morning after their 5:45 A.M. Mass, Mother Teresa's sisters and novices left the convent on Lower Circular Road to return to their places of work. The city's poor and suffering knew the routes they took. At every moment hands reached out to them, mothers held out their starving babies, lepers tugged at the hems of their saris. They passed through a corridor of poverty, endlessly counting off their *Hail Marys*. So insistent was Mother Teresa on the benefits of reciting the rosary that the sisters measured distances not in miles or the time it took to walk them, but in the number of rosaries said. For Ananda, the former leper girl from Benares, and for Sister Alice, the appointed companion of her journeys, the door to the home for the dying was located 280 *Hail Marys* from the mother house.

At first, Ananda had been amazed at all the time wasted on these comings and goings when the minutes lost could have been used to relieve others' suffering. But it was not long before she, too, began to appreciate the value of such prayer, which had only seemed monotonous at first. She remembered what Bandona, her benefactress from Benares, had said. Now she knew how to waste her time for God, how to love Him in a disinterested way and without ulterior motive, how to say to Him: "I am reciting this rosary for the sole pleasure of being united for a few moments with you, like a wife with her husband."

Ananda's first days in the home for the dying in Calcutta had put her severely to the test. As she had feared, neither the crucifix pinned to her shoulder, nor the rosary strung from her waist, nor the pure white novice's sari, nor the blue apron of a servant of the poor, nothing had been able to obliterate the stigma of her birth. It was not long before the Hindu residents figured out the origins of the newcomer looking after them. Everything about her, from the very dark color of her skin to her somewhat abrupt manners, from the way she walked to the coarse intonations of her voice, still betrayed her status as an untouchable. Some of the dying were seen to push away the charitable hand held out to offer them a spoonful of food. Ananda never insisted. Forcing back the tears, she would move on to another destitute person, a Muslim this time or a pariah like herself, or someone still too weak to recognize the hand that succored him. Nevertheless these rebuffs did hurt the young woman where she was most fragile: If these men were really her brothers, and if, as Mother Teresa claimed, Jesus Christ was present in each one of them, then why did they reject her? Neither Sister Bandona nor Sister Paul could give her a satisfactory answer. Time alone might possibly soothe the wound. It was much more painful for a poor person than a rich one to suffer the humiliations inflicted by the poor.

*   *   *

That winter, an unexpected incident would disrupt the nursing team in the home for the dying. In the three years that she had been helping Sister Paul in the running of the hospice, twenty-eight-year-old Sister Domenica had become one of the most popular figures in the old building. Originally from the island of Mauritius, she had retained the island's lilting accent and characteristic exuberance. With her feline movements and very light skin, this tall, stately woman brought a hint of exoticism into the austere world of the Place of the Immaculate Heart. Even Sister Paul drew courage and comfort from the calmness and the gaiety of this companion.

Whenever Sister Domenica appeared in a bay, heads turned automatically in her direction. Ever ready to bend over a dying person, give him something to drink, take his hand, wipe his forehead, she knew how to communicate peace with a few kind, reassuring words.

Nothing in her background had prepared her for such a ministry. The daughter of rich Hindu merchants, she had grown up in a vast pillared home overlooking the ocean that washed her native island. It was on arriving in Bombay that she caught her first glimpse of poverty. Her parents had sent her to a convent boarding school there to complete her education with a view to marriage. She was fifteen years old. Every day, she set aside a piece of bread for the beggar crouching at the school entrance. One Sunday, not finding him in his usual place, she set out to look for him in the slum that stretched out in all its wretchedness just behind the convent. The discovery of that neighborhood would leave a lifelong impression on her.

Four years later, to the despair of her parents and despite offers of marriage from the most glittering suitors in Mauritius, Domenica had announced her intention of going to Calcutta to don the white-and-blue sari of the Missionaries of Charity. It was a decision she had never regretted, even if at times she yearned to have a more direct influence on the causes of poverty rather than on its effects.

"I would have liked Mother Teresa to attack more the injustices that create poverty," Domenica would later say, "to use her charisma and prestige to force governments and people of influence to take radical steps." Toward the end of the twentieth century, almost half a billion Indians still did not know the basic satisfaction of a full stomach. Hundreds of thousands of children stagnated in sweatshops, enslaved to perform inhuman tasks. Millions of landless peasants still struggled to survive in the nightmare of the slums. Nor was such a state of affairs unique to India. Who could take up the challenge if not the woman who in the eyes of humanity was the very embodiment of the ideal of charity? The woman who had set up her dispensaries, her orphanages, her hospices, all over India and the world, from the heart of the two Americas to the heart of communist countries. Wasn't she the woman who came running every time a catastrophe wrought death and desolation in some corner of the globe; the one who defended the right to life on all the world's podiums, whom universities and governments showered with honors and distinctions; whom the Nobel Prize for peace had distinguished as a symbol of love and human compassion?

Domenica was not the only one to dream of seeing the illustrious old lady raise the flag of rebellion in the name of the poor, the flag of nonviolent rebellion, obviously. Why didn't she stage a hunger strike outside the Indian prime minister's, Indira Gandhi's, door? Other spectacular activities abroad might be conceivable, outside Buckingham Palace, in front of the seat of the United Nations, at the Kremlin, in Paris, Rome, or Peking, anywhere where people in authority could intercede on behalf of the downtrodden.

This unfulfilled ideal remained hidden in the young Mauritian girl's innermost being. For the moment she was content to wash the dying, give them their meals, help them to smoke a cigarette, alleviate their suffering with the help of an injection, a smile, and a few words of comfort. Her medical knowledge was too limited to do much more. She regretted that. But the sisters' vocation was not so much to cure as to relieve and comfort. This she did so well that the occupants of the home for the dying made no secret of their preference for the gentle, beautiful Mauritian girl. Her fellow sisters sometimes took umbrage. Domenica pretended not to notice.

That winter, a particularly disturbing inner conflict was troubling the young nun. Was it the unusually biting cold that eventually eroded her morale? Or the feeling of frustration brought on by the presence of the foreign volunteers who were better medically trained than she and therefore more effective? She asked herself more and more questions. "Is God only asking me to do these humble tasks? Hasn't He got some other plan for me to serve the poor more usefully?"

*　　*　　*

The answer came in a guise as unvarnished as it was unexpected. With his blond locks tied in a ponytail at the nape of his neck, a small diamond lodged in the lobe of his left ear, two blue-and-pink butterflies tattooed on his forearms, and his heady smell of after-shave, the German doctor Rudolf Benz, thirty-two, did not exactly conform to anyone's image of an apostle of charity. Yet the team in the home for the dying knew that this man had dedicated his life to the cause of India's disinherited. During his first stay in Calcutta two years previously he had presented himself at the door to the old building and offered his services as a volunteer for several weeks.

Horrified at the sisters' amateurishness when it came to medical procedures, he had undertaken to teach them the rudiments of hygiene and asepsis. His efforts would prevent many a death and contribute to diverting the home from regarding the accompaniment of the dying as its only vocation. The team pledged their undying gratitude to this providential friend. On his return to his own country, Rudolf Benz had given talks, written articles, and shown slides in clubs and schools. Convinced that action should primarily be directed at the source of the problem, he conceived the idea of an irrigation system for ten villages in an impoverished area of the Ganges delta that could provide the peasants with rice and lentils all through the seasons. He founded a body to finance the project. Soon the German organization Work and Rice for a Thousand Indian Families had five thousand donors. The first channels could be dug without delay. Rudolf Benz stopped over in Calcutta to receive the funds transferred from Germany. Such formalities were still complicated in a country where bureaucracy is particularly petty. The wait gave him the opportunity to visit his friends at the Place of the Immaculate Heart and bring them up to date on the venture, while working alongside them for a few days.

The arrival of the German doctor swiftly revived Sister Domenica's doubts about the usefulness of her work in the home for the dying. It became a catalyst for all her frustration and made her look for some way in which she, too, could tackle the root causes of poverty. One morning, Sister Paul noticed the young novice's absence. Worried, she telephoned the mother house. She was informed that Domenica had gone out as usual that morning after Mass and breakfast. A letter found shortly afterward on her missal was to provide the explanation for her disappearance. It was addressed to Mother Teresa.

Very Holy and Respected Mother,

  I know what pain my departure will cause you. Do not see it as an act either of impulse or rebellion but only as a need to serve the cause of God's poor in a different way. I am taking

with me the ideal you have taught me and I will strive to show myself worthy of it. In my heart I am still a Missionary of Charity. God is calling me to carry out his will in other ways. I shall come and see you as soon as you get back. Pray for me.
    Your faithful, devoted and ever affectionate,

Domenica

Domenica was not the first Missionary of Charity "the saint of Calcutta" had lost. The rigorous discipline, the harsh physical conditions, the temptations presented by a life in close contact with the world, inevitably led to some desertions. But they were so few in number that the constant influx of vocations more than made up for them. All the same this precipitous departure caused consternation among those caring for the dying in the Place of the Immaculate Heart. Ananda was perhaps the most affected. Domenica had been both an elder sister and a model for her, the one who had quietly mastered every situation and who had never allowed any taboo to daunt her.

30

An Epic in a Former Washhouse
Paris, France: Winter 1983

The name "Rabies Building" had remained unchanged since the days when Louis Pasteur used to inject rabbits there with lethal germs to obtain a serum to save the victims of rabies. Unlike African and Asian countries where this terrible disease was still common, France had scarcely known any cases for a long time, so the premises were now taken up with other activities. One of the rooms on the first floor was a former washhouse in which the peeling walls had solely resounded with the whir of sterilizers. Only the floor with its gray and gold tiling contrasted with the banality of the decor. On the door a small notice would soon denote the "Bru room," a name not intended to honor any scientist or particular scientific achievement. "Bru" was simply the first syllable of the surname of the Parisian fashion designer Frédéric Brugère whose piece of infected lymph node had been submitted to Luc Montagnier for research into the virus suspected of being responsible for AIDS.

The small team that was now expected to find this virus was made up of two experienced research scientists and two technicians. They had made a specialty of the very delicate technique to test for retroviral activity in cells. Since evidence of this activity could not be obtained by direct means, it was actually the reverse transcriptases that had to be located, the famous enzymes that retroviruses used to introduce themselves into the host cell nuclei. The first task confronting the four team members in the Bru room was thus that of bringing these enzymes to light.

Their chances of success might well seem slim. Unlike Robert Gallo's powerful American symphony orchestra, the modest French quartet did not have all that much experience in the field of human retrovirology, nor had its work led as yet to any major discovery. Paradoxically this relative inexperience was to be its greatest asset because it embarked on the venture without being overly confident and without preconceived ideas. It decided to approach this particular piece of research by starting from scratch and proceeding one step at a time.

*   *   *

The leader and the only male in the group was a solid Parisian of forty-two who had worked hard to achieve his science doctorates and force his entry into the Pasteurian citadel. Brought up by his mother—a seamstress by day and a theater usherette by night— Jean-Claude Chermann, a former rugby player, owed his introduction to the medical world to a motorbike accident. Suffering from multiple fractures and deprived forever of his sense of smell, he had had to undergo numerous surgical operations, one of which had resulted in a severe *Staphylococcus aureus* infection. The experience had awakened in him a desire to be a doctor. Feeling himself to be too poor to complete such a long course of study, he opted instead for a science degree at the University of Paris. Having obtained his science doctorate, he had landed one day in a lecture given by the future Nobel Prize winner Jacques Monod. "It was like an instantaneous bolt from the blue, total, irresistible," he would later comment. "DNA, genes, heredity . . . all the links in the chain of life were suddenly laid out before me by a genial sorcerer. The way was lit. But when you were without means or connections, you might just as well dream of conquering the moon as hope to become a research scientist."

It was in a small café on the Rue Princesse opposite the dispensary attached to the Paris police headquarters that fortune chose none-theless to smile upon this dream. His mother had taken over managing the establishment in the hope of helping her son to pay for his studies. One day, just when Jean-Claude Chermann despaired of meeting anyone capable of opening the doors of a research laboratory to him, a customer who had overheard him scribbled a name on a scrap of paper.

"Here you are, young man. Go and see this gentleman for me. Tell him his friend Dr. Juin from the police headquarters sent you."

The young man rushed to the address indicated and found himself outside the gates of the Pasteur Institute, where the "gentleman" in question, Prof. Marcel Raynaud, was one of the principal immunologists. He took Chermann onto the staff and put him in the hands of his best collaborator. Everything Jean-Claude Chermann knew today he owed to Monique Dijeon, "a forty-five-year-old spinster, slightly bigoted but magnificent all the same, and madly in love with science." He owed her everything, from scientific precision to the cult of truth. Eighteen years of in-depth study into viruses had turned the young researcher into one of the most eminent French experts on the invisible killers. Following promotion after promotion, he was now director of the small laboratory linked to Luc Montagnier's viral oncology unit.

* * *

With him worked a brilliant and beautiful young blonde of thirty-five who also happened to be a cordon bleu cook. Dr. Françoise Barré-Sinoussi was just as capable of rustling up a traditional blanquette of veal or a Grand Marnier soufflé as she was of lovingly cultivating her fragile lymphocytes. Her favorite reading matter ranged from the major Anglo-Saxon medical reviews to the Larousse book of gastronomy. "Every recipe is an opportunity to look for variation, to invent," she used to say. Her first guides along the paths of science had been her childhood companions: her cat Pussy, her white mouse, and her parakeet. They had provided her with "the observations that had inspired such enthusiasm for the treasures contained in the great book of life." Instinct, species, heredity: what mysteries there were to be explored when you had a keen appetite to know and understand everything. Françoise Barré-Sinoussi had preferred the acquisition of an impressive array of certificates to fashionable holidays at Club Med. Her industry had one day earned her a probationary seat in a research laboratory in that holy of holies of French scientific research, the Pasteur Institute. She had just turned twenty-three. Jean-Claude Chermann, the man in charge, immediately took her under his wing. "You can have me do anything you like," she announced to him, "but I warn you: I shall never lay hands on an animal."

Twelve years later, the AIDS adventure did not frighten Françoise at all. In 1979 she had taken a course in the United States including several weeks in Robert Gallo's Bethesda laboratory, where she had learned the latest techniques of retroviral research. The celebrated American was not exactly given to praising his French counterparts to the skies, but he had nonetheless been impressed by the pretty Parisian girl whose tinted glasses concealed the beautiful eyes of a Mata Hari eager to learn everything.

* * *

Great scientific epics almost invariably begin in a commonplace way. All the same, the examination, that morning of January 4, 1983, of the five flasks Luc Montagnier had prepared would produce a certain amount of excitement in the former laundry now converted into an experimental laboratory. Jean-Claude Chermann had chosen these premises on purpose. No one had ever handled any kind of parasite there. No virus found in their test tubes could be attributed to environmental contamination. The Bru room team's excitement was not without foundation. Chermann had drawn his associates' attention to the dangers of the enterprise. "We don't know what we're going to find and the bastard could be fatal," he had explained. They had all accepted the risk quite calmly. In the few innocuous-looking drops contained in those flasks lived millions of white cells, any one of which might be harboring the killer agent of the new epidemic.

They had very little information about it other than that, like the human HTLV and animal retroviruses already known, it could remain inactive for a long time in the bosom of its prey before actually setting about devouring it. Some form of external activation seemed to be necessary before its murderous instinct was unleashed. Simple cellular reproduction could be enough. In splitting and multiplying, the cells awaken the viruses dormant in them, and the latter take advantage of the process to reproduce themselves in large numbers before going into action. The scientists in the Bru room were counting on making use of this process in order to overcome their first decisive difficulty: that of having a large enough quantity of the virus at their disposal to be in a position to identify it. In other words, they must induce the diseased lymphocytes from the Parisian stylist to generate the widespread production of the virus that the cells were suspected of containing. There was only one way of achieving the desired result: the cells would have to be coddled, pampered, and gorged on sweets so that they divided and multiplied generously. Françoise Barré-Sinoussi was all too well aware that it would not be easy.

She believed cells are living organisms with their own personalities, tastes, phobias, and above all, a need for tender loving care. Treating them like objects was out of the question. They needed to be swathed in gentleness and kindness; they must be listened to and talked to properly. Many an overly hasty apprentice researcher had been rejected from the world of tubes and cell cultures because of his or her failure to sense the need for this very special relationship.

The success of any approach was dependent on extensive knowledge of the mechanics governing the growth and reproduction of cells. It is known, for instance, that the human body secretes certain substances that activate the cells and promote their multiplication. As soon as they are taken out of their natural environment and put in test tubes, cells find themselves deprived of this indispensable leavening. They become like fish out of water. They wilt, go into a decline, and eventually die. Although food as sophisticated as a serum from a fetal calf can delay their demise, it cannot actually stop it. For a century this phenomenon prevented biologists from successfully cultivating lymphocytes under laboratory conditions.* This obstacle was overcome, however, in 1975 when Robert Gallo and his team isolated interleukin-2, the cellular growth substance

---

*I.e., *in vitro* as opposed to the natural growth of cells *in vivo*.

produced by the human body, which meant that scientists could now induce their cultures to grow and flourish in their test tubes for a long time.

Of course, interleukin-2 was not sold in pharmacies. However, through his contacts in other research laboratories, Luc Montagnier was able to get hold of some for his team in the Bru room. Françoise Barré-Sinoussi hurriedly divided the precious product between the various flasks containing the Parisian designer's infected lymphocytes. She could already envision them, thus stimulated, waking suddenly from their torpor, breaking out into myriads of brand-new cells that would activate the millions of viruses lurking in their nuclei. Here was a dream that must somehow become a reality if they were going to make the murderous virus take off its mask and reveal its identity.

Conscious of how much was at stake, the team left nothing to chance, approaching each obstacle methodically, one at a time. One of the hurdles was the propensity of lymphocytes to secrete an antiviral substance at the first sign of viral attack. The usually beneficial effect of this substance, known as interferon, might in the present circumstances prove inauspicious. In fact, as soon as they were stimulated by the addition of the interleukin-2, the sick man's lymphocytes could begin to produce powerful doses of interferon to combat the very virus the scientists were actually trying to cause to proliferate. True, interferon could not by itself free the white cells of the virus infecting them—if it could, there would have been no AIDS. All the same, there was a chance of its hindering the multiplication of the viral stock.

There was only one way to avert this danger, and that was by neutralizing it. Luc Montagnier and Jean-Claude Chermann, who had worked a good deal on interferon in connection with cancer, had just developed a serum capable of resolving the problem. To obtain a few doses of it, the Bru room team had a sheep injected with human interferon. Under attack from this foreign body, the animal's blood immediately reacted by secreting millions of antibodies. All they had to do was to introduce a few drops of this serum packed with antibodies into the test tubes containing the Parisian designer's lymphocytes to prevent the interferon they were producing from effectively fulfilling its antiviral function. The scientists in the Bru room hoped, by means of this stratagem, to make the virus emerge from the cells.

The hardest part, however, was yet to be accomplished: that of finding the villain lurking in the depths of their test tubes and proving that it was responsible for the dreadful epidemic.

31

Another Disaster with Each New Day

New York, USA: Winter 1983

The young doctor grabbed his gabardine raincoat, ran out of the hospital, and made a dash for the yellow car.

"Drop me outside any cinema on Broadway," he directed as he let himself flop onto the backseat of the taxi.

Dr. Jack Dehovitz, aged thirty, assistant head of the department for infectious diseases at New York's St. Clare's Hospital, got out a handkerchief and mopped his forehead, his thin cheeks, and balding head. He surrendered to the urge that had been consuming him all that afternoon and wept. He had sensed it for several days now: he was in the process of cracking up. "It was too much and too quick. I wasn't ready for it," he would say of the situation that so brutally confronted him.

The spread of the epidemic was affecting more and more American practitioners, most of whom were as inexperienced as he was in treating this unusual epidemic. The Atlanta CDC's bulletin was reflecting a reality that grew more unrelenting with every passing week. At the beginning of that year, 1983, four new AIDS victims were being identified every day, and statistics showed that the rate was likely to increase. "The symptoms of the disease were so horrifying I could hardly believe my eyes," Dr. Dehovitz would later acknowledge.

*   *   *

This admission was one that weighed particularly heavily on the son of a family of doctors from St. Louis, Missouri. At the end of his medical studies, Jack Dehovitz had decided to embrace the only specialist field apart from surgery that, in his view, would almost always enable him to cure his patients. "You take cardiology," he would explain. "Someone has an infarction. Of course you can control the attack, but the muscle has been affected. The patient will have another infarction. Take nephrology: someone suffers from kidney failure. Of course you can put him on dialysis three times a week. Sure, he'll live, but always with the sword of Damocles dangling over his head. The same goes for pulmonary diseases and in a general way, for all chronic infections for which medicine can only apply a palliative. What I wanted was to be in a position to cure the illnesses I dealt with definitively."

The miracle of antibiotics had served his ambition. For nearly half a century, antibiotics had in fact reigned triumphant over a vast area of human pathology, those diseases classified as infectious. "Even though many of them were still difficult to treat," Jack Dehovitz would confide, "what a relief it was to know that none of them was fatal." Like his Parisian colleague Willy Rozenbaum, he had been attracted further by the enormous possibilities that this branch of medicine had to offer in relation to the well-being of the general public. Keeping the population informed—the prevention and control of infection and epidemics—there were so many areas of activity that went far beyond the case of any one isolated patient. Dehovitz used a dramatic example to show how epidemiology worked. "Even if you contract a nice attack of syphilis with some whore," he explained a bit cynically, "at least you can make sure your wife doesn't catch it."

But now this comforting pattern had been shattered. The apocalypse had struck. In New York, only a few hospitals would take the first victims of the new plague. There were times when the lack of precise information about the disease and the terror it therefore inspired in the medical staff compromised the quality of care. Newspapers reported instances of hospitals where food had been left at the doors to rooms, where nurses would not go near patients' beds unless they were dressed in sterile gowns, masks, and gloves. The wildest rumors were in circulation at the time. There were claims that a mere verbal exchange could be enough to transmit the disease. The fact that the illness affected categories of people on the margins of society—gay men and drug addicts—contributed to the ostracism to which victims found themselves subjected. In the end the authorities were moved. "Even if sin is to be condemned, we have no right to abandon the sinner," John O'Connor, archbishop of New York, would declare, in a statement that did not please the gay community.

The prelate had the idea of creating a specialist unit for AIDS patients in the old St. Clare's Hospital funded by his archdiocese. Highly motivated doctors were engaged. Dr. Jack Dehovitz was one of those chosen. Two floors were rearranged to take some twenty AIDS victims. The press applauded this initiative and patients were quick to arrive. At last, New York had a hospital where AIDS was treated as an illness like any other. This state of affairs was as providential for its victims as it was for the defective finances of an establishment founded years ago by a nun to provide medical care for the poor immigrants on the West Side. But it subjected its medical staff to a process of torture that no one had predicted.

Dr. Jack Dehovitz's Story

Every day thrust me into some new catastrophe. One morning, I saw a couple of about thirty. He was an English teacher at a college on the outskirts of New York; she worked in a travel agency. They were intelligent and apparently responsible people. He was in a very bad way. I arranged to speak to the wife, one to one, because she had to be made to realize her husband was going to die within forty-eight hours. I explained to her that there was no point in putting him through the agonies of some emergency treatment that wouldn't ultimately do any good. It was too late. Above all I tried to make her understand that she herself was in danger. I asked her if she had recently taken any tests. "Yes," she replied, almost aghast. "My gynecologist had me undergo some tests. He told me I was probably carrying the virus, but that I didn't have to worry, that I'd be all right." She had a two-year-old son and in all probability that child had been infected during pregnancy. They would most likely both develop AIDS, but that woman was quite oblivious. It was staggering to find so much ignorance in so-called responsible people. I insisted on the need for extensive biological tests. We arranged an appointment for the next day. She never came back. Sure enough, I learned that her husband had died two days later.

Telling patients they have a terminal illness is a difficult task even for doctors more hardened than I am. There are no ready-made formulas for informing some poor guy that his "bronchitis" is actually *Pneumocystis carinii* and the violet pustules on his face are Kaposi's sarcoma. In short, that he has AIDS. Once, while I was a student, I had been assigned to explain to a patient that he had lung cancer. He was a sixtyish black man, a heavy smoker, a nice guy. He had at most six months to live. The prospect of breaking the fact to him terrified me, but at least there I could wrap the news up in a batch of reassuring words about all the weaponry medicine had at its disposal: surgery, chemotherapy, radiotherapy. Against AIDS, all I could offer were meaningless words. Sometimes I would wait four or five days before I could bring myself to speak.

The interview would vary according to individuals and personalities. With homosexuals it was usually easier because they were already aware how serious AIDS was. They had seen their friends die around them. They were ready for the worst.

Still, the young gay public relations man from Baltimore to whom I had to break the truth the other day reacted unexpectedly. I shall not forget that conversation.

"We've just had the results of your bronchoscopy," I told him. "They confirm that what you have is pneumocystis pneumonia."

"What does that mean, Doc?"

"That your immune system is in a bad way," I tried to explain, "which is what has allowed this infection to set in."

Usually, after that explanation a patient asks the crucial question: "Doc, have I got AIDS?" But this particular patient didn't ask anything. He remained silent. I had to actually spell out to him myself that it could be concluded from that diagnosis that he had AIDS. He listened without moving. I saw him just curl up like a fetus in the hollow of his bed. It was heartrending. After a long pause he raised his head again.

"Doc," he said, "I'm only thirty. It's tough to know that I shan't make forty."

You poor fellow, I thought to myself. *You won't even make thirty-one*. I gave my little speech about the general mobilization of medical research. I told him thousands of scientists were working all over the world to identify the causes of the disease and that significant discoveries would be made within a matter of months. I tried to instill in him as much hope as possible. But he still didn't react at all. He showed very little sign of life either that day or the next. I began to be alarmed. My concern was all the more acute by the fact that I could imagine my own reaction in similar circumstances. We were the same age. In his shoes I was quite sure that I, too, would withdraw into myself like a larva and not want to speak to anyone.

That patient hadn't finished surprising me. On the sixth day, as I was examining him, he took my hand. "Don't just give up on me, Doc, I'm going to give your bloody little illness a hard time."

32

Eleven Monks in Israel to the Rescue of Two Little Servants of the Poor

Latrun, Israel: Winter 1983

Philippe Malouf surveyed the three stamps on the envelope at length. It was as if the whole of India with its emblems and symbols had just erupted onto his sickbed. Next to the figure of a peasant woman in a sari, driving a cow, with a jug of water on her head, and the futuristic bulb of Asia's first atomic reactor, he recognized the large protruding ears and shining skull of Mahatma Gandhi, around which the Calcutta postmark had traced a curious halo.

The envelope contained a letter several pages long and two photographs. The first was the famous portrait of Mother Teresa holding a baby in her arms. It looked like a picture of the Virgin and Child painted by some master of the Renaissance. The photo was accompanied by a verse from Isaiah: "See! I will not forget you. I have carved you on the palm of my hand. I have called you by your name. You are mine. You are precious to me. I love you." Underneath, Mother Teresa had inscribed her wishes at the beginning of that year 1983 for the paralyzed young monk in Israel who was offering his suffering to support the work of one of the Missionaries of Charity. "Happy new year, dear Brother Philippe," she had written. "Keep loving others as Jesus loves you. May He protect and bless you. M. Teresa, M.C."

The second photograph showed a sister in a white sari and blue apron feeding a skeletal man. Philippe could see other similar bodies on mattresses next to him. The lens had succeeded in capturing the intensity of what passed between those two people: the nun smiling tenderly as she held out a spoon brimming over with rice to the starving man, who received the food with an expression of gratitude. Philippe Malouf realized this must be Ananda, the little Indian sister to whom he was spiritually married. He examined in minute detail her face, her delicate hands, her frail build, the setting that surrounded her. He tried to imagine the sounds and the smells. He thought of the improvised hospital in war-torn Lebanon where Christians cared for their wounded. No one in this photograph had on bandages. All you could see were those unfortunate, desperately thin people and the smiling little Indian women busy feeding them.

For some strange reason, the letter was not signed by Ananda but by the sister in charge of the home for the dying in Calcutta where she worked.

Dear Brother Philippe,

I have to give you some very sad news [wrote Sister Paul]. *Our dear Sister Ananda has been the victim of an accident and we are afraid the Good Lord may take her from us. The other morning, when they got to the home for the dying with Sister Alice, they were both badly bitten by a mad dog.*

There are lots of stray dogs in our neighborhood. They are attracted by the scraps from the animal sacrifices carried out in the enclosure of the nearby Hindu temple. Every day families bring goats or chickens which they ask the temple officials to decapitate in a ritual to persuade the goddess Kali to grant their requests. The animal that bit our Sisters had already attacked two children. It was foaming at the mouth and howling horribly. The men of the neighborhood attempted to catch it with a sack but it got away from them. It had taken refuge underneath a sweet vendor's cart, just outside the door to the home for the dying, when it jumped out at a little girl who was passing by.

Our two Sisters rushed to try and protect her. That was

*when the animal bit them on their hands and face. A rickshaw-
puller hurled himself after it but the dog disappeared. Later,
it was caught down by the river where the Hindus burn their
dead. A police van came to fetch it and took it away.*

*That afternoon, two policemen came. They brought a cer-
tificate from the veterinary department at the town hall, stating that the dog's brains were indeed "those of an animal
infected with rabies." I immediately called for one of the taxis
standing outside the temple and took our two injured to the
emergency ward at the Government Hospital myself. But they
had no antirabies serum. They referred us to another hospital.
They didn't have any serum there either and we were sent to
a third hospital. . . .*

Sister Paul went on to relate in detail the odyssey that had taken
her from hospital to hospital with Ananda and Alice, in quest of
the indispensable serum. Not one nursing center in the whole of
that vast city seemed to have any that day. Finally, somebody had
advised them to try an establishment by the name of the Pasteur
Institute on Convent Road. Apparently a few sheep were raised
there for the specific purpose of producing a little of the precious
serum. But they found only an abandoned building, the roof and
walls of which had been wrecked by the monsoon. A neighbor
informed them that the institute had long ago closed its doors and
that the staff had eaten the sheep one by one before leaving. The
three nuns had ended up going back to the convent on Lower
Circular Road where a doctor had come to examine the injured. In
the absence of Mother Teresa, who was traveling abroad, her assistant had sent a telegram to New Delhi to ask for the urgent
dispatch of some serum. By the time Sister Paul had written to
Philippe, it had still not yet arrived.

We are very worried [she concluded], *because as you know,
rabies is a fatal disease. Once it breaks out, there is nothing
we can do. If the serum doesn't get here within the next forty-
eight hours, it may perhaps be too late.*

Dear Brother, we have pressing need of your prayers.

Philippe Malouf looked for the date at the top of the first page. The letter had been written twelve days previously. In his distress he asked for the father abbot to be called.

"Father," he told the bearded old man, "read this letter quickly. Our community is being urgently called upon to show that the community of saints is a living reality."

Having read it, the monk did not utter a word but went swiftly to the monastery bell and summoned all the monks to chapel. Without waiting for vespers, the ten Trappists in the Monastery of the Seven Agonies in Latrun added their chanting and their prayers to their bedridden brother's offering of his suffering "in order that two little Indian sisters in saris who had given their lives to relieve the misery of mankind might live."

33

A Race Against the Clock to Save the Murderous Virus
Paris, France: Winter 1983

It was such a beautiful sight that Françoise Barré-Sinoussi could hardly take her eyes off it. No goldsmith could ever have created or even conceived the fluorescent mosaic made up of myriads of golden balls and rods that coated the glass slide under her microscope. She had studied billions of cells in the course of her career, but she never tired of marveling at nature's ability to deploy so much harmony in the creation of these infinitesimal elements.

All the same, there was so much at stake that winter's afternoon that the young biologist could not give free rein to her aesthetic appreciation. She had an urgent job to do. She must check the lymphocytes swimming about in the nourishing liquid of her test tubes to be sure she had the right quantity of cells. She knew that too strong or too weak a concentration of the liquid could prevent the lymphocytes from growing normally. The slide on which she had deposited her sample was scored with a fine cross-hatching that made it possible to count them. When next she looked up, there was a dimple in the hollow of her cheeks. The squares of her slides were filled.

"That's fine," she said to herself with a smile.

For several days now, in the confined atmosphere of the Bru

room at the Pasteur Institute in Paris, they had all been busying themselves over their tubes and centrifuges. They were preparing for the decisive operation that would confirm whether or not there was a retrovirus in the white cells of the Parisian designer's infected lymph node. The challenge lay in unmasking the transcriptase enzyme that served as the Trojan horse by which the virus introduced itself into the cells' nuclei. Here was one of the most delicate and complicated operations in cellular biology. Françoise Barré-Sinoussi placed the test tubes in a centrifuge rotating at a thousand revolutions a minute. This was a process designed to make the healthy lymphocytes fall to the bottom of the receptacles and allow her to capture the viral particles floating in the surface liquid. Then she made these viral particles into a concentrate by rotating them in a small flask for a second time, this time at a hundred thousand revolutions a minute. Next she placed this concentrate behind the safety screen of a hood with a stream of sterile air and added a few drops of ordinary detergent. If all went according to her expectations, the detergent would make the viral cells split and simultaneously liberate the reverse transcriptase enzyme that acted as intermediary for the retrovirus. It then remained for her to prove the presence of the reverse transcriptase and measure it. To do so, she would add to the flask a light-green mixture containing various ingredients that would activate the enzyme.

The young woman left the task of concocting these ingredients to no one else. She made up several variations, sometimes adding manganese, at others magnesium or some other substance. The key element was always a special preparation kept in the freezer and known, in laboratory jargon, as the "primer." This primer is a transparent solution, containing a perfect genetic baiting device, a fiendish kind of lure made up of a small quantity of DNA, complementary to the cells' genetic code. The enzyme finds itself irresistibly attracted to the DNA. Caught in the trap, the enzyme reveals itself and the retrovirus's signature can thus be detected by introducing a radioactive substance into the preparation to "mark" a specific secretion from the enzyme.

Having added her subtle concoction to the virus concentrates, the biologist placed her flasks in the sockets of a shaking incubator. Like the mixing of a milk shake, the movement of the oscillator would bring about the complete integration of the various elements.

Now the operation was reaching its critical stage. It was now or never that it would be possible to prove the presence of the enzyme by means of its radioactive secretion, provided of course that the test tubes actually contained the sought-after retrovirus. The incubator oscillated for over an hour. The crucial moment was drawing near. The solution must now be set out to dry like pancakes on a series of small circular filters the size of a communion wafer. With the help of her teammates, Françoise Barré-Sinoussi put each of these pancakes into an oven for approximately ten minutes at 206°. This baking process completed, she moved the pancakes to glass dishes into which she poured a few drops of a liquid that would make the enzymes scintillate. Then, all she had to do was put the glass receptacles into an electronic machine equipped with a digital counter, which would measure the presence of the enzyme. This would be the final verdict on whether a retrovirus was present or not.

The entire team took its place in front of the greenish screen in the hope of seeing reflected there the dramatic figures showing the radioactivity that would indicate that the culprit responsible for AIDS was indeed a retrovirus and that the researchers at the Pasteur Institute had just identified it. But the screen remained desperately virginal and the printer silent. The process had failed. As with Robert Gallo in Bethesda, the mystery of the cells refused to reveal its secrets. They would have to start again from scratch, modify the composition of the DNA bait, check the processes used to detect the stubbornly silent enzyme, check for possible procedural errors. In biological research such setbacks were far from rare. They were all well aware of that. However, on that icy January evening, the successors to Louis Pasteur were nonetheless beset with disappointment.

*   *   *

"No, still nothing. No sign of radioactivity on the counter."

Luc Montagnier gloomily replaced the receiver for the umpteenth time. For fourteen nights now his frustrated associates had given him the same response. Yet they had done everything they could, and with exceptional tenaciousness, to try to make their test tubes speak. If it was really a retrovirus that had infected the Parisian designer's cells, it hardly seemed possible for the killer agent to have remained incognito after so long a hunt. Doubts began to assail the team in the Bru room. Were they technically equipped to take on an adversary of this sort? What if there was no virus? What if it was just an invention, a figment of imagination created by medical practitioners and epidemiologists to clear themselves of their inability to subdue the disease?

It was in this baleful atmosphere that, on the morning of the fifteenth day, a cry of joy rang out. There, on the screen of the electronic counter, the figure 3,000 had just appeared. True, it was still a pretty pathetic number, but it was the first intimation of the presence of a radioactive substance in their test tubes, possibly the first manifestation of the enzyme that could prove the existence of the hypothetical AIDS agent. The scientists still needed further confirmation. It came three days later. This time the counter showed 6,000 radioactive counts a minute. Three days after that, the figure rose to 9,000. Luc Montagnier came rushing over to congratulate his colleagues. Their euphoria was just about to sweep away all the doubts of the previous week when disaster struck.

It happened in the course of a routine check of the lymphocyte cultures. The check was of such prime importance that Françoise Barré-Sinoussi carried it out herself several times a day. The white cells taken from the designer's lymph node had to be regarded as an invaluable asset because they were suspected of containing the infamous AIDS agent. Up until that day they had enjoyed admirable health and had been a source of pride, and a basis for all the biologist's hopes. Given the necessary time and constant attention, the young woman had been quite sure these cells would reproduce in sufficient numbers to create the simultaneous replication of the killer retrovirus contained within their nuclei, thus making identification possible. However, the scene of desolation she found under the light of her microscope obliterated this hope. The cells were dying before her very eyes. The sumptuous mosaic of fluorescent balls and rods, so often the source of her delight, had given way to an image of doom. Some of the cells had blown up like dirigible balloons and were on the point of bursting. Others had merged to form grotesque giant amalgams. Instead of sparkling like the facets of a diamond, their membranes had turned black. They were granulous, breaking up into small pieces, bristling with asperities, the indications of their imminent end.

Consternation struck the French scientists. What had caused such a disaster? What was the explanation? Where had they gone wrong? In the cultures' nutrition, in the warming of them or their respiration? Had some foreign body been able to contaminate the pipettes, tubes, or filters? Jean-Claude Chermann and Françoise Barré-Sinoussi checked all the possibilities, one by one. They could find no accidental cause. It was then that they had an idea: What if the retrovirus itself was responsible for the catastrophe? The one whose existence they had been slaving away to prove through the presence of the reverse transcriptase enzyme. The possibility made their heads swim. If the agent that was even now killing their white cell cultures was indeed a retrovirus, it must be an unknown retrovirus, because it behaved in the opposite way to the first human retrovirus discovered by Robert Gallo and to all the retroviruses found in animals. Instead of causing the frenzied and anarchic proliferation of the white cells detected in leukemia cases, this retrovirus quite simply killed them.

Was it possible that there was a human retrovirus that belonged to a totally different family than that of the retrovirus that the American scientists had discovered? If only this hypothesis could be confirmed, what a bomb it would drop on the medical research competition! What a sanctioning of the Bru room team it would be! And what a source of anxiety, too! "The death of the young designer's lymphocytes was in danger of depriving us of the very object of our discovery," Jean-Claude Chermann would explain. "It was inevitably going to bring about the destruction of the virus the lymphocytes were harboring. No more cells; no more virus." To avert this catastrophe, they must urgently try to prolong the life of the dying cultures by introducing other, healthy cells.

A laboratory's incubators and freezers are permanently stocked to overflowing with cell cultures destined for the various research projects in progress. That winter, Jean-Claude Chermann's stock included a considerable number of cells from mice, mink, and other furry mammals. Would the sick designer's virus come to life again when brought into contact with these animal cells? Would it want to lay siege to them? Would it be in a position to force its entry, infiltrate their nuclei, make them reproduce it? But all attempts with animal cells ended in failure. Only the introduction of human cells might, it seemed, avert the disaster.

The history of medical research will not preserve the names of the Parisians who presented themselves at the Pasteur Institute's blood transfusion center that January 24, 1983. Which of those donors could ever have dreamt that his blood might be used to resurrect several thousand viruses responsible for the worst scourge of the modern age? The anonymous donor's blood was welcomed with open arms by the team in the Bru room. Françoise Barré-Sinoussi swiftly isolated the lymphocytes, which she then immersed in a solution of vitamins and growth factors. As a special precaution, the biologist poured half of her preparation into a sterile test tube. "We had to check that the donor was not by some remote chance already carrying the virus we were looking for, or some other virus that might set us off on the wrong track," she explained later. Then she tipped the rest of the preparation into test tubes containing the dying lymphocytes from the diseased lymph node. She would have to wait patiently for several days to know the result of this attempt at revival.

34

"Do Not Resuscitate"
New York, USA: Winter 1983

While the French scientists waited for their cells to revive, the tragedy continued to spread. "It was like in the fable of the blind men and the elephant," Jack Dehovitz, the young doctor in charge of the care unit at St. Clare's Hospital, New York, would say. "The scientists with their test tubes were touching a different part of the 'animal' from those of us in the thick of it, and so our perceptions of its reality were different. To the scientists the AIDS elephant was just a virus concentrate at the bottom of their test tubes; to us it was a death mask on a white pillow with two great haunting eyes already staring death in the face." Dehovitz carried unbearable images away with him each evening. They were there when he went home, to a restaurant, to the cinema, out in the streets, on the subway; images that haunted him even when he was making love or reading the *New York Times*. "I couldn't shake them off even when I'd left the hospital. Too many patients were the same age as me, from the same background, or had something about them I could identify with. The memory of the guy from Baltimore who had literally gone to pieces before my very eyes when he discovered he had AIDS haunted me constantly."

The requirement that American doctors obtain the consent of

their patients prior to giving certain forms of treatment did not make things any easier. Any consent or refusal had to be endorsed with their signature on an official form. Thus each one's medical file contained a slip entitled "Living Will." Everyone called it the DNR, an abbreviation for "Do not resuscitate." Although each person had the right to choose whether or not to cling to life with the aid of modern revival techniques, doctors had to explain this choice to their patients and obtain their decision.

At the beginning of 1983 this became an ever more frequent duty for young Dr. Dehovitz. "This catastrophic epidemic was forcing us to improvise constantly," he would explain. "There were no universally acceptable ways of asking someone if, when the time came, he wanted to be linked up to a load of machines to prolong his life at all costs. We had to adapt ourselves to individual personalities even if the essential message remained the same: for the time being all's well, but the possibility exists that one day your condition will deteriorate and a decision will have to be made as to the appropriateness of continuing the fight. In case you are not then in a fit state to make your wishes known, it would be as well to be on the safe side and determine now whether or not you would want in such circumstances to be moved to the intensive care unit. I tried to deliver this message as gently as possible and without exerting any influence either way. I even advised my patients to think about it for a few days, to discuss it with their families, with other members of the medical staff, other patients. But in my heart of hearts, I always hoped that their decision would be in favor of giving up a hopeless struggle."

Whenever this was in fact the case, Dehovitz would take the small slip marked with the initials DNR out of his overall pocket and ask his patient to sign. Afterward he would complete the document by entering a summary of their conversation. Sometimes, before reaching a decision, patients wanted to see what was actually meant by emergency treatment. There were always one or two patients in the intensive care unit at St. Clare's. The sight of the impressive skein of tubes and pipes that linked the bodies of these unfortunates to the battery of bottles and appliances that kept them artificially alive nearly always eradicated all desire to cling to existence. The shock was sometimes such that patients gave specific instructions to their families or the person closest to them to put a stop, if necessary by judicial means, to all attempts to prolong their life under similar circumstances. Such measures were a source of worry to doctors, who were aware that they might be accused of homicide if they did not fight to the very last.

*   *   *

Jack Dehovitz was amazed at the different reactions his administrative obligation provoked. Some patients refused to talk about it in their state of exhaustion. Others cursed him, demanding every possible form of treatment, even going as far as to threaten him with legal action. In some cases, the disease had affected the brain, which made these exchanges even more complicated.

The doctor found he made the best contact with members of the community first affected by the scourge. Socially and culturally, gay men were an elite in the St. Clare's unit. The victims of frequent infections, most of them had already spent time in hospitals and were therefore familiar with medical procedures. They knew their rights, including the right to refuse a particular medicine. The directions for use relating to proposed remedies did not escape their vigilance, and especially not the small print indicating possible side effects. Jack Dehovitz would often have occasion to regret patients' priorities that seemed to him ridiculous in view of the seriousness of their condition. If they found some piece of information they did not like, they might reject the whole treatment.

The doctor would never forget certain confrontations. One day, one of his patients, whose virus was threatening his eyesight, discovered that the remedy prescribed to delay impending blindness could cause minor lesions on his genitals. No sooner had he spotted the word "testicles" as a side effect on the label than he reared up in his bed like a cobra about to strike.

"Doc, I'm not having anyone interfering with my balls," he raged.

"John, it's to save your sight," pleaded Jack Dehovitz.

"To hell with my eyes!" he yelled. "It's my balls that matter!"

The sophisticated manner in which some other patients expressed themselves surprised the doctor more than once. "You'd tell some young guy you were going to put a drip in his chest and he'd answer: 'No, Doc, I don't want a perfusion inserted in my subclavian artery,' which was the correct term for what you proposed doing." The refusal to have certain forms of treatment also amazed Jack

Dehovitz. "You'd think all patients in danger of dying would be keen to let you do absolutely anything you thought necessary. Not true. Many gays had their own way of looking at things. For the most part they were primarily concerned with safeguarding the quality of their life and staying in command of their faculties. They didn't want anything to do with the tubes that kept you alive only as a vegetable."

This attitude was not shared by another category of New York patients that St. Clare's began to accept in growing numbers. Drug addicts showed scarcely any interest in their last moments. They even refused to discuss them, preferring to take refuge in a state of open rebellion, which did not make the task of their doctors and nurses any easier. Before treating them for AIDS, the doctors had first to try to detoxify them. Weeks, sometimes months, went by before they could be drawn into a tentative conversation, before a shred of trust was formed. "Their behavior was the cause of more than one of the unit's nurses leaving," Dehovitz would remember. "To men obsessed with the lack of drugs, the suffocating effects caused by fungal *Candida* or the disfiguring lesions of Kaposi's sarcoma were secondary. Raising the circumstances of their death with them, suggesting that they should renounce artificial resuscitation in advance, was like trying to discuss the colors of a rainbow with a blind man."

*   *   *

There were many deaths at St. Clare's that winter of 1983. The first patient to pass away was the young publicity man from Baltimore. Despite the support of his companion, who was constantly present in his small room full of flowers and music, and despite Jack Dehovitz's assiduous care, he had been unable to keep his promise to "give your bloody little illness a hard time." He died peacefully, surrounded by his mother, brother, and friends, and leaving on his bedside table a thick marketing handbook that he had not had the time to finish reading.

Strangely, the young doctor saw neither this death nor any of the others as defeats, which was surprising for a man who had embraced the ideal of medicine purely for the joy of making people better. "The effects of the disease are so awful that in the end it almost made me love death," he would admit. "Death in such circumstances is not, in my view, a failure but a triumph over suffering. No one can take people suffering like that for too long. I found myself actually willing the death of a patient, even while I fought like an alley cat to bar its way. One other thing was a source of comfort to me. I knew that one day soon death would not be the unavoidable outcome, that treatment would get the better of the 'bloody little illness' that had taken the life of the young man from Baltimore. That went without question.

"It was that burning conviction that helped me to hold out that winter. And to hope that my experience as a medical practitioner up to my neck in the daily tragedies of AIDS would help in some small way to win the war against the terrible disease."

35

Hundreds of Thousands of Retroviruses in a Boeing Jet
Paris, France: Winter 1983

For three days and three nights the team members in the Bru room had done everything they could to make the radioactivity counter register a significant number. Fearing that the Parisian designer's moribund viruses might not sufficiently be revived by the blood donor's lymphocytes alone, Françoise Barré-Sinoussi had rushed to the nearest maternity hospital. With their exceptional capacity to proliferate, the cell stocks in blood from a newborn baby's umbilical cord would make ideal food for her declining white cell cultures.

A little before midday on January 27, the biologist took a test tube containing her latest preparation to the electronic counter set up in the corridor. Interminable seconds went by. Then came a click and a figure appeared on the counter. Behind her thick glasses, the young woman's eyes opened immeasurably wide.

"Eighteen thousand!" she gasped.

It was double the best result previously achieved.

"The culture's going again!" cried Jean-Claude Chermann.

"Yes. The baby's breathing!" exclaimed Françoise Barré-Sinoussi, lighting one of the Marlboros she chain-smoked.

The French had certainly found something, but what? Apparently a retrovirus, as indicated by the activity of the signature enzyme reflected on the radioactivity counter. But what retrovirus? Could it be the same as the one Robert Gallo had identified in rare leukemia cases, which was still to date the only retrovirus to have been found in humans? Could it be a member of the same family, like the one Prem Sarin, the American's Indian collaborator, was expecting to find? Or was it instead a completely different retrovirus? Jean-Claude Chermann and Françoise Barré-Sinoussi were in no doubt whatsoever: their retrovirus had nothing in common with Robert Gallo's. His had caused lymphocytes to multiply; theirs killed them. Cousins, no matter how distant, could not behave in such a diametrically opposite way.

*   *   *

After the euphoria came a further bout of anxiety. The French knew their discovery would be condemned to oblivion if they failed to produce startling evidence of it for the benefit of the international scientific community. A formidable prospect. Who was going to believe a team of virtually unknown virologists? Certainly not the American researcher who was working hard to defend a different thesis and who reigned like a king over world retrovirology. In his heart of hearts, Robert Gallo was convinced it was still "his" retrovirus the well-meaning "Pasteurians" had just sighted in their test tubes, but he was far too clever not to show interest in the results of his competitors' labors. He lost no time in sending them two strains of cells producing his HTLV, together with some samples of its particular antibodies. In this way the French would be able to compare the viral agent that they thought they had discovered with the American retrovirus and realize for themselves that they were one and the same virus.

Passengers on board Air France flight 021 taking off from Dulles Airport in Washington that evening had no idea in what strange company they were crossing the Atlantic. Inside two small boxes —one packed with cotton wool, the other full of ice—were two flasks containing a slightly opaque liquid. In the first, protected by the cotton wool, swam hundreds of thousands of cells carrying the highly carcinogenic American retrovirus, and in the second, kept cold in ice, were as many antibodies capable of recognizing those agents of death.

Françoise Barré-Sinoussi rushed to open the precious package herself as soon as it arrived in Paris. Its contents had the potential either to shatter all the hopes of the Bru room team or to propel it to the front of the Nobel Prize lineup. Robert Gallo's dispatch would indeed provide a decisive tool for verification. The French would bring together face-to-face Gallo's HTLV retrovirus and the Pasteur's antibodies taken from the infected lymphocytes of the Parisian designer. If these antibodies attacked the American retrovirus, this would be proof that they belonged to the same family. Then the agent uncovered by the French scientists would, in fact, be identical to the first human retrovirus discovered by Robert Gallo. If, on the other hand, the "partners" refused to interact, that would be an indication that the two retroviruses were not of the same kind.

There were two ways of setting about this test. While Luc Montagnier used one initial method, Jean-Claude Chermann and Françoise Barré-Sinoussi entrusted the implementation of a different method to one of their best technicians. The art of immunofluorescence held no secrets for the attractive twenty-seven-year-old Marie-Thérèse Nugeyre. Working with the delicacy of a harpist, her long fingers equipped with a pipette would mix on one glass slide specimens of American lymphocytes carrying Robert Gallo's virus with the specific antibodies that had previously been colored with a rosy dye called fluorescein. Then, on a second slide, she placed some dyed American antibodies with the French lymphocytes harboring the Pasteur's retrovirus. All she had to do now was wait patiently for the results of these arranged marriages.

That evening, the young technician felt suddenly as if her heart were leaping out of her breast. On the first slide, a sparkling agglutination of mingled cells and viral particles had appeared in the hazy light of her fluorescent microscope. Like a shining emerald brooch, the cells infected with Robert Gallo's retrovirus blazed with a thousand flames. The contrast with the second slide was astonishing. On that slide, the cells infected by the French retrovirus had remained completely black. The American antibodies had not enveloped them with their luminous green spangles. Like an organ rejecting a graft, they had refused all contact with the unfamiliar viral particles. Marie-Thérèse Nugeyre rushed out into the corridor.

"Come and look!" she cried.

Everyone came running to take a look at the unforgettable sight. Montagnier, usually so austere and reserved, assumed the light-hearted air of a schoolboy at a football game. Such was the euphoria around the microscope that "we could have danced in a circle around it," Françoise Barré-Sinoussi would remember. In his imagination, Jean-Claude Chermann could already see "Gallo's face when he heard he wasn't the only one to have discovered a human retrovirus."

*   *   *

Decisive as this demonstration was, the team in the Bru room knew that it was only the opening act. Before announcing their discovery to the international scientific community, they would have to establish the characteristics of this new human retrovirus, determine its morphology, its density, analyze its different proteins, specify its molecular weight, identify its genes; in short, gather all the information necessary to give the retrovirus an identity. To succeed in this undertaking the French would need the assistance of a number of people, none more vital than a jovial, modest little man who had spent all his professional life in the artificial light of a tiny windowless room in the Pasteur Institute.

36

A Little Indian Sister's Agony
Calcutta, India: Winter 1983

Sister Paul had moved heaven and earth to get some antirabies serum. While they waited for the lifesaving ampules, the nun had dispatched the two novices bitten by the rabid dog to bed, with the instructions that they were to have complete rest. The infirmary she had chosen, however, was hardly in a place conducive to inactivity. It stood immediately next to the long building that housed one of the main centers created by Mother Teresa to relieve the poverty of the inhuman metropolis.

The name of the center sprawled in enormous black letters across its yellow-painted facade: PREM DAN—GIFT OF LOVE. It had been given to the foundress of the Missionaries of Charity in 1975 by the British Imperial Chemical Industries corporation, whose local staff had refused to put up with the pestilential smells from the nearby tanneries. With its luxurious setting of tropical greenery, from a distance the long structure could have passed for some tourist paradise. The hovels that surrounded it on all sides could almost be forgotten. Now the laboratories, workshops, and offices that had harbored the previous occupants swarmed with a piteous humanity. Many of these waifs had lost their sanity, which made this place the largest lunatic asylum in Bengal. Yet Prem Dan was not just a dumping ground for broken, vanquished people. Under the sisters' influence the establishment hummed with life and activity. Here, some of the residents were singing as they made mats. There, others were weaving bags and making rope out of the fiber from coconuts recovered from public refuse dumps. The idea of relieving the city of some of its rubbish and simultaneously providing her protégés with work had come from Mother Teresa. She called it "turning garbage into gold." Farther on, people handicapped as a result of poliomyelitis were taking part in a physical reeducation session. A kindly instructor guided them one step at a time between two parallel bars. Elsewhere, an American volunteer was trying to introduce some mentally sick people to the sonorousness of her guitar while other young paralytics meticulously deloused the hair of a group of old people.

Tired of doing nothing while they waited for the serum to arrive, one morning Sister Ananda and Sister Alice broke their vow of obedience and went to help the occupants of the home. The gaiety of one wizened woman immediately attracted the attention of the former leper from Benares. Her laughter and liveliness brought an atmosphere of surprising joy to the enormous dormitory. She caught hold of the young novice's hand and indicated that she wanted to be massaged. Ananda knelt down beside the stunted little body and began to knead her gently. She discovered the woman had been found several years earlier by a hunter in the depths of a Himalayan forest. It was thought she had been raised by bears because she only moved about on all fours. It had taken months for her stomach to get used to human food, and for a long time she would only eat off the bare floor. With patience, the sisters had taught her how to stand upright and place one foot in front of the other. Her existence in the wild had deprived her of the power of speech. She only expressed herself in growls. Being massaged seemed to give her the greatest delight. The sisters couldn't help wondering whether bears' tongues had introduced her to this pleasurable sensation.

The unexpected arrival of Sister Paul put a premature stop to the two novices' escapade. The nun had received the antirabies serum at last. She had brought with her a young English doctor who was working for a while at the home for the dying so that he could give them their first injection immediately. This treatment, reputed to be especially painful, had to be repeated every twenty-four hours for fourteen days. In this particular case the delay in initiating the course meant there was no guarantee of success.

*   *   *

Three weeks later, Brother Philippe Malouf at the Monastery of the Seven Agonies at Latrun, Israel, received an envelope from England containing a small sheet of the Missionaries of Charity's stationery together with an accompanying letter signed by a Dr. Williams. The monk's heart missed a beat when he recognized Sister Paul's handwriting.

Dearest Brother Philippe,

I have to tell you of our sadness [he read with impatience]. *Doubtless we did not pray enough. The good Lord has taken our little Sister Alice from us. Dr. Williams, who is returning to Europe this evening, will tell you in what horrifying circumstances.*

Fortunately, Sister Ananda, your spiritual link, does not to date have any of the disease's early symptoms. But she is still in great need of the support of your prayers and the offering of your suffering.

Deeply upset, the monk paused for a long moment before finding the resolution to read Dr. Williams's letter.

The two patients were enduring their treatment courageously when Sister Alice started to show signs of agitation and anxiety. She began to chatter incessantly in a rapid, jerky way. She lost her appetite, suffered from insomnia, headaches, respiratory problems. After two days, the characteristic symptom we had all been dreading showed itself. She was uncontrollably repelled by the smallest drop of liquid. Though racked with the desire to drink, the slightest attempt to absorb so much as a drop of water paralyzed her respiratory muscles for several seconds. Soon the mere sound of water running was enough to cause violent attacks of suffocation. Sisters Paul and Ananda, some of the other Sisters, together with myself and two Indian doctors, kept up a constant relay at her side to support her in the hope of giving the serum time to work. But the disease continued to wreak destruction.

Sister Alice became terribly sensitive to any external sensation such as bright light, a noise that was the least bit loud, a draft of cool air. Convulsions began to shake her body. The attacks of suffocation grew more frequent. Every exhalation was accompanied by a kind of rattle. She sounded like an animal groaning. The terror of swallowing her own saliva made her spit out streams of foam. Her teeth started to chatter so violently that she looked as if she wanted to bite. It was dreadful. There was nothing human anymore about a face that had once been so beautiful and serene. On the fourth day an attack of suffocation worse than the previous ones put an end to her torment.

The British doctor went on to explain briefly how anxiously the sisters and doctors were watching over Ananda's condition. He was able to confirm that nothing had given cause for alarm to date, but they would have to wait several weeks, possibly months, before they could be certain the disease was not going to declare itself. His letter concluded with a long postscript.

All through poor Sister Alice's agony, a dog did not stop barking in the courtyard outside the infirmary. That dog looks so fierce the Sisters have, very aptly, nicknamed it Kala Shaitan—"the Black Devil."

The Black Devil's jaws inspire as much fear in the Sisters obliged to pass his kennel as they do in thieves. He has bitten several of them. But no one asks that he be sent away for fear of upsetting Mother Teresa, because Mother is particularly fond of this watchdog, who returns her affection. As soon as he sees her, Black Devil becomes as gentle as a lamb. He goes rushing up to her with his tail wagging, asking her blessing in the form of a pat.

37

Eyes That Were Wonderstruck by a Small Black Sphere
Paris, France: Winter 1983

Luc Montagnier pointed to the small flask he had brought with him.

"You're bound to find it in there. We've managed to show traces of its enzyme. Now it's your turn to have a look."

Charles Dauguet, known as Charlie, aged fifty-four, ran a sturdy hand over the thin rim of gray beard that formed a halo round his face. The suggestion could not but delight the jovial little man who had but one passion in life: photography. His laboratory's mission was to supply the scientists at the Pasteur Institute with documentary evidence to confirm the validity of their hypotheses. He was the photographer in charge of supplying visual proof.

Dauguet adjusted his bifocals to examine the little bottle.

"Be careful!" Montagnier went on. "It's only right that I should tell you there's an extremely dangerous virus in there. You're quite at liberty not to want to touch it."

"Don't worry," responded Dauguet with his habitual calm, "I taught the little bastards to respect me a long time ago."

For twenty-six years, in a tiny room on the first floor of the Pasteur Institute's venerable Rabies Building, Charles Dauguet had been photographing the invisible germs that attack men, animals, and plants. Few killers from the realms of the infinitely microscopic had eluded his lenses. Sometimes Dauguet would have to track his prey for weeks before capturing them on film. He had photographed thousands of viruses responsible for hepatitis B, rabies, polio, smallpox, herpes, shingles, and a multitude of other infections, many of them fatal. They came in an infinite variety of forms. Some looked like golf balls, others like car wheels, paving stones, owl's eyes, half-moons, packets of macaroni. Charles Dauguet had so frequently been amazed by the malice and originality of the viral disguises that the walls of his lab were covered with the trophies of his career, his most remarkable shots.

*   *   *

His passion for photography went back to his tenderest child-hood. He had scarcely been three years old when his grandfather, a Norman garage owner, had given him his first camera. That had been the first of a collection that now comprised about a hundred extremely rare models patiently unearthed from flea markets and innumerable scrap-metal sales. As a teenager, his leisure time had been spent scouring the Paris wholesale food market, his picturesque neighborhood of Les Halles, with his eye glued to his viewfinder. "It gave me so much pleasure to capture the moment a quarter of beef was sold," he would say, "or an armful of roses, to freeze on film even the most insignificant event at the very second it occurred. Afterward it would give me quite a thrill to look at those snapshots of life and say to myself: 'That happened at such and such a moment and I actually saw it.'"

For a young high school boy, the Paris uprising and liberation from German occupation in August 1944 had been an opportunity to take some unforgettable shots: extraordinary moments of popular activity and rejoicing. He had even involuntarily immortalized a horrific scene when a Paris insurgent executed a pro-German po-liceman. The man had been caught firing on the crowd from the rooftops. His clothes had been torn off. An insurgent had bran-dished a gun with a bayonet. "Take a photo, lad!" he called out to Charlie. Terrified, the boy had automatically flattened his eye against the viewfinder and depressed the shutter's release.

Dauguet owed his real success to an infinitely more banal piece of paper—a photo of a flea magnified forty times over. It was a fine brown-colored female flea with the legs of a high jumper, a coiled body, and a serrated proboscis capable of piercing the toughest of skins. To photograph the flea, he had mounted one of the cameras from his collection on the lens of a small German microscope his parents had given him for Christmas.

As destiny would have it, his portrait of a flea came under the scrutiny of the woman in charge of the brand-new laboratory for electronic microscopy at the Pasteur Institute. Mlle. Croissant was so impressed that she invited the young amateur photographer to come and work for her. Charlie blessed his flea and was quick to accept, a decision he would never regret. "Spending my life surveying an invisible world trying to unearth its mysteries and take pictures of them for those who can advance the progress of science—what could be more exciting?" And yet his universe was austere indeed: devoid of fresh air, sunshine, or light, with a large throbbing cylinder like a submarine periscope for his only companion. With its compressor, its water cooler, its high-performance lenses, its ion fluxes, its electronic counters and cathode screen, the Siemens 101 in Charles Dauguet's laboratory made such huge enlargements possible that a single cell could be made to assume the dimensions of the Eiffel Tower. Sometimes it would take Charlie's probing eye an entire week to explore the microuniverse of a few white cells on a glass slide in its entirety. Through his camera a monochrome expanse in gray and white would become a geographic panorama, traversed by thousands of islands, promontories, rivers, deltas, craters, and mounds. And suddenly, after days of searching, a strange mark, an abnormal protrusion, an odd black sphere: a virus would loom before him. Then the photographer's fingers would tighten their grip on the knobs of the microscope to line the suspect area delicately up on the screen. He would vary the contrast in the lighting, increase the magnification, seek out the most favorable angle. "A photo should speak louder than words," Dauguet would claim. He had applied this formula so successfully to his own work that scientists could recognize his mark on any photographic document at a glance.

After so many years of exploration at the heart of the infinitely small, Charles Dauguet now nurtured a new dream. "God willing that I reach retirement," he would say, "I shall join the ranks of an amateur astronomers' club. I'd like to go on to examine the infinitely large and make the connection between the cell world and the star world." Charlie was already working on the means to this ultimate conquest. In the miniworkshop he had set up at home in the Rue Lecourbe, the first skeleton model of his future telescope was beginning to take shape.

* * *

The Dauguets made an endearing couple. Their love had been born in the most unromantic of places: the laboratory at the Pasteur Institute where Charlie photographed his viruses. Claudine washed the cell samples there, before centrifuging, drying, then "fossilizing" them in cups of resin.

Less than three hours after Montagnier's visit, the blocks of resin containing the virus were ready. They had only to be cut into very thin slices. To perform this delicate operation, which he made a point of doing himself, Charlie used a rare goldsmith's tool that he placed under lock and key whenever he had finished using it. The tool in question was a diamond knife, one and a half millimeters in size, with a cutting edge so fine and so true that there were only two or three cutters in the world capable of fashioning such a jewel. Set in a special electric cutting device, the blade made it possible to make incisions that were "beyond reality," impossible to see with the naked eye. Charlie was especially proud of his diamond. It came from a mine in Venezuela and had cost the princely sum of $1,000.

Put on a grid punctured with tiny holes, each shaving would be studied under the microscope with a view to detecting the sought-after viral particles and photographing them. "A diabolical game of hide-and-seek," was how Charles Dauguet would define the relentless hunt he then began at the controls of his Siemens 101. As usual, he set the apparatus to his favorite level of magnification of fifty thousand. "With an electronic microscope it's better always to stick to the same magnification because the relative sizes of the virus and the cells tell you quite a lot in themselves," he would explain. Each shaving of resin contained about fifty cells, which could take several hours to examine or sometimes an entire day. Since his diamond sliced a good hundred shavings of each block of resin, every new piece of research meant a titanic effort. After ten or eleven hours of staring uninterruptedly at his luminescent screen, Charles

Dauguet would reel like a blind man when he reentered the outside world.

It was shortly before six, on the evening of Friday, February 3, 1983, that the eagerly awaited event occurred. As he recounted: "I was about to stop the microscope compressor and switch off the screen after one last look at a vast cellular delta when something made me start. I had just spotted a small black sphere breaking out of the surface of a lymphocyte. Although it hadn't quite emerged from its coat, I could tell quite clearly from its structure that it was a foreign body that didn't belong to the cell. I clasped Claudine in my arms and yelled out, 'That's it. I've got the bloody virus!'"

Luc Montagnier's secretary jumped as Charlie burst into the professor's office. He was like a "bull escaped from the ring." He was yelling at the top of his voice, "I've found the virus, I've found the virus!" In her boss's absence, the young woman wanted to be the first to congratulate him. "Bravo, Charlie, bravo," she said over and over again in her excitement. Since Jean-Claude Chermann and Françoise Barré-Sinoussi were not there either, Charlie went running back to his laboratory to record the sight his wonderstruck eyes had just discovered on a gelatin film. It took him only a few minutes to fit up his plates, adjust his camera, and set the time interval for the shutter stop and the regulator for electron flow. Then, with the same depression of his index finger that had previously enabled him to immortalize a flea, he pressed the electronic shutter release to take history's first photographs of the AIDS retrovirus.

This international scoop would not in any way interfere with Charlie and Claudine's usual routine. It was nearly midnight when they left their laboratory to go back to their car parked beneath a chestnut tree. As on any other Friday night, they made for their native Normandy to indulge in their favorite hobby: shrimping.

*   *   *

At eight o'clock sharp on the following Monday morning, Charles Dauguet switched on his Siemens and its electronic screens again. News of his success had already made the rounds of the building. Luc Montagnier and the entire team from the Bru room gathered in his laboratory to admire the first pictures of the killer virus. They saw for themselves how totally unusual its appearance was. At first sight, it did not look like Robert Gallo's or like any known animal retrovirus. To be absolutely certain and able to give official confirmation, they would need further proof. Working on cell samples taken from other patients, Charlie made up new cuts. Once more he began his patient research. The same triumphant cry, the same hug for Claudine, greeted each new discovery. Luc Montagnier and his associates were sent ever more precise photographs with each passing day.

To demonstrate irrefutably the absence of any structural relationship between Robert Gallo's HTLV and the retrovirus discovered at the Pasteur Institute, Charlie had Claudine make up some blocks of resin containing cells infected with the American virus. Photographs made it possible to draw a direct comparison between the two agents. There could no longer be any doubt about it: neither their form nor their structure nor the way in which they formed expansive bumps on the cells were identical.

This time the French scientists were convinced they were viewing the culprit responsible for AIDS.

38

"Sam, Is There Any Risk of This Virus Affecting the Children?"

Bethesda, USA: Spring–Summer 1983

Small, thickset with a neck like a bull's and a determined face lined by a thin handlebar mustache, Dr. Samuel Broder, the forty-one-year-old director of the clinical oncology program of the National Cancer Institute at Bethesda, was the perfect example of a man who liked to meet the world head-on. From his childhood in Poland where his family of Jewish partisans had been hunted down by the Nazis, to his brutal encounter with the AIDS tragedy, his entire life had been a succession of confrontations.

After arriving in America with a handful of Polish survivors of the holocaust, Broder had grown up in the streets of an industrial suburb of Detroit, the American car capital. He had spent his weekends and holidays serving hamburgers and cokes at Mary's, a luncheonette run by his parents on the corner of Dexter and Boston streets. The establishment had burned down in 1968 during the race riots triggered by the assassination of Martin Luther King. The young Broder, who had never intended to make a career out of the family business, was not unduly sorry. His ambitions lay elsewhere. Very early, during his years at the local Ferndale High School, he had realized that a scientific career was one in which it was possible to succeed without having a fortune or social standing. It was a discovery that would shape his destiny.

Sam Broder worked hard to achieve the top marks in science subjects that would earn him a scholarship to the University of Michigan, one of the most prestigious universities in the United States. "Barely an hour's bus journey from Detroit, for me it was like going into a different universe. Most people at home had as their aspiration that they would become mechanics or plumbers. Here I shared my room with a friend who wanted to be a composer—and from my standpoint it was like announcing that he was going to the moon."

Within a few months, the attraction of the onetime fast-food waiter to science had been transformed into a real vocation. "How could I fail to be spellbound by so many new ideas with such fantastic implications? For example, the idea that a simple drop of nucleic acid could be the carrier of the whole hereditary patrimony of a living creature. Or that you had only to analyze a person's genetic code to predict his behavior. Or that the day would come when it would be possible to modify that behavior by working on this or that gene . . . wasn't there material enough there to trigger the imagination of a young immigrant thirsting for knowledge?"

He found his hero in a book. In the novel *Arrowsmith*, the great American writer Sinclair Lewis had painted the portrait of a doctor from a small town in the Midwest with an all-consuming passion for scientific truth. This doctor found himself, at the end of the last century, at the head of one of the country's most renowned institutes for medical research. His noble ideals clashed with too many old habits and too many interests. The scientist was finally obliged to opt for a life of solitude and heroic deprivation in which to pursue his quest for truth. "The prayer of the scientist" that the author offers his readers at the end of the book had such an impact on young Broder that twenty years later every word remained engraved upon his heart and memory:

God give me unclouded eyes and freedom from haste. God give me a quiet and relentless anger against all pretense and all pretentious work and all work left slack and unfinished. God

> *give me a restlessness whereby I may neither sleep nor accept*
> *praise till my observed results equal my calculated results or in*
> *pious glee I discover and assault my error. God give me strength*
> *not to trust to God!*

In an attempt to emulate the example of Dr. Martin Arrowsmith, Sam Broder enrolled at the University of Michigan's prestigious medical school. One of his microbiology teachers, Prof. Frank Whitehouse, spotted a student eager for knowledge and opened the doors of his laboratory to him. There, Broder would undergo the decisive introduction to what would become the inspiration for his whole professional life: cancer. "I shut myself away for evenings and whole weekends, learning how to produce antibodies to combat cancerous cells. My efforts weren't always productive, but I did come to realize there that cancer was going to play a fundamental role in biological research, that the mastery of numerous pathologies was necessarily via a better understanding of the behavior of cancerous cells. Even my failures, I felt, were not entirely useless. They made me appreciate that research is above all a question of method, that the difference between a great scientist and a mediocre researcher derives from the fact that the one knows how to ask the right questions, the other doesn't; that one is capable of making use of the most advanced technology, the other isn't."

*   *   *

At first sight, the Clinical Center, where Sam Broder worked, looked like a five-star luxury hotel with its rooms decorated with reproductions of the works of contemporary artists, its corridors lined with thick, brightly colored carpeting, and its bay windows overlooking the verdant countryside of Maryland. Behind these luxurious appointments, the National Cancer Institute, anxious to link research and treatment as closely as possible, had created a unique establishment where, in order to develop new treatments, doctor-scientists could have access to both patients and experimental laboratories at the same time. Not everyone with cancer could hope to be hospitalized in this forward-looking unit of which Sam Broder was now the director. The only cases admitted were those that corresponded to research work, either planned or already in progress, together with patients whose pathology was so rare or exceptional that they became subjects for study.

The young cancer specialist was aware that he enjoyed a degree of freedom that was almost miraculous for the Bethesda campus, so often paralyzed by crushing government bureaucracy. He alone was responsible for the choice of research subjects and the treatment of patients. The fact that he was daily confronted with the tragedy of illness imbued his scientific approach with an acute sense of the urgent need for discovery. His impatience verged on the morbid. "The big difference between Robert Gallo and me," he would explain, "is that in his laboratory he is never actually confronted with death. Whereas I feel obliged to get concrete results as quickly as possible, especially as my failures are more numerous than my successes." The failures in no way changed the line of reasoning he imposed on his associates. His philosophy could be summed up in the single sentence: "There is always some more effective medicine to be found."

The AIDS outbreak was a traumatic ordeal. "At first the most unbearable part about it was our inability to understand the disease, and the way in which most scientists were frightened of it. They reminded me of people who hear a noise in the cellar of their home and try to convince themselves it isn't a burglar." The announcement that a retrovirus was the most likely cause of the epidemic had not failed to reinforce this skeptical attitude, inducing a number of scientists and doctors to take refuge in a convenient fatalism. This kind of ostrich reaction provoked such anger in Broder that he swiftly acquired a reputation on the Bethesda campus for being an *enfant terrible*. All his attention was directed toward finding a medicine capable of stopping the development of the disease. It was the duty of scientists to spur their laboratories on to discover the causes of the illness; it was his duty to devise a suitable remedy to put an end to the agony of the living dead who filled his ward. "There was nothing conjectural or speculative about my conviction that AIDS could be held in check," he asserted. "We already had chemical products that could inhibit the effect of viruses in the laboratory, and we had enormous experience to draw on in the art of developing anticancerous substances. All we needed was time, more knowledge, a lot of work, a good measure of discipline . . . and a little bit of luck."

*   *   *

A pretty, dark-haired woman of forty, a lawyer by profession, still remembers the anxious expression on Sam's face that evening in the spring in 1983. In nineteen years of marriage, Gail Broder had had time to get used to her husband's taciturn moods. Since cancer treatment was not inherently a field conducive to optimism and joie de vivre, she knew how to read the daily defeats in Sam's face or the tone of his voice. She could hear in his intimations of the day's experiences of some battle lost at a patient's bedside, of the failure of some promising medicine he had prescribed. Gail knew how to soften these blows and open, at just the right moment, the bottle of Riesling or Traminer she always had ready in the refrigerator.

On that particular evening, no Rhine wine could smoothe the cancer expert's brow. What he had to say to his wife and their two daughters, aged fourteen and seventeen, was too serious.

"He told us he had just made the decision to tackle the virus suspected of causing AIDS by researching a medicine that would inhibit its effects," Gail would recount. "He stressed the fact that it was a dangerous undertaking because no one could assess the risks involved in handling significant concentrates of living viruses under laboratory conditions. He tried not to alarm us too much, but even so, he had to admit that two out of five of his researchers had already left the laboratory. I should say that at that time Sam's team was the only one to have agreed to work on such quantities of living viruses.

"I took a long look at our two innocent daughters with their schoolgirl's braids and came up with the only question that really mattered to me.

" 'Is there any risk of your bringing the virus home with you and having it affecting the children?'

"Sam nodded his head several times. 'There is a risk,' he replied."

39

Crimes of High Treason Against the Retrovirus King
Cold Spring Harbor, USA: Spring 1983

Lawns stretching down to a beach of fine sand, rose-laurel walk-ways, old Victorian houses, tennis and volleyball courts, low modern buildings providing a venue for cafés, guest rooms, auditoriums, libraries, laboratories, workrooms, and even a printing press: Cold Spring Harbor looks both like a university campus and something of a tourist complex. A little port nestling on the north coast of Long Island, it is famous for its mussels and clams but also for quite another specialty. It is one of the world's shrines of molecular biology. Every year for the last half century, in the high season between April and September, symposiums, conferences, and lectures have brought scientists to its campus from all over the world.

It was there that, in June 1946, the brand-new discipline of molecular genetics had received its letters patent; there that, one day in June 1953, James Watson, a future Nobel Prize winner aged only twenty-four at the time, had brought to the attention of the world one of the century's most important discoveries, the structure of DNA, the molecule that carries the genetic code. There, in 1966, the largest gathering ever of microbiologists, geneticists, and virologists had definitively codified the principles of heredity. There, in 1972, three other prospective Nobel Prize winners, the biologists

Dominique Lapierre

David Baltimore, Renato Dulbecco, and Howard Temin, had demonstrated the role of the reverse transcriptase, the signature enzyme of the retrovirus. The list of papers presented at Cold Spring Harbor seminars was synonymous with the greatest biological discoveries of the last half century. So prestigious were these gatherings that the honor of taking part in them or simply of being present was courted by all the world's scientific elite, particularly by the young staffs of basic research laboratories. Cold Spring Harbor had also become a "brain market" to which leaders came to recruit the future crack members of their teams.

That Monday, May 9, 1983, a young French woman who was virtually unknown to the international scientific community arrived at the campus to attend a conference on retroviruses. Because of the Pasteur Institute's meager travel allowance, she found herself the only representative of the celebrated Parisian laboratory at this important event, whereas Robert Gallo's group and most of the other American research units had turned out in force. Françoise Barré-Sinoussi, who had possibly just collaborated in the discovery of the AIDS retrovirus, was there only in the capacity of observer. The issue of AIDS and the achievements of French retrovirology had still not aroused the curiosity of the Cold Spring Harbor delegates that spring, so she was not due to present any of the eighty papers planned for the conference agenda. Determined to break through this indifference, she besieged the office of the conference organizer, the biologist Malcolm Martin of the National Institutes of Health, in an attempt to convince him of the importance of the results she and her team had obtained in the search for a new retrovirus. To support her argument, she showed him five slides that provided graphic illustrations of the Bru room's work. The fifth slide finally stimulated action from the American.

"Interesting," he declared. "I can give you five minutes on Friday at the end of the session. Five minutes and no more. It's up to you to convince us of the value of your conclusions."

Françoise Barré-Sinoussi was "thrilled." She knew that the right to take the floor at this prestigious conference depended on the goodwill of a committee of experts more inclined to give recognition to the delegates from large American research centers than to obscure scientists from abroad. Subjects normally had to be submitted more than six months in advance, and candidates whose topics were selected took weeks preparing themselves for their important ordeal. The young woman trembled at the thought of it. She knew that the five minutes she had been granted could well create a storm. Was she not about to attack the dogma laid down by the powerful Robert Gallo? Wasn't she to take issue with his findings that there were no other human retroviruses apart from his HTLV? How could she take on a scientist who dominated world retrovirology so completely? How was she to proclaim the existence of a new family of human retroviruses found in a patient with AIDS symptoms?

"I didn't sleep at all before the fateful day," Françoise Barré-Sinoussi would remember. "When I climbed onto the podium in the packed auditorium to give my commentary on the first slide, I was so nervous I dropped the pointer on David Baltimore's head. The famous codiscoverer of the reverse transcriptase enzyme happened to be sitting in the front row."

Apart from François Jacob, André Lwoff, and Jacques Monod, the three Nobel Prize–winner specialists of the bacteriophages, those viruses whose hosts are common bacteria, few French people had earned the privilege of mounting that podium in the fifty years of conferences held at Cold Spring Harbor. Yet the young Frenchwoman at once managed to engage the sympathy of her demanding audience. The appreciative reaction to her last slide encouraged her. The cream of world biology were suddenly gazing at the photograph taken by Charles Dauguet in his Paris laboratory. The experts present could make no mistake about it: with its small and very eccentric nucleus, this particle's structure was in no way similar to Robert Gallo's celebrated HTLV. All that remained to be done was to produce proof that it was indeed the AIDS agent the French had isolated and not some parasite arising out of the illness or out of some laboratory accident.

As soon as the lights came back on, scientists began to fire questions.

"Have you cloned your virus? Have you sequenced it?"*

Françoise Barré-Sinoussi had anticipated these questions and prepared her answers. She formulated them with the most disarming of smiles.

---

* Cloning and sequencing are complex biological processes designed to determine the genetic structure of a virus.

"Do be patient," she said. "We discovered the activity of our virus's reverse transcriptase in January. We identified the virus itself in February. We photographed it in March. It's only May now. Be so good as to give us a little time in which to do the rest!"

Laughter and applause greeted this response.

The young Frenchwoman had hardly left the auditorium before she was accosted by all those whose appetites had been whetted by her all too brief presentation. One of the men in charge at the American Institute for Allergies and Infectious Diseases invited her to come and address top scientists working on the Bethesda campus. The head of the virology department at the Centers for Disease Control begged her to make the journey to Atlanta to speak to his colleagues about this crucial discovery. Even the representatives from Gallo's laboratory pressed her to come to Washington to explain the Pasteur team's discovery to their leader in detail.

*   *   *

The leader in question already knew all about it. Nothing ever happened in the small world of retrovirology without Robert Gallo being instantly informed. There was not one single research laboratory, even in the most remote of countries, where he did not have some contact, someone who was obligated to him, an informer. The enormous budget his own center enjoyed made it possible for him to dispense bounteous grants in America and abroad. Therein lay the source of many allegiances. His fame as a scientist, his consummate skill as a communicator, his irresistible charm, had also won him countless political and scientific connections. His sovereign grip on world virological research was in fact so absolute that no major discovery could hope to be recognized without his having approved it himself. "For any research project, we needed the great god Gallo's blessing," the Frenchman Jean-Claude Chermann would say. "It was the only way we would be taken seriously by our own bosses and wrest the necessary finances from them. Poor backward creatures that we were, we needed American sanction. At that time, French, even European medical research, only put in the commas while the Americans supplied whole sentences."

To aspire to attack the infallibility of one of the most illustrious of these scientists was like committing a crime of high treason. If Luc Montagnier and his team wanted to bring their discovery to the attention of the international scientific community, they must risk the wrath of the "god Gallo." Yet it was this very "god" in person who suggested to the French the choice of vehicle for their communication and the date of publication. Montagnier recalls: "As a matter of fact, Gallo told me that he was going to publish a study showing how his HTLV was implicated in AIDS in an edition of *Science* of May twentieth, 1983, and that it would be accompanied by a text by the veterinary biologist Max Essex, who had just found the HTLV retrovirus in thirty percent of a group of AIDS patients." The American suggested that his Parisian colleague publish a paper in the same issue describing the results achieved by the team at the Pasteur Institute.

Had Robert Gallo seen the opportunity to defuse the French discovery? Not only did he undertake to have Luc Montagnier's article accepted for the same edition of *Science*, he also wrote the introductory summary. This was an act of "generosity" that would enable him to exploit to his own advantage a lamentable blunder on the part of the French in their designation of their retrovirus. Since the latter essentially infected the T lymphocytes,* they had christened it the "human T-lymphotropic virus," which meant that it had the same initials, HTLV, as Robert Gallo's "human T-cell leukemia virus." This confusion served to reinforce the conviction Gallo persisted in maintaining. He was quick to announce that as the French had given their virus the same surname as his HTLV, they must themselves consider it to be a close relative.

This piece of deviousness astounded the Pasteur team. That summer they immediately rechristened their virus "lymphadenopathy-associated virus." Its three initials—LAV—could also stand for "lymphadenopathy AIDS virus." The French LAV versus the American HTLV: within a matter of weeks this battle of initials would make the headlines of the world's press.

---

*The lymphocytes that come from the thymus.

40

"We Shall All Be Mounting the Victory Podium Soon"
Paris, France–Bethesda, USA: Spring–Summer 1983

They called it "the Saturday service." Every Saturday of that spring of 1983, at precisely ten o'clock, the whole team from the virology laboratory at the Pasteur Institute would gather around Luc Montagnier in his vast office cluttered with files, reports, and medical journals. The work of these ten men and women, almost all under forty, was expected to confirm that the retrovirus found in the Bru room test tubes was, incontrovertibly, the agent responsible for AIDS. Apart from the "Pasteurians" Luc Montagnier, Jean-Claude Chermann, and Françoise Barré-Sinoussi, this group of ten included two virologists from the Claude-Bernard Hospital, Françoise Brun-Vézinet and Christine Rouzioux, the clinicians Willy Rozenbaum and Etienne Vilmer, the immunologists Jean-Claude Gluckmann and David Klatzmann, together with an epidemiologist from the Ministry of Health, Jean-Baptiste Brunet. The French retrovirus had been discovered in a lymph node taken from someone who only had the precursory symptoms of AIDS. Its presence had still to be proved at the more advanced end of the disease, and demonstrated in all categories of patients whether they were gay men, drug addicts, hemophiliacs, Haitians, or Africans. In science, every claim must have an opposite: the researchers also had to show that the virus was not found in healthy subjects. The prospect was far from easy.

Finally, in a gay man afflicted with Kaposi's sarcoma, the team managed to isolate the LAV retrovirus for a second time. Its morphology and its immunological and biochemical characteristics were in every respect similar to those of the first virus found in the Parisian designer. A third identical virus was found in the lymphocytes of an adolescent hemophiliac. The blood of a young woman from Zaire who was undergoing treatment at the Claude-Bernard Hospital and who would die of AIDS ten days after the sample was taken provided a fourth specimen. Other viruses of the same kind, stemming from very different patients, would soon find their way into the Bru room's cold storage. Luc Montagnier and his team felt they were on the right track: all these viruses from different sources had a common foundation: the same proteins and the same tendency to destroy T lymphocytes.

The consistency of these results made it possible to launch a decisive stage in the battle against the fatal disease. Although these researchers offered no hope of prevention by vaccination or treatment in the short term, they did at least give rise to innovative measures to restrict the spread of the epidemic. Within a few weeks, "the Saturday service" team would manage to come up with a test to reveal the presence of the antibodies produced by the organism in the event of viral attack. Called ELISA,* this test makes it possible to detect an individual's "sero-positivity," in other words, to say whether or not he or she has been infected by the AIDS agent. One of the immediate advantages of this system of detection was in relation to the control of blood being used for transfusion. It put an end to the nightmare that haunted Jim Curran, the head of the Atlanta medical detectives, who had failed to convince the American blood banks that they should adopt urgent measures to protect their country's blood stocks.

The manufacture and sale of ELISA test kits involved considerable financial interests. The American authorities were alarmed at the prospect of this lucrative, multimillion-dollar market's slipping away from them. Robert Gallo swiftly broadcast the alleged limitations of the French invention. Seeing this as a move designed to

---

*ELISA: enzyme-linked immunosorbent assay

make them give up its exploitation, the French stood their ground, and the Pasteur Institute announced the production of the ELISA test on a commercial basis. In April 1984 they placed an application for the patent before the American authorities. A short while later, the Americans did the same thing with a test they had produced by a different process. This patent would be granted within a few months; the French would have to wait for two years.

In the meantime war was already being waged between French and American scientists.

*   *   *

Stung by the unexpected success of the small French team devoid of any great resources, the American giant bestirred himself. One morning in April 1983, Robert Gallo assembled all his staff under the neon lighting of the conference room on the sixth floor of block 37 at Bethesda.

The eminent scientist's staff meetings were almost always major events for his associates. They were an opportunity to meet the leading lights in the research world, who came to lay their work before Gallo as a matter of priority. Privileged in this way, his research scientists did not have to wait for the appearance of scientific publications to be kept informed of what was happening across the world. "A great advantage at a time when research is taking giant leaps forward all the time," Gallo liked to say.

No one would have wanted to miss the meeting that took place that day in April 1983. They were a prodigious group. This disparate band of young Americans, Japanese, Germans, Indians, Chinese, French, Swedes, and Finns gathered around their high priest—a concentration of gray matter forming a matchless research team. Yet thus far their leader had not known how to use his resources to rise to the greatest challenge of the end of the millennium. The timid Indian biochemist whom, nine months previously, he had chosen to uncover the agent responsible for AIDS had been so poorly prepared and so poorly motivated that the resulting fiasco was hardly surprising. As Robert Gallo himself would acknowledge, it was "with a sense of shame that I stood up in front of my team that April morning. I wouldn't have admitted it for the world, but it's true: I was ashamed. Ashamed that we hadn't discovered that blasted virus before the Pasteur people. We had the means to succeed. How many times had Popovic* come bursting into my room, protesting that I should never have put Sarin on the job and that it was my fault that we had wasted so many months. Popovic felt he would have identified the culprit virus long ago! And he may have been right. My mistake was not to have given enough credence to the magnitude of the AIDS cataclysm right from the start. I had made up my mind to acknowledge my sins."

From then on everything was to change. A few days earlier a summit meeting held in the office of Dr. Vincent T. DeVita, director of the National Cancer Institute, had decided upon the creation of a task force to discover the causal agent of the disease as swiftly as possible. This initiative marked a fundamental turnabout in the American health authorities' policy. This time, they were declaring war on the epidemic in earnest. The sum of $40 million had suddenly been allocated for research.

The direction of this special task force had naturally been entrusted to the distinguished discoverer of the first human retrovirus, together with a substantial portion of the financial resources. Robert Gallo was given carte blanche. Not only could he involve the best members of his own team in the venture, but he was also in a position to engage any other research scientists he wanted, both from America and abroad. A special budget for honoraria and travel expenses had been set aside for the purpose.

*　　*　　*

That April morning, looking even more relaxed than usual with the knot of his tie undone and his shirtsleeves rolled up, the celebrated scientist announced that he had decided to pour all his resources into the fray. Phil Markham, Mikulas Popovic, Zaki Salahuddin, M. G. Sarngadharan, Flossie Wong-Staal, his crack people were to give up the work they were currently engaged in immediately. "I want each one of you to think about the best way of conducting this fight, and let me have the fruits of your reflections in writing," he told them. He had already chosen the outside collaborators he wanted to incorporate in his strike force, notably Bill Jarrett, an eminent specialist in retroviruses who was working in

---

*The Czeck biologist Mikulas Popovic had developed a line of cells particularly susceptible to infection by and reproduction of the AIDS virus.

Scotland, and Wade Parks, a distinguished research scientist at the University of Miami.

This mobilization would have served no useful purpose, however, had Gallo not supplied his troops with the ammunition they needed to fight. Inconceivable as it might seem in a country as organized as the United States, the scientific community was sadly lacking in organ, bone marrow, and blood samples taken from suitable patients, accompanied by detailed medical dossiers. Their research was fatally delayed because of this. One of the reasons for the shortage was the lack of contact and collaboration between scientists and medical practitioners. The latter tended to regard their patients and their observations as exclusive personal property.

Robert Gallo also knew that in the particular case of this latest epidemic, the geographical location of his laboratory was a handicap. With the exception of the nearby anticancer center directed by his colleague Sam Broder, virtually no Washington hospital had yet had to treat victims of the new epidemic. For one thing, AIDS was manifesting itself primarily in New York and California; for another, homosexuality was such a taboo subject in the puritanical American capital that no one dared to talk openly about "the dread disease" even in medical circles.

Robert Gallo promised his collaborators he would fight like the devil to see that everyone had access to all the biological material they needed. If necessary, he would turn himself into a traveling salesman. He would go to the New York hospitals and enlist the help of the doctors fighting the disease at their patients' bedsides. He would send an SOS to Dr. Michael Gottlieb, the man who had discovered the first AIDS cases in Los Angeles. He would call upon the assistance of Drs. Marcus Conant and Paul Volberding, who were already treating several dozen cases in San Francisco. "One thing's for sure," he affirmed. "We shall all be mounting the victory podium soon."

The results of his efforts did not take long to appear. Parcels containing precious samples accompanied by detailed medical dossiers began to pour in from all directions. "Some even turned up at my own front door in the middle of the night," Zaki Salahuddin, the Pakistani tissue culturer, would recount.

Robert Gallo was too circumspect not to take other precautionary measures to guarantee his team's success. Although quite sure that the viral agent found by the French belonged to the same family as his HTLV, he asked Luc Montagnier to send him some specimens. His associates—under the leadership of Popovic and Salahuddin—would have no difficulty in demonstrating that the French retrovirus was none other than a cousin of his virus. His presumptuous competitors would then be reduced to admitting their defeat.

41

Pilgrimage in Pursuit of a Miracle

Latrun, Israel: Summer 1983

"Philippe!"

"Sam!"

The two names rang out in the same delighted tone. The American and the young monk from Latrun had not seen each other for nearly two years. Sometime after his accident, Philippe Malouf had learned that Sam Blum and Josef Stein, the two archaeologist friends who had been with him when he fell into the Gezer excavations, had left the team at the dig and gone back to the United States. He had received several postcards—from Mexico, Haiti, Paris. Then there had been no more news from the two Americans, as if they wanted to wipe from their memories all trace of their paralyzed companion in his hospital bed.

Sam Blum did not have time to run and embrace his friend. He saw the wheelchair bearing down upon him like a dodge'm car at a carnival, skillfully maneuvered by Philippe, who wore the triumphant expression of a child who had just successfully played a trick on someone.

"See, my body isn't a total loss anymore. I can get about with all the grace of a gazelle."

They both burst out laughing, and the monk agreed to give an account of his metamorphosis. It had begun a few months after his accident with an unexpected twitching in his shoulders. This phenomenon had immediately caught the doctors' attention. If Philippe managed to recover even partial use of his arms, it would make a radical difference to his invalid state. He would only have to undergo an operation devised by a Swedish surgeon that would enable him to hang by his arms. He would then be able to get himself unaided from his bed into a wheelchair. This relative autonomy would change his living conditions. After twelve months of exercises to build up his deltoid muscles, the surgeons in Jerusalem proceeded to carry out what they called "a transposition of the muscles." They moved the lower muscles of the deltoids from his shoulders to his useless elbow joints. After a while, thanks to these new connections, Philippe Malouf could move, stretch out, and bend his arms. A second operation on the wrists furthered the rehabilitation: this time the young monk could hold a spoon between two fingers, press a button, tap the keys of a typewriter. For all practical purposes, he had been resurrected.

Sam Blum listened to his friend with a shudder of emotion. He saw again the scenes of the accident: the recovery of the dislocated body, the race to Jerusalem, the surgeon's ghastly expression as he emerged from the operating room. Superimposed on Philippe's happy voice, he could hear the doctor's words in response to the questions whether their companion would be paralyzed for life: "To the best of our present knowledge, I'm afraid so."

Sam clasped the monk's hand in both of his.

"You've won, man," he said, full of admiration.

Philippe reversed his wheelchair a few paces.

"Josef isn't with you?" he exclaimed, suddenly abashed at having talked about himself before asking this question.

A shadow passed over the American's face. He took off his glasses and wiped them slowly with his shirttail. "Josef's sick."

The monk grimaced. "Is it serious?"

Sam nodded his nearly bald head several times. "Some sickness the doctors don't know how to treat," he said.

Philippe Malouf did not know that a strange epidemic was in the throes of decimating so many young Americans. He had never even heard the word "AIDS."

"A year . . . perhaps a bit longer. In any case, he's had it," Sam went on. Forcing a smile, he added with a sigh, "Unless some sort of miracle happens!"

It was in the hope of precisely such a miracle that he had undertaken, at his friend's urgent request, to journey to Israel. His visit coincided with the Jewish Passover. Tomorrow he would go to the Wailing Wall in Jerusalem. Between two stones, he would slip the small piece of paper on which Josef had written his supplication to the God of the Jews. Having accomplished this mission, he would stop off again at the Monastery of the Seven Agonies in Latrun to say good-bye to Philippe en route to the airport.

* * *

A vestige of the foundations of the temple originally built by Solomon, the long facade constructed out of enormous blocks of stone is Judaism's most sacred place. Shining, glazed, smoothed out at its base by the time-honored touch of foreheads, lips, and hands, the Wailing Wall is the concrete expression of the Jewish people's hope for divine mercy. The thousands of bits of paper slipped into its cracks and chinks are as many expressions of fidelity to Almighty God, prayers imploring His blessing on a newborn son, a sick spouse, a failing business, or peace in the land of Zion. Twice a year, on the day of Yom Kippur, the festival of Great Forgiveness, and at Passover, the wardens of the wall devoutly collect all these supplications and put them in large sacks. In accordance with the law of the Talmud that forbids the discarding or destruction of anything bearing the name of God, these sacks are deposited in a vault in the ancient Jewish cemetery on the Mount of Olives, among the tombs of generations of Jews who rest there in eternal peace.

On the eve of that Passover, hundreds of men in black frock coats and large round hats trimmed with fur swayed their upper bodies. Next to them, women with scarves covering their heads joined them in time with the rhythm of their chanted prayers. Tightly knit groups of visitors and tourists crowded together in front of the imposing wall, closely watched from the surrounding terraces by soldiers of the Israeli army.

Sam Blum stopped dead in his tracks, his breath taken away by the rediscovery of the spectacular scene at the end of the narrow alleyway. He thought of the happy hours he and Josef had shared on that esplanade, of those Sabbath eves spent in the same pink light of dusk, of the festival mornings filled with farandoles, singing, and the sound of shofars. It seemed like only yesterday, as if at any moment he might again hear Josef's deep voice intoning the Shema Israel in front of the largest stone. Slowly he made his way down the steps and passed through the barrier that encloses the area reserved for prayer. As ritual prescribed, he covered his head with the violet velvet skullcap his mother had embroidered for him and draped over his shoulders the prayer shawl he had brought with him from New York. Then he carefully knotted two small black leather cases round his left arm and round his forehead. These phylacteries, reminders that all manual work and prayer should be constantly dedicated to God, contained tiny scrolls of parchment on which were inscribed the foundations of the Jewish faith. "Hear, O Israel," proclaimed one of the verses. "The Lord our God, the Lord is one . . . Thou shalt love him with all thy heart, with all thy soul and with all thy might . . . These words which I command thee this day shall be upon thine heart. Thou shalt bind them for a sign upon thine hand and they shall be frontlets between thine eyes."

The adornment on his forehead made the American look like a Cyclops. He drew near to the largest block of stone, the one before which Josef used to stand to say his favorite prayer. It was one of the psalms of David, a cry of love and hope, an appeal that the people of this earth had been sending up to their creator for thirty centuries. "Hearken unto my voice, O Lord," recited Sam fervently, swaying his torso rhythmically toward the wall, "that my prayer may be like incense in Thy sight and the raising of my hands like an evening offering . . ." Then, paraphrasing Moses' appeal to God to cure his sister who had leprosy, Sam implored his Creator to put an end to the modern leprosy from which his friend was suffering. "O God, I beg you, heal Your servant Josef," he repeated passionately several times. Then he took out of his wallet the small, carefully folded slip of paper on which Josef had written his petition and slid it among the other messages in a fissure between two stones.

From beside him there rose the repetitive prayer of the faithful. The call of an Arab muezzin rang out into the still air above the Wall. The American could feel on his shoulders the last warm caresses of the sun setting over the new Jerusalem. He remained there mediatating for a good while longer, his eyes full of the vision of his sick friend. Gradually the esplanade emptied. Soon he found himself all alone but for two or three venerable rabbis. It was the beginning of Passover. All around him in the noisy confusion of the old quarter and throughout the Jewish Jerusalem, families were preparing the seder, which commemorated the deliverance of the Jewish people from the torment of their exile.

Next day at dawn, while Israel was recovering from its festivities, Sam Blum took a taxi to Tiberias in Galilee. There he had another pilgrimage to complete in pursuit of a cure for his friend. Tradition actually ordains that Jews in distress should turn to the great saints of their history and ask them to intercede with the Omnipotent One. One of these saints was a doctor who lived in the twelfth century. Moses Maimonides was also one of the most celebrated theologians of Judaism. For eight centuries his writings, such as the famous *Guide for the Perplexed,* had been a beacon and a recourse for Jewish consciences. His mortal remains are laid to rest on the shores of the lake where Jesus calmed the tempest and walked upon the water. Sam prostrated himself before the humble white stone tomb and begged Maimonides "to use his sanctity to intercede with God that Josef might be restored to health." Then he went and addressed the same request to Rabbi Meir Ba'al Haness, an eleventh-century saint buried not far away. He, too, had been a doctor of the Law, a scholar and a humanist. Every spring a great festival held at his tomb attracted thousands of the faithful.

As promised, before catching his plane for New York, the American went to say good-bye to Philippe Malouf in his monastery. The paralyzed monk had been waiting for his arrival with an impatience that was visible on his face. He motioned with his head to an envelope on his bedside table.

"I've typed a note for Josef," he said. "It's nothing really, just a few lines of comfort and friendship."

Sam took the envelope and slipped it into his bag. "That'll please him a lot. He often talks about the happy times we spent here together."

Philippe looked worried. "Josef is going through a really rough time. I wouldn't want to hurt him in any way. I'd like you to know what's in my letter."

Sam adjusted his glasses and began to read softly:

Dear Josef,

When I discovered I was going to be paralyzed for life, I rebelled. It went on for weeks, months. I insulted God. I was horrible to the good Father Abbot, who had the effrontery, when he was in such radiant good health, to exhort me to seek a meaning in my suffering. He told me that if he had invited the whole community to pray for me, it wasn't just to ask God to cure me but above all that I might discover that my life as a handicapped person had meaning. Poor Father Abbot! My rebellion remained complete.

Gradually, however, stuck there in my bed, I began to understand that I was still a man. And that if I was still a man, then I could still have a role as a man, that I wasn't a vegetable, or an animal, but a being fully able to have a useful life.

The monk went on to tell of how two surgical operations had gradually brought him back to the land of the living, then how circumstances had put him in touch with a young Indian sister working with the dying in Calcutta.

She is eighteen years old and her name is Sister Ananda. That means Sister "Joy." She is doing the work for me. She is my arms and legs. As for me, I offer my suffering and my prayers for her. That gives her the strength to act. It's wonderful: every day we're in touch with each other across a distance of thousands of miles simply through the power of prayer.

In the name of the meaning I have found for my life, you can be sure, Josef, dear friend, that from now on I shall offer my suffering for you also, that you, too, may have the good fortune I have had.

42

Violet Lesions for an Opera Addict
New York, USA: Spring–Summer 1983

Josef Stein's Story

It all began one day last winter with an unusual feeling of fatigue. I
who was used to walking thirty blocks on Fifth Avenue and back or
jogging for two hours on Sundays on the roads through Central Park
found myself suddenly incapable of climbing the two flights of stairs
to my apartment in one shot. Every ten steps I would have to stop
and get my breath back. A few days later I felt a burning in my chest.
I started to cough. A small, dry cough like someone who smokes
too much. And yet I'd never smoked. The cough disappeared as
spontaneously as it had arrived, and I put the incident down to the
level of pollution in the air. The streets are narrow in Greenwich
Village. On the rooftop of the house just opposite me there's a
chimney that spews out great black wreaths of smoke night and day.
Despite my persistent tiredness, I tried not to change my way of life
in any way. On my return from Israel I had given up archaeology
altogether to move to New York where Sam Blum was living. I had
found a job with a large travel agency in Manhattan. At first I worked

in the business-travel department, then I was put in charge of business conferences and conventions. In that capacity I traveled a great deal both in the United States and abroad.

I was very happy living in New York. Apart from my attraction to lost civilizations, I have another passion that the city enabled me to satisfy every week. I'm an opera addict. I never missed a production at the Metropolitan or Lincoln Center. Moreover it was the evening I went to hear *Samson and Delilah* that I got the news, during the interval after the famous aria of the first act in which Delilah sings: "Springtime approaches, full of hope." While other members of the audience rushed for the bar and their glasses of white wine or champagne, I dashed to a phone booth to call my doctor.

My fits of coughing had started again and sometimes I found myself waking in the night bathed in perspiration. At first, I thought it was just an ordinary chill or the flu. No one with a cold wants to think it might be something else. All the same, as the cough persisted, in the end I went to see my doctor. Dr. F. is very small and bald. He looks like the actor Mickey Rooney with his large tortoiseshell glasses and his bow tie. He examined me thoroughly and prescribed antibiotics. He didn't seem the least bit worried. Shortly afterward, the cough and the night sweats disappeared. But I still felt as tired as ever. Soon, when I got dressed, my clothes seemed to hang off me. I must have lost weight, and yet I hadn't lost my appetite. Several weeks went by. I got used to living at a reduced pace, feeling a bit like a car with half its pistons missing.

One morning, at breakfast, I had difficulty in swallowing. I took a look at the back of my throat and discovered that my tongue was covered with small bluish bruises that were insensitive to the touch. I thought it might be aphtha. Next day, the rash had receded, but I still had difficulty swallowing. I saw the doctor again and he referred me to a dermatologist. After a scrupulously detailed examination that left him puzzled, he took some samples off my tongue and asked me to telephone my general practitioner a week later for the results.

I tried not to think about it too much until I called Dr. F. that momentous evening at the opera house. The telephone rang interminably and I was just going to hang up when at last I heard his voice on the other end of the line. He seemed a little disconcerted.

"The news is not very good," he ended up saying to me. "The

biopsy of your tongue indicates something serious. It may be a very rare infection that doesn't usually affect people of your age. Other tests will be necessary before it can be confirmed."

I asked what this illness was. The doctor gave me a name I didn't understand. He repeated it and spelled it out: *K* for kilo, *A* for America, *P* for Providence . . . *Kaposi*, I noted it down on the corner of my program. Already the opera house bell was calling the audience back to its seats. I quickly made an appointment for the following day and ran back to my place. I forgot everything, caught up in the joy of rejoining the beautiful Delilah in her climactic moment of the second act when, having discovered the secret of Samson's Herculean strength, she ruthlessly cuts off his hair.

A few days later, further tests confirmed the diagnosis of my oral infection. In the meantime, I'd tried to find out more about this illness with the bizarre name. I had discovered that this disease of Kaposi's was one of the forms in which the epidemic that had just broken out in New York and California manifested itself, and that it hit homosexuals in particular. My doctor confirmed that it was indeed a case of what they called AIDS, a disease of unknown origins but suspected of being a virus transmitted sexually or through the blood. AIDS destroyed the body's immune system, thus prompting the appearance of infectious lesions such as the pustules on my tongue.

Dr. F. set about finding the reason for my immunodepression. He asked me all sorts of questions. Some of them were really embarrassing. Essentially, he was interested in my sexual behavior during the past three years. Did I go in for homosexual practices? How many partners had I had? Did I frequent bathhouses? Etc., etc. He took notes. I'm afraid my answers didn't really satisfy him.

In fact, I was living alone. With Sam I only had sporadic relations. Although bound by a deep affection, we allowed each other total freedom. Until the age of eighteen, I had only been out with girls, without experiencing any undue sexual urges. I discovered my homosexuality in a train, between Salt Lake City and Chicago. For a while, I felt horribly guilty. I had had quite a strict religious upbringing and knew that the Torah condemned all carnal relations other than those within marriage. While we were still very young, my father had made my brother and me learn by heart the famous commandment in Leviticus that proclaims: "You shall not lie with a male as with a woman; it is an abomination." I hesitated for a long time before transgressing that directive because I'm a believer. It was only when I went to do my advanced studies in San Francisco that I finally succumbed.

Even so, I hadn't exactly gone in for many excesses since I left the family laundry business in Pittsburgh. I met an artist and we lived together for three years on a virtually monogamous basis. Sure, every now and then I would go and have a drink in a bar, a disco, or one of the bathhouses in the Castro, but it was more out of curiosity than to satisfy my libido. I even found the scene there a bit depressing. Nor was I tempted by the orgies in the many New York establishments in the Village. Only my stay in Israel had led me astray a few times. Should I put that down to the climate, or the excitement of being in a country where every way you turned your imagination was excited? Did it stem from the exoticism of certain fortuitous meetings with some young Arabs? I don't know. In any case, it doesn't much matter. If I had the chance, I'd do it all again.

$$* \quad * \quad *$$

Rigorous treatment with vinblastine-based chemotherapy got rid of Josef Stein's oral infection. However, at the end of the particularly torrid summer that New York was experiencing that year, fresh violet pustules similar to those that had overrun his mouth began to break out on various parts of his body, notably on the sole of one foot, above his knee, on the side of his nose. This cruel spreading of the illness from which he thought he had recovered coincided with the reappearance of the dry cough, fever, and extreme fatigue that had weighed him down the previous winter. This time, his doctor suspected pneumocystis pneumonia, one of the very serious infections that can be unleashed when the immune system is weakened. He had his patient urgently transported to the Bellevue Medical Center, whose twenty-six stories towered over the East River. There was no bed available there, so Josef Stein was directed to another hospital in the Bronx. A dreadful experience.

I don't know whether it was out of horror of gays or terror of AIDS, but they left me practically without nursing care or food for two days [Josef Stein would recount]. They left my meal trays in the

corridor. No one would come into my room to empty my bedpan
or tidy up. The rare nurses who brought me my medicine had masks
on their faces, gloves on their hands, and were dressed in special
clothing. They looked like astronauts. Not one single doctor examined the Kaposi's lesions on my legs and arms. They caused me terrible
discomfort. My skin had become so hard, my limbs so rigid, I was
in desperate need of a massage. No one dared to touch me. During
those two nightmarish days I heard not a single word of comfort,
not one expression of sympathy. I was treated worse than an animal.

Sam Blum came and snatched his friend away from that hellhole
to take him somewhere where they cared in a humane way for people
stricken with this new plague. He pointed the ambulance driver in
the direction of the Manhattan skyscrapers emerging out of the mist.
"To St. Clare's Hospital!" he directed before giving the address
of the old building in the Italian-immigrant quarter on the West
Side where Dr. Jack Dehovitz and a handful of volunteer nurses
were practically the only people in New York at the time trying to
relieve the distress of the victims of what many Catholics were still
calling "the wrath of God."

43

Ruthless Competition Across the Atlantic
Bethesda, USA–Paris, France: Spring 1983–Winter 1985

As precise and unrelenting as a train timetable, each week the modest bulletin from the Centers for Disease Control in Atlanta reported the inexorable worsening of the epidemic. The statistics it published on June 22, 1984, were enlightening. In three years, 4,918 Americans had been diagnosed with AIDS. Nearly half, 2,221, were already dead, and the proportion of deaths among patients diagnosed before July 1982 had risen to three-quarters. The situation in Europe was just as alarming. In its November 2, 1984, issue, the CDC revealed that in eight months the number of cases had increased by 100 percent. France topped this sad ledger for the number of patients, and Denmark for the percentage of victims per million inhabitants.

It would be reasonable to think that a tragedy of this kind would bind all the scientists and researchers of this world together in holy union. Far from it. The new plague gave rise to regrettable conflicts of personality and interests, and to heated rivalry. No one would ever have imagined the duel that went on between the American Robert Gallo and the Frenchman Luc Montagnier behind the scenes, a duel in which sword thrusts were exchanged under the guise of the most brotherly collaboration and everlasting friendship.

The two scientists and their teams visited each other, telephoned each other, wrote to each other, welcomed their respective technicians, shared with each other their chemical secrets, their viruses, their results. They wined and dined together in Washington's Italian trattorias and in the Auvergne bistros of Paris's Left Bank. They received each other in their homes or met at airports and saw each other off again. Occasionally, they splashed about like schoolboys in the swimming pools at the hotels where their conferences were held.

Behind this facade, a ruthless contest was going on. Once Robert Gallo finally launched himself into the race, he had shown himself to be an implacable adversary of the French. On the strength of his incontestable supremacy in matters of retrovirology, he was convinced it was only right that he should be the one to put his name to the discovery of the agent responsible for AIDS. By daring to contest this privilege, Luc Montagnier and his team were treading on Gallo's toes, an act of audaciousness that the distinguished American scientist was firmly resolved not to tolerate. A skillful strategist, he was careful not to clash head-on with his competitors. Instead, he sought to soften them up, lull them into a false sense of security, charm them with his legendary enthusiasm, his good nature, his friendly condescension. After all, had he not gone so far as to send the French some specimens of his own HTLV retrovirus so that they could compare it with their own retrovirus "discovery" to help them recognize their mistake?

He crossed the Atlantic at the beginning of June 1983 to give his French partners a better hearing and continue their "love story." True, he raised some objections. In his view, the virus from Jean-Claude Chermann and Françoise Barré-Sinoussi's test tubes was definitely a close cousin of his HTLV. Didn't they have the same properties? Both were transmitted through the blood, through sexual contact, and through congenital infection. Both attacked the same T-4 lymphocytes, the mainstays of the immune system. His sincere warmth, his promises of help, the strength of his conviction, were such that the French had no reason to distrust him.

Robert Gallo invited Luc Montagnier to come to Bethesda to give an account of his results to members of the special NIH task force set up by the American health authorities. The Frenchman landed that summer with a small box of dry ice in his suitcase containing a sample of the virus isolated at the Pasteur Institute. Montagnier was expecting Gallo and his collaborators to study it at their leisure and recognize its unique character. But the master of Bethesda had, it seemed, no intention of admitting his mistake. He buried the gift at the bottom of one of his freezers and only gave his guest a few minutes, not even allowing him the time to implant a seed of curiosity in the learned assembly of scientists Gallo had brought together.

Humiliated and disappointed, Luc Montagnier returned to France firmly set upon taking up the challenge. If the elite of American retrovirology were refusing to take any notice of the French discovery, he would make a fresh appeal to the media. In August 1983, he offered an article to the scientific review *Nature* describing the specific affinity of the LAV* virus for the T-4 lymphocyte regulators of the human body's immune system. But Robert Gallo's influence extended throughout the scientific press. The scientific journal declined the French offer: "The virus you claim may only be the result of contamination in the laboratory," objected its chief editor. He suggested that the French laboratory "wait a little while before making your results officially known. Follow Gallo's example. He worked for two years before publishing his findings on the first human HTLV retrovirus."

An article by a British journalist in the *Journal of the American Medical Association* in August 1983 helped to ease the French team's frustration. It was the first time the abbreviation LAV had appeared in the international medical press. But Gallo had not let it catch him off guard. He had managed to mute the impact of this publicity. Another article, by the same journalist in the same issue, sang the American scientist's praises and claimed that his HTLV virus was the prime candidate as the principal AIDS agent.

As if to allay his competitor's fears, Robert Gallo in late summer directed his specialist in retrovirus cultures, the Czech Mikulas Popovic, to ask the team at the Pasteur Institute to send new specimens of the LAV virus. Popovic humbly conceded that he had been unable to make the samples of virus that Luc Montagnier had brought them in July grow in his cell cultures. Before granting this

---

*Name given by Pasteur Institute team to its retrovirus discovered in the Bru room—lymphadenopathy-associated virus.

request, the French scientist asked for a signed document in which the American laboratory agreed not to use the Pasteur Institute's LAV virus other than for basic research purposes and never for commercial ends. Mikulas Popovic was quick to provide the requisite guarantee on Gallo's behalf, a guarantee that would prove to be worth no more than the paper on which it was written. Later, when the day came for Gallo to announce his own discovery of the AIDS agent, Robert Gallo would claim never to have used the specimens provided by the French.

*   *   *

However, in the fall of 1983, Gallo continued to feign the most cordial collaboration. The American invited Luc Montagnier to come and talk about the LAV at a conference he was organizing for September 15 and 16 at Cold Spring Harbor, the campus where some months previously Françoise Barré-Sinoussi had unveiled her slides of the retrovirus. Once more, Montagnier found that the meeting was a well-orchestrated tribute to the greater glory of the master of Bethesda. "I wasn't given the opportunity to speak until the very last evening session," he would later complain. "Half the participants had already left and I was allotted barely twenty minutes!" The reduced audience greeted his presentation with a barrage of critical questions. Gallo himself displayed particular virulence, even going so far as to cast doubt upon whether the LAV belonged to the retrovirus family at all.

Astounded, Luc Montagnier called upon his host to explain his animosity.

"You have punched me out," the American allegedly replied.*

Robert Gallo had realized that the French discovery was beginning to shake certain American scientists' convictions as to the role of the HTLV retrovirus in relation to AIDS. His ascendancy over his colleagues was such, however, that no one dared as yet to press the matter. "As far as America was concerned, the LAV was still just a rank outsider," Montagnier noted angrily.

No amount of slide presentations seemed to help. A conference in a château in the Loire Valley, an international meeting in Paris,

---

* Luc Montagnier, *Vaincre le sida, Entretiens avec Pierre Bourget* (*Conquering AIDS, Conversations with Pierre Bourget*), Editions Cana, Paris, 1986.

a convention sponsored by the World Health Organization in Geneva, and finally a huge congress on the ski slopes of Park City, Utah, all were held in late '83 and early '84. Each meeting provided opportunities for the French to pursue their relentless crusade to have the validity of their work recognized. Without much success. One year after the French discovery, most virologists on the other side of the Atlantic were still refusing to admit that the virus isolated in Paris could be the AIDS agent. At Park City, however, the French did find a few chinks in the hostile front. Brilliantly defended by Jean-Claude Chermann, the Pasteur Institute's thesis seemed to interest representatives from the Centers for Disease Control. They requested further specimens of the LAV for their study. Two months later, a dramatic turn of events would shake the research world. In an April 1984 interview with the *New York Times*, James Mason, director of the CDC, announced that "the Pasteur Institute's LAV is the most likely AIDS agent."

*   *   *

The French were shrewd enough not to celebrate too quickly. Sure enough, the ink on the venerable New York daily was still wet when another, even more sensational piece of news broke: "Prof. Robert Gallo has isolated the real AIDS virus!" The American declared that this new arrival belonged to the same family of retroviruses as his previous discoveries, the HTLV-I and HTLV-II. So he baptized it HTLV-III. This latest addition to the family made a thundering entrance into world scientific circles. Wanting to obtain maximum advantage from this discovery, the American government chose as its godmother Margaret Heckler, the U.S. secretary of Health and Human Services, a charming redhead full of good intentions but ill-informed as to the nuances of international scientific rivalry. Some seven months away from the 1984 presidential elections, the political powers considered the advent of Robert Gallo's "baby" providential. The announcement of this victory over the terrifying disease could only influence some gays to go Ronald Reagan's way. What was more, the Gallo announcement provided the glowing proof that the dollars allocated to AIDS research had not been spent in vain.

Proclaiming "the triumph of science over the dread disease," the Health secretary officially announced at a press conference held in

Washington on April 23, 1984, that "Prof. Robert Gallo and his team have discovered a new virus, the HTLV-III, and furnished proof that it is the AIDS agent." She also claimed that within seven months the researchers at Bethesda would have a test to eliminate all risk of contamination of the blood stocks used for transfusions. And she promised that within two years a vaccine would be available. She breathed not a word about the French virus, confining herself to a vague reference to "other research scientists in the world who have achieved results in this field." In particular, she cited "the efforts of the Pasteur Institute in France who have worked in part in collaboration with the National Cancer Institute."

One journalist dared to ask a rude question.

"Isn't your virus the same as the French one?" the impertinent individual inquired.

Robert Gallo neatly sidestepped this embarrassing question.

*　　　*　　　*

Luc Montagnier could not contain his indignation when he heard about what had been staged in Washington. "From the point of view of scientific ethics, the official announcement of this discovery was highly questionable," he would later write. "Having received the samples of our retrovirus, the American scientist should have compared the one he had just found with ours and himself published the comparison, in the same way that we had compared it with his HTLV-I retrovirus. Did he think the French, as he would tell a New York paper, wouldn't stay the distance, that they would bend before the American steamroller and resign themselves to calling their virus HTLV-III?"

Everything was for the best in the best possible of worlds for the venerable master at Bethesda. A few hours before the Health secretary announced that Gallo had developed his own detection test for the AIDS virus, U.S. government lawyers were applying for the patent. This precautionary measure had the effect of barring from the American market the ELISA test the Pasteur team had developed one year previously. If the French wanted to assert their rights, only one recourse remained open to them: they would have to take the United States government to court.

The appearance of four articles in the May 4, 1984, issue of *Science* magazine would further poison the Franco-American rivalry. The scientific literary offensive in question had Robert Gallo as its leader. One article, cosigned by Gallo, was illustrated with spectacular photographs allegedly depicting the HTLV-III virus at the various stages of its development. Two years later, the American scientist would be forced to acknowledge that the documents published under his name did not in any instance show his virus, but quite definitely the French scientists' LAV. He would exonerate himself by claiming that it had been a stupid mistake on the part of the photographer working in his laboratory.

In June, one month later, Luc Montagnier would discover that the official report of the conference he had attended at Cold Spring Harbor had been amended. At the conference Gallo had not breathed a word about his HTLV-III, for the excellent reason that he had not yet identified it. In the official report of the proceedings, Gallo added an introduction describing the retrovirus as if it had been discovered earlier. "That wasn't the first time that Robert Gallo, considering himself to be the uncontested master of medical research, had allowed himself to make people believe in the earlier occurrence of results he had only later achieved," two highly regarded Dutch journalists would write.* Luc Montagnier, for his part, would confine himself to adding one more melancholy line to his long list of grievances: "In defiance of all the rules of scientific ethics, Gallo rewrote history to suit himself."

*   *   *

In the end, Gallo's methodology aroused certain suspicions. Members of the American scientific community began to ask themselves a few questions. Was this HTLV-III virus heralded with such a role of drums really a new retrovirus or simply the one the French had already discovered a year ago? Was it irrefutably the cause of AIDS? These two fundamental queries would induce Gallo to stop trying to make Nobel brownie points and become once more the outstanding virologist he really was. He dispatched the Indian biologist M. G. Sarngadharan, one of his best researchers, to compare the proteins of his virus with those of the Pasteur Institute. This

---

*"Mécanismes de concurrence et de défense dans un conflit scientifique" ("Techniques of competition and defense in a scientific conflict"), by Johan Heilbron and Jaap Gondsmidt, *Actes de recherches en sciences sociales*, September 1987.

study revealed that they were similar on all counts. Meanwhile, the Atlanta headquarters of the Centers for Disease Control asked the two rival laboratories to provide blood samples containing their respective viruses. To avoid any possible bias, both specimens were studied under an anonymous code. But the results were the same. The two viruses were identical twins.

In fact, one final comparison, this time at the molecular level, was necessary to confirm their identical composition beyond all debate. This molecular analysis made use of extremely sophisticated techniques. The first step, known as cloning, consists of the introduction of genetic elements from the virus into bacteria. When the latter multiply, they make it possible to obtain significant quantities of the virus. This leads to the second operation, called sequencing, which is intended to decipher a virus's genetic code. It is a question of establishing the exact sequence of the nucleotides, the chain of the elements that in a determined order make up that code. Infinitely complex and detailed, this molecular work required people who were real artisans with a high degree of know-how. With all its vast experience and greater number of specialists, Robert Gallo's group had a clear advantage over the French researchers.

The two laboratories launched themselves into a frantic race. It was the Chinese-American woman Flossie Wong-Staal, one of the exceptionally gifted biologists on the Bethesda team, who first succeeded in cloning the American retrovirus, beating the French researchers by several weeks. The French would have their revenge. On January 21, 1985, in three pages of the prestigious review *Cell*, they described the chain of 9,139 nucleotides that made up the genetic code of the LAV they had discovered nearly two years previously. Five days later, it was the Gallo team's turn to publish results on the genetic code of his retrovirus in the review *Nature*. The article was signed by twenty authors from three different research centers, whereas only five biologists, all of them from the same laboratory, had signed the French text.* "Does that mean one Frenchman is worth four Americans?" Luc Montagnier would inquire, delighted to be able to make up for some of the humiliation he had suffered.

What was truly important was the exact similarity of these dif-

_____
*Marc Alizon, Stewart Cole, Olivier Danos, Pierre Sonigo, and Simon Wain-Hobson.

ferent results. Now no one could be in any doubt: the American virus and the French virus were definitely one and the same. The deciphering of their genetic code illustrated furthermore that this was a new virus, without any of the family links Robert Gallo had believed it to have with the first human retrovirus he had discovered. Above all, the detailed identification of its genes confirmed what everyone had been waiting impatiently to know: yes, the HTLV-III/LAV was indeed the fatal agent of AIDS.

*   *   *

Thereafter, on both sides of the Atlantic, a totally virgin experimental field would be opened up to the scientists researching AIDS. By fathoming the secrets of the virus's genes one by one, they would come to a better understanding of its part in the illness. In the short term they would be able to perfect diagnostic tests, and in the near future, one hoped, vaccines.

This burst of hope for the future was curiously oblivious to the tragic reality of the present. AIDS victims were suffering and dying in greater numbers every day without the enormous sums invested in research bringing them the slightest relief. People talked theoretically about tests and vaccines, but hardly ever about treatment, as though it were a matter of more pressing necessity to settle the score with the killer than to repair the personal damage it had already done.

To Dr. Sam Broder, confronted daily with the suffering, despair, and death of the patients in his hospital, this oversight was unacceptable. It was his duty as head of the oncology program at the National Cancer Institute to put an end to it.

44

A First Light in the AIDS Darkness
Bethesda, USA: Autumn 1984

It would take all the stubborn dedication of a survivor from the terror of the Nazis to tackle this challenge head on. Dr. Sam Broder assessed the enormity of the task ahead. All previous efforts to develop antiviral medicines had produced very limited results. The ability of retroviruses to conceal themselves in the genetic heritage of the cells makes them particularly difficult targets. All the more so for the fact that they could remain inactive—hence undetectable—for years. How could they be destroyed without the risk of the white cells that harbored them being wiped out by the same process? It all came down to the question of devising a remedy with what doctors call "an acceptable therapeutic indication," in other words a remedy that wasn't more toxic than the disease.

Since the AIDS virus infected a wide variety of tissues and cells, the problem was even more complicated. It could, for example, lodge itself in the central nervous system, in which case it would be protected by specific defenses that few pharmaceutical compounds were capable of penetrating. And if, by any chance, a medicine did manage to cross that barrier, the cells already affected by the virus would probably never recover. Other complications from AIDS, such as Kaposi's sarcoma and certain aggressive malignant tumors of the lymphatic system, were not completely curable either. The complexity of these devastating effects represented, by the American cancer expert's own admission, "an exceptional, virtually insurmountable challenge."

All the same, scientists were not totally defenseless. They might not as yet have had the time to dwell upon the retrovirus in human form, but scientists had been working for a long time on animal retroviruses. They had already tried out a large number of chemical substances against them. Sam Broder knew of at least five compounds that had produced some notable successes. Might not agents that were effective in mice or sheep be equally so in humans? In the light of the urgency and the absence of any alternative, it was an attractive idea. But then, as only a trial on live patients could provide the answer, the issue came up against an obstacle of a different kind. The all-powerful federal agency, the Food and Drug Administration, must recognize and approve any medicine before it can actually be tried on a human being in the United States, regardless of whether he has volunteered or is at the point of death. The approval procedures involved are so complicated that they can take months, even years. "How could I wait for that sort of delay," Sam Broder would say, "when every day patients were crying out to me in their agony: 'Hurry up, Doctor!' "

The medical researcher was thus reduced to looking for other ways. In the belief that therapeutic treatments already approved by the FDA for other viral infections might also prove to be effective against AIDS, he set his collaborators on a systematic search through the pharmaceutical and medical literature of recent years. This was a formidable task requiring painstaking research, a job that was completed in record time thanks to the computers at the National Medical Library located less than five hundred yards from his laboratory.

Spurred on by the same sense of urgency as Jim Curran, his equally indefatigable colleague at the Atlanta CDC, Sam Broder became an impatient taskmaster spurring on the team of virologists assembled on the Bethesda campus. For several months, he had been bombarding them with a flood of biological matter taken from the most infected cases among the patients in his care. To add to the attractions of these samples of lymph node, blood, and bone marrow, he would often go and deliver them personally. Only five minutes away on foot, Robert Gallo's laboratory on the 6th floor of block 37 was a favorite port of call. At first the eminent scientist and his collaborators were astonished to see the head of the NCI's clinical oncology program taking the trouble to come in person. "They very quickly realized I wasn't just going there to take them a few bits of organ or a drop of infected blood," Sam Broder explained. "My presence underlined the fact that this situation was exceptional and demanded their immediate and total commitment."

In the end his persistence paid off. In one of the scientific reviews kept in the National Medical Library, his collaborators discovered the existence of a compound with surprising properties. Few Americans now suffered from the disease that, for sixty years, had been treated with suramin, a pale-pink sulphonic salt that kills *Trypanosoma gambiense*, the African parasite that causes sleeping sickness. It was a very different property of this salt, however, that had caught the attention of Sam Broder's investigators. According to the publication's authors, suramin was capable of inhibiting in animals the activity of the reverse transcriptase, the specific enzyme that enables the retrovirus to lodge itself in the genetic heritage of the cells. By a stroke of good fortune, this medicine had long ago been given the approval for human use by the FDA.

Several other studies, one of which was extracted from the yellowing pages of a journal of tropical medicine half a century old, would nevertheless reveal that suramin had serious toxic side effects on the functioning of the kidneys, and additionally, involved a risk of coma. "But at least this remedy had the advantage of already being in existence," Sam Broder would say. "All we had to do was telephone its manufacturer, Bayer, in Germany, and we'd have something to treat our patients with at once." Having tested its effectiveness in the laboratory, he published an article in the October 12, 1984, issue of *Science* stating that "in vitro tests of suramin showed that it protected white cells brought into contact with the AIDS virus." Immediately exploited by the national press, this information had created an enormous stir. The very day of the publication, dozens of calls paralyzed the Bethesda hospital switchboard. Patients from San Francisco hopped on board the first plane to Washington in the hope of being included among the volunteers Sam Broder was going to inject with the first doses of suramin. Clinicians, reduced to despair by their inability to help the ever increasing number of their patients, poured in from New York, Los Angeles, Miami, Houston, and all over the country. Others offered Broder the opportunity to test his new treatment directly in their hospital wards.

One of the most ardent supporters of any attempt to discover a cure was Michael Gottlieb, the young immunologist from the University of California at Los Angeles who, in June 1981, had told the world of the existence of the new epidemic. "My desire to cure my patients made me fanatically attentive to any research that was going on to try and find a remedy," he would say. "I kept a particular eye on the various therapeutic programs being tested out on the Bethesda campus. For practitioners like me brought face-to-face each day with the horror, Sam Broder was the incarnation of our hope of one day emerging from the nightmare."

Like Sam Broder, he had explored medical literature, examined reports of experiments from the great virology laboratories, and taken the opportunity at scientific conferences to question anyone working on antiviral substances. At one point, as he was sipping a Campari with the French scientist Jean-Claude Chermann, looking out over the romantic bay of Naples, he had learned of a medicine developed by the Pasteur Institute by the name of HPA-23, which sounded very promising. The medicine in question was made up of mineral molecules and chemical elements that had, like suramin, the capacity to prevent retroviruses from introducing themselves into the cells. Its toxicity seemed so weak that Michael Gottlieb had been quick to send his Parisian colleagues his most illustrious patient. Thanks to injections of HPA-23, the actor Rock Hudson had enjoyed a spectacular remission that had made it possible for him to complete the filming of a role on the famous series *Dynasty*. Alas, it was not long before the inexorable disease overcame him despite his being treated for a second time with HPA-23 at the American Hospital in Neuilly. A few days after his return to Los Angeles, the actor passed away in the arms of the helpless Michael Gottlieb. Reported nationally with front-page headlines, the death of Rock Hudson shocked America. For the first time the AIDS tragedy had a face, the face of one of its Hollywood demigods.

The French HPA-23 having slipped into oblivion, Gottlieb set about looking for other curative substances. Like Sam Broder, he had fallen upon the trail of the pink powder that cured sleeping sickness and inhibited the reverse transcriptase in animal retroviruses. As soon as Broder announced the preparation of clinical tests for several dozen patients, Gottlieb volunteered. He selected twelve of his AIDS patients at random, and a dozen others with only a pre-AIDS condition, and began giving them a weekly dose of suramin. Six other hospitals across the United States joined in the experiment.

Sam Broder was exultant. His efforts had made the medical community acknowledge that treatment was actually feasible. For the first time, doctors had agreed to band together to study the best way of putting it into practice. The notions of clinical experimentation, monitoring, therapeutic programs, in short the prospect of a cure, was suddenly sweeping away skepticism.

Paradoxically, this hope raised a general outcry in the gay community. They protested: "If there's a medicine, the government should distribute it as a matter of urgency to all patients without exception, and not secretly reserve it for a privileged few!" Furious at being deprived of this first opportunity to do something, numerous gay doctors in Los Angeles and San Francisco went and got their suramin straight from the German manufacturer, Bayer.

In November, at the beginning of the eighth week of treatment, Sam Broder called all the doctors taking part in his clinical trials together in Washington. He wanted to assess the first results. "We were in a state of utter euphoria," Michael Gottlieb would recount. "We were all so keen for this blasted suramin to work that we'd lost all our scientific objectivity. One of our colleagues, Dr. Alexander Levine from the University of Southern California, had even brought photographs of his patients undergoing treatment. They looked so happy and in such good health that there was no doubt in our minds: suramin was effective."

One discordant voice would temper the general enthusiasm of this first meeting, however. Dr. Peter Wolf, a clinician from Los Angeles, put forward the idea that the remedy was far from harmless. He had found violent skin eruptions in several of his patients at the end of the sixth week of treatment. It was not long before his fears were confirmed by other toxic reactions in patients. At the beginning of the tenth week, several centers carrying out the clinical trials were reporting cases of coma. Soon they were registering the first deaths. Finally all their hopes were dashed: suramin was not the panacea they had hoped for. It turned out to be even more toxic than Sam Broder had feared. In a few weeks it caused the general destruction of kidney functions. Far from curing, it was proving to be a faster killer than AIDS. Trials being carried out on patients had to be stopped immediately.

Despite his disappointment, Sam Broder remained convinced that he had lost a battle and not the war. "Cruel as that setback was, it was far from useless. Paradoxically, it even represented the first victory over the illness. Suramin was definitely a product ill suited to the struggle against AIDS, but fruitless though it had been, the use of it had at least shaken the medical world out of its inertia. The idea that the disease could be treated had asserted itself decisively. Now everyone knew that one day we would have a medicine to cure AIDS."

PART THREE

Scientists and Saints – Torchbearers of Hope

45

Pharmaceutical Virus Killers
Research Triangle Park, USA: Spring 1984

It is probably the most important private research complex in the world. In an area as large as the Grand Duchy of Luxembourg, Research Triangle Park in North Carolina harbors several advanced technology establishments in which twenty thousand research scientists and technicians are employed. The boundaries of this enormous triangular campus are marked by three cities—Raleigh, Durham, and Chapel Hill. Its expertise is supplied by three of the best universities in the South—Duke, North Carolina, and North Carolina State.

The American branch of the British-owned Burroughs Wellcome Co., one of the giants in world pharmaceutical production, had implanted itself in this landscape of flat open country and pine groves worthy of a hunting scene by Thomas Gainsborough. It had set up its general headquarters in a futuristic building that looked like the decks of an ocean liner. Here, 1,450 experts in all disciplines—doctors, biologists, chemists—prepared and experimented with the remedies that earned the firm its reputation. Two American pharmaceutical inventors, Silas M. Burroughs and Henry S. Wellcome, had founded the firm in 1880 in London. They had chosen as its emblem the unicorn, the mythical creature that, according to legend, protects against poison and cures all ills.

Sure enough, the ninety-three medicines now manufactured by their successors claimed to take on the whole gamut of human pathology. They provided treatment for cancerous tumors, cardiovascular infections, rheumatism, malaria, gout, and Parkinson's disease, as well as a whole host of viral infections. In fact, this last specialty had built the reputation of the establishment at Research Triangle Park. Its researchers had recently developed the first effective treatment against herpes. The experimental development and manufacture of this special medication, acyclovir, had alone involved an investment of one hundred million dollars. The Burroughs Wellcome laboratory might therefore be regarded as, in its way, one of humanity's benefactors. Each day, millions of sick people used its products to restore themselves to health.

Apart from its scientific discoveries, the laboratory had a sense of the human adventure that had made it a pioneer. It was armed with survival kits stamped with its unicorn emblem that the explorer Henry M. Stanley had tackled the hazards of the Congo River, that Admirals Robert Peary and Richard Byrd had braved the dangers of their conquest of the North Pole, that Theodore Roosevelt had been able to resist the fevers of the Amazon, that Charles Lindbergh had defied the vastness of the Atlantic in his single-engined aircraft *Spirit of St. Louis*. Equipped with Burroughs Wellcome antihistamines and antibiotics, on July 20, 1969, men had landed on the moon, and later, other astronauts had circled in space with these products aboard the spaceship *Skylab* and the shuttle *Columbia*.

With this spirit of adventure and its experience in fighting viruses, the North Carolina laboratory seemed destined to play a key role in the researching of a medicine to combat AIDS. That at least was the hope of the young immunologist Michael Gottlieb. As early as autumn 1983, he had gone to make the Research Triangle Park scientists aware of AIDS and its opportunistic infections. He had even suggested an original line of research to them. Since the causal agent of AIDS was a retrovirus and retroviruses needed the intermediary of a reverse transcriptase enzyme, why not look for a substance that would act directly on this enzyme? Apparently his proposal had met with only polite interest.

There were several reasons for this reluctance, but the primary motive was financial. The development of any pharmaceutical product cost tens of millions of dollars. To guarantee the profitability of any such investment, the directors of Burroughs Wellcome had established precise criteria. Any new medicine must be directed at a potential market of at least 200,000 patients. Below this level, a pathological infection was regarded as an "orphan disease." With only 5,000 victims on record at the time, AIDS did not measure up to the company's—or the pharmaceutical industry's—commercial criteria.

In fact, the California immunologist's visit had more impact than it might have seemed. His vibrant appeal made the prestigious laboratory take an indirect interest in the unusual epidemic. For some time now, its young vice president in charge of research, Dr. David W. Barry, had been amazed the way sales of certain products marketed by his firm were rocketing. These were medicines used to treat various sexually transmissible diseases, such as genital herpes or shigellosis, a violent bacterial dysentery. Since these infections were evidently linked to the pathology of AIDS, David Barry recognized that his company was already involved in the treatment of certain manifestations of the new disease. This fact was not likely to displease a man of science who had devoted his life to waging war on viruses.

Originally from the East Coast, having emerged with honors from Yale University, a former cum laude student of the Sorbonne, forty-year-old Dr. David Barry had begun his career as head of the Food and Drug Administration's general virology department. An intrepid rider, avid reader of French classics, and chain-smoker of long Winstons, this blue-eyed multilinguist, who was always immaculately dressed, personified the new breed of managerial scientist. A member of numerous medical societies, author of more than a hundred scientific articles treating subjects as diverse as viruses in green monkeys in Africa, influenza in mice, the rectal treatment of infectious pneumocystis pneumonia, or tolerance of vaccines in old people, he now ran the department for research and development of new medicines at the celebrated Research Triangle Park laboratory.

It would not be long before other facts emerged to reinforce

David Barry's interest in the disturbing epidemic. Burroughs Wellcome manufactured an amyl-nitrite-based medication that millions of Americans suffering from angina and other vascular deficiencies were quick to inhale or place under their tongues at the slightest cardiac pain. This product had the capacity to dilate the blood vessels almost instantaneously. It was the same substance as was contained in those slender ampuls that went "pop" when broken, christened "poppers" by a category of users rather different from that envisioned by the austere pharmaceutical code. Gays had been quick to discover in amyl nitrite a means of dilating the blood vessels of the penis and the anal membranes. These poppers became so popular that the medical detectives from the Atlanta-based CDC had wondered at one point whether they were not the direct cause of AIDS. "Frankly it was not long before our position became a delicate one," David Barry would confide. "Certain newspapers dared to make us responsible for the epidemic. It was unbelievable: in San Francisco and Los Angeles, gays were even parading in T-shirts decorated with slogans proclaiming 'We have a good time thanks to Burroughs Wellcome poppers!' " The young doctor/executive understood that his laboratory could no longer remain uninvolved in the health crisis that was shattering America.

It was then that Françoise Barré-Sinoussi arrived from Paris, on June 1, 1984, in the stifling humidity of a Carolina summer. She had come to inform the American pharmaceutical industry of the discovery of the LAV, whose genetic identity card she and her colleagues at the Pasteur Institute had managed to put together. For one of her listeners, Dr. Sandra Lehrman, head of virological research, "the Frenchwoman was describing an experiment which in my view was as phenomenal as that of her compatriot Pasteur when he discovered microbes." For her colleague Phil Furman, a doctor of biology, "the visitor was suddenly providing us with proof that the mysterious virus was not just pie in the sky but something truly real!" For the chemist Janet Rideout, "the time had come for us to dig into our reserves for a substance that could wipe this monstrosity out." For Marty St. Clair, a young twenty-eight-year-old virologist with the naive expression of a little girl behind her thick glasses, "that Parisian woman's revelations called on us to get our test tubes and our incubators moving." For David Barry, to whom fell the onerous responsibility of deciding the expediency of such a mobilization and organizing it, "the picture painted of the disease by the one who had identified the culprit called on us to stop being so cautious."

Other arguments in favor of the mobilization of the Burroughs Wellcome laboratory arrived from Bethesda a few weeks later. An auditorium packed to the bursting point paid tribute to Robert Gallo, the flamboyant master of retrovirology, who had come to offer his prestige and his encouragement to the research scientists of Research Triangle Park.

But it was from another authority that David Barry hoped to receive the decisive support that would convince his company directors. He was not disappointed. More than ever, Dr. Sam Broder considered the commitment of private laboratories a key asset in the crusade he was conducting for the urgent discovery of a medicine to treat AIDS patients. "Sure, I could sense that the people in charge of Burroughs Wellcome were still hesitant about joining the dance," the young cancer specialist would recount. "They were afraid of not getting the necessary finances from their directorship to see that kind of venture through to its conclusion. And even if they managed to come up with a drug, they weren't a hundred percent sure that the operation would one day be commercially profitable. I couldn't hold it against them. More than anything else, I wanted that enterprise to be profit-making. Not because of any personal devotion to capitalism, but for the simple reason that a commercial failure would have the effect of putting all the other pharmaceutical laboratories off researching an anti-AIDS medicine. There was another reason for their reticence. There were safety considerations involved. They would willingly test their chemical compounds on animal retroviruses, but not on the human AIDS agent. I reassured them by suggesting a solution that would give them all the necessary safety guarantees. They would send me the substances they found effective on their animal viruses, and I would try them out on the AIDS retrovirus in my own hospital's laboratory at the National Cancer Institute. 'If we find one that works,' I told them, 'we'll inject patients with it and I shall supervise the operation myself.' "

This proposal enabled the Burroughs Wellcome laboratory to enter into an ideal partnership. Its researchers would consult their computers to ascertain the most effective antiviral compounds, then test them on their animal retroviruses.

Of course, there was still one unknown factor: Would a remedy that killed an animal retrovirus be equally effective against a human retrovirus? The answer would come from the test tubes at Bethesda.

46

A Honeymoon Off to a Bad Start
Research Triangle Park, USA: Autumn 1984

Marty St. Clair was excessively fond of her house. She had drawn up the plans herself. Then she and her husband, a land surveyor, had actually built it with their own hands, from its foundations to its majestic central fireplace. Made entirely out of wood, the building looked as much like a high mountain refuge as a Jules Verne space capsule. Most of all, however, its bulbous shape reminded Marty, the young Burroughs Wellcome virologist, of the particles that monopolized her professional life: a virus.

That last Sunday in October 1984, the inhabitants of the St. Clairs' "virus house" were in a state of unusual excitement. A preparation on the eve of battle. Tomorrow, the prestigious pharmaceutical laboratory to which Marty belonged would officially throw itself into the AIDS venture.

What a challenge for the farmer's daughter from Oregon, born with a passion for science. While her classmates worshiped their rock idols, she had written to one of the most celebrated American virologists to ask him to take her on at his laboratory at Duke University. Dr. Dani Bolognesi had agreed to her request, and Marty had been able to fulfill a dream. She had found herself on the campus and earned her promotion to research scientist before being taken on by Burroughs Wellcome. David Barry had been charmed at once by "an astonishing slip of a woman with her hair cropped so short she looked like a boy." Here was a headstrong individual capable of working for thirty-six hours at a stretch without uttering a sound, an ascetic who ate nothing but vegetables and whose hands bore the calluses created by the work she had done on her unique house.

To Marty St. Clair went the honor of opening the celebrated laboratory's onslaught against AIDS. David Barry gave her the task of obtaining the base elements indispensable for researching any medicine, in this case samples of various animal retroviruses and the strains of cells they liked to infect. It was only by bringing this biological material into contact with antiviral substances that they could hope to discover a cure.

Finding the requisite viruses and cells presented no particular difficulties. Such items are bought and sold like horticultural nursery products. There is even an official bank of cell tissue, the American Type Culture Collection, which for the moderate sum of twenty to thirty dollars, will mail frozen and guaranteed samples of virtually every kind of cell culture biologists have ever invented. On the whole, however, researchers prefer to use suppliers they know. The scientists at Burroughs Wellcome were lucky to be able to do their shopping in the deep freezer of their virologist neighbors at Duke University.

With its vast hospital specializing in infectious diseases, its brilliant medical school faculty, its research centers, and its battalions of handpicked doctors and researchers, Duke University was an amazing reservoir of skills. Yet this temple of knowledge had very nearly not existed at all. Its founder, a multmillionaire tobacco planter, had actually originally intended to bequeath his fortune to the great Northern university Princeton. He had set one condition to his legacy: the building of a belfry similar to the one at Yale University, but higher by one foot. When Princeton rejected this proposal, the planter had turned to the modest institution in his home state and offered it his millions. He had built the Gothic tower of his dreams there, given it his name, and made it the most renowned center for medical instruction and treatment in the South.

Dani Bolognesi, the leading virologist at Duke, had no difficulty finding in his freezers the animal retroviruses Marty St. Clair requested. Like a solicitous horticulturalist wanting to give a client his best sprouts, he picked out two of his favorite retroviruses. The first caused cancerous tumors in mice, and the second, leukemia in chickens. Next he selected some of the cell cultures that the little monsters liked. Marty stored the lot in the safety of the arctic cold of her own laboratory freezers. She would be ready to proceed as soon as her chemist colleagues supplied her with their antiviral substances.

"How many viral substances do you think you'll be able to test?" David Barry inquired anxiously.

The young woman smiled. "Thousands if you can find them!"

* * *

The real difficulty lay in selecting the substances to be used in her tests. The cupboards, drawers, shelves, flasks, and test tubes at Burroughs Wellcome bulged with tens of thousands of organic and chemical compounds. Every year, chemists, pharmacologists, and enzymologists added between a thousand and fifteen hundred new formulas to this incredible stock. How were they to determine among such riches which molecules were capable of killing the AIDS virus? David Barry decided to select first the components of antiviral medicines his company had already commercialized and then go on to those that were part of research programs in progress. "The fact that the first lot had already been tested on humans at least eliminated the problems of toxicity," he would say. That made a good fifty samples with which to keep Marty St. Clair's experimental zeal satisfied for the time being.

The history of science will not record either the date or the time of the first anti-AIDS operation carried out on the Research Triangle Park campus. That day, Marty went through the same procedures as usual. First she deposited in dozens of small round plastic containers placed on trays a few drops of a blue-tinted solution containing in some instances the mouse cells and in others the chicken cells provided by the virologist at Duke University. After adding to this preparation a liquid full of growth factors and minerals intended to promote the growth and multiplication of the cells, she placed each tray under her sterile-air-cleansed safety hood. Thus protected, she could pour into each container a few drops of a second solution containing the retroviruses that caused either cancerous tumors in mice or leukemia in chickens. After an hour in the incubators at 100°, the containers were then ready to receive the antiviral agent that was actually being tested. To increase the odds, Marty had prepared different concentrations of this product for each series of containers. This last step completed, she returned the trays of containers to the incubators. Then all she had to do was wait for nature to take its course. In exactly seven days' time, the young virologist would examine with her naked eye the bluish film remaining at the bottom of each receptacle. If it was studded with tiny holes, it would show that the cells had been killed by the virus. If, on the other hand, the bottom had kept its blue color uniformly, it would indicate that the cells were intact, that they had been protected against the onslaught of the viruses by the antiviral substance being tested.

At the end of each week, the young woman would be filled with feverish anticipation. But not one of the first fifty compounds tested deigned to show an aggressive reaction to the virus. She would have to get hold of others. Fortunately the resources at Burroughs Wellcome were virtually inexhaustible. "Every single one of our scientists kept several antiviral preparations he'd invented along the way, pampering them in the firm hope that they would one day make him famous," David Barry would recount. A new series of tests produced this time a few timorous results with which to appease the impatience of Sam Broder, who was bombarding Barry with phone calls from Bethesda nearly every day. Marty hastily sent him the most promising of her compounds, but she knew full well there was not one in the batch that would provide the desired panacea.

The Burroughs Wellcome chemists went back to their computers. Again, they sifted through their registers and foraged in their storerooms. David Barry organized group inquiry sessions aimed at helping his associates to remember whether they had ever worked on a molecule, formula, or chemical or organic compound that had shown signs of any antiviral properties, no matter how imperfect.

"We got together at every possible opportunity to rack our brains and force them to come up with some clue. Anytime, anyplace, we would have an orgy of coffee and cigarettes to stimulate some bright ideas," Barry recalled.

One day, Janet Rideout, head of the organic chemistry department, banged the table with her fist and exclaimed, "I think I've got it. What we need is five oh nine!"

Her colleagues looked at her, flabbergasted. They were used to identifying their products by number, but 509 didn't call to mind any particular compound.

"Don't you remember? It's that nucleoside whose antibacterial properties gave rise to such great hopes three years ago," she explained. She went on to remind them of the tests of 509 as an antiviral agent, their lack of success, and finally the dispatch of the 509 compound to the British branch for more thorough experimental trials on animals. She had heard no further news since then.

This information caused a stir among the team. David Barry called the staff of the toxicology department together. He wanted to know as a matter of urgency the results of the work carried out in Great Britain. What effect did 509 have on British animals? Had it killed them, cured them, or allowed them to die of their bacterial infections? The Burroughs Wellcome headquarters in England replied by telex that 509 had been tested on chickens, pigs, and newborn calves with infectious complications. Its effect had been judged moderately satisfactory, but its toxicity had proved to be perfectly acceptable. It was enough to set the scientists at Research Triangle Park back on the trail of 509.

They made inquiries at once into its pedigree. Who had invented it? For what purpose? Was it readily available? The answers would have provided material for a scientific soap opera. The product owed its designation to the fact that it was the 509th substance synthesized in 1981 by the Burroughs Wellcome chemists. Its real name was azido-thymidine, or AZT. Its structure was that of a nucleoside similar to the components of DNA, the constituent acid of the cell nucleus. In 1964, an oncologist at the Michigan Cancer Foundation, Dr. Jerome Horovitz, had tried to use its analogous cell structure as a decoy to lure cancerous cells and thus halt the machinery of abnormal reproduction. The attempt failed and Horovitz discarded his AZT work. Ten years later, a German laboratory resuscitated the substance and tested it against a virus found in mice. Despite the fact that that particular trial had achieved a certain success, the product had been abandoned for a second time.

In 1981, the Burroughs Wellcome chemist Janet Rideout had tried to drag AZT back from the scientific dustbin. As she and her colleagues had previously done in the development of the herpes medicine acyclovir, she had tried to strengthen the properties of AZT by adding a particular enzyme. The concept—known as "the suicide remedy"—was an extremely ingenious one. It consisted of forcing the virus to act as its own executioner by triggering the chemical actions that would destroy it. This strategy of antiviral manipulation had been devised by Howard Schaeffer, one of the leading research scientists at Burroughs Wellcome. At that time, AZT-509 did not live up to Janet Rideout's hopes. Although endowed with indisputable power against human bacterial infections, the range of its effectiveness had eventually been found too limited to justify further tests. That was why the American chemist had handed it over to her British colleagues for them to carry out more extensive experiments.

Three years later, did she still have a few milligrams of AZT-509 left in her storeroom to be used for further tests? The young woman rushed to her computer register without too much hope. There were approximately 1,500 compounds synthesized each year at the laboratory. Once experiments were completed, all that was left was an identification slip and a lab report. AZT-509 was not a readily available product: it required herring sperm to obtain the thymidine, which was one of its components.

* * *

The honeymoon of the Burroughs Wellcome laboratory and the head of the clinical oncology program at Bethesda's National Cancer Institute had gotten off to the worst possible start. Dr. Sam Broder had never seen his Japanese-born associate Hiroaki Mitsuya, known as Mitch, so completely lose his usual Oriental calm. A biologist of the highest caliber, Mitch was director of the small laboratory at the hospital where Sam Broder had undertaken to test antiviral substances on living strains of the AIDS retrovirus. Together they had conceived and developed an original scheme of experiments designed to achieve rapid and reliable results. Mitch had already started work on several products suggested by Sam Broder when the first package bearing the unicorn emblem arrived from North Carolina, followed shortly afterward by others.

"Poison! All they've sent us is poison!" Mitch grumbled. "Poison that kills all our cells every time. It's a disaster!"

Sam Broder felt a wave of anger. He looked for some explanation. "Perhaps we've made a mistake in the conception of our experiments," he ventured.

Mitch shook his head, pointing to a test tube half full of a transparent liquid.

"Everything they send us is soaked in this damned stuff. Formaldehyde!"

"Formaldehyde?" repeated Sam Broder, astounded, as he furiously punched out the telephone number for Burroughs Wellcome.

None of the staff at the Research Triangle Park laboratory dared to tell him how such a mistake could have been made, or whose fault it was. But the fury of the man from Bethesda raged for a long time through the Carolina campus like a tropical hurricane.

"No doubt it was an accident," Sam Broder said later. "They were trying too hard. They immediately replaced the defective specimens and regularly sent us other substances as they went on testing. Mitch carried on relentlessly, giving them to his cells infected with the AIDS retrovirus. Sometimes there were a few faint signs of positive action. When this was the case, I would call David Barry or one of his assistants to urge him to develop the product in question as a matter of urgency. But every time I did, I came up against it. They weren't there to be philanthropists. First they had to be certain they'd come up with the real McCoy. Only then would they agree to spend the millions of dollars involved in transforming a few milligrams of powder into an effective medicine."

47

"Perhaps One Small Step Toward Victory"
Research Triangle Park, USA: Autumn 1984–Winter 1985

It required the artistry of a goldsmith, the drudgery of a convict, the indefatigability of an ant. There were no such things as evenings or weekends anymore. Marty St. Clair deserted her husband and their virus-shaped house. For twenty hours a day, she camped out in her lab at Research Triangle Park, endlessly putting her round plastic containers into incubators. The discouraging results of her first tests and Sam Broder's repeated outbursts of anger on the telephone set the whole team at the laboratory on edge. Almost every day someone would burst in with a new chemical or an organic compound to be tested. In six weeks, Marty had subjected more than two hundred products presumed to be anti-infectious to the onslaughts of her mouse or chicken retroviruses. Less than twenty showed faint antiviral activity. When they did, she sent a specimen to Sam Broder for him to try on the human AIDS retrovirus.

After the enthusiasm of the initial weeks, the young woman was suffering as a result of this uninterrupted series of setbacks. Despite the proximity of Christmas, an atmosphere of general moroseness prevailed. Even David Barry was seized with doubt. One late Friday afternoon in December, Marty was on the brink of tears, exhausted and discouraged. She had just examined more than four hundred containers, checking the holes that punctured the thin bluish film at the bottom of the receptacles. Each hole represented a defeat, the gap left by the cells that the antiviral substance had failed to protect from the virus's lance. Each hole signified the presence of the virus. Since that morning, she had counted thousands of holes. Not one of the various concentrates of the twenty-two substances under experiment that day had been effective. There was still another tray with two lots of fourteen containers to check. Once she had counted their holes, Marty would only have to lock up the freezers, switch off the light, and go home, with despair in her heart.

The young woman had difficulty reconstructing precisely what happened next. All she would remember was taking the last trays of containers out of the incubators. Mechanically she prepared to count the holes in the last batch of the day. First she methodically referred to their references to find out the code number for the antiviral substance being tested. She had written it down herself seven days previously in felt-tip pen on the lid of each container. Suddenly she asked herself, "Was it some kind of hallucination that I was seeing through eyes red with fatigue?" As she took off each lid, she would not believe what she saw. There was not one single hole in the bluish skin that coated the bottom of the receptacles. Out of habit, she noted the time of the check. It was 4:57 P.M. on Friday, December 20, 1984. Marty slumped down on a stool, took off her glasses, and buried her head in her hands. "It's not possible, it's not possible," she murmured several times. "I must be mistaken. Could I have forgotten to put the virus in this lot of containers? No, it was unlikely. Why would I have made a mistake with these fourteen containers only, and not with the others?" All at once she felt like Christopher Columbus sighting the New World in his spyglasss. She ran into the office of her boss, Phil Furman.

"Phil, come and look!" she begged, pulling the young Ph.D. out of his chair.

Together, they examined the bottoms of the fourteen containers. There could be no doubt about it: not the smallest pinhead of white punctured the blue surface.

"Do you think I could have forgotten to put the virus in these containers only?" Marty asked softly.

Phil Furman shook his head. "The only way to find out is to run the experiment again. In seven days' time we'll know." He placed a friendly hand on the young woman's shoulder. "Don't worry. In seven days' time, this blasted epidemic will still be with us."

He was already on his way back to his office when he turned around. "By the way, what compound were you testing in those containers?"

"Five oh nine."

It was the AZT molecule with the herring-sperm base. By some miracle, Janet Rideout had managed to find a few grams of 509 in her storeroom.

*   *   *

"That was the longest Christmas week of my life," Marty St. Clair would later reflect. In the absence of freshly available cells, she had to wait until the following Monday to make up new preparations and put them in fourteen new containers. There was so little 509 left that she decided to dilute some concentrates to minute doses, at the risk of diminishing the chances of getting a result comparable to that of the previous experiment. She decided to take David Barry into her confidence. Soon the whole laboratory knew what was happening. An anxious vigil began all through the long building's four stories. Resorting once more to a childhood habit of hers, Marty bit her nails as she watched over "her bloody incubator that had to keep my containers locked up for so long."

The fateful day arrived. Everyone heard the victory cry that went up from the young virologist. The blue film at the bottom of the fourteen containers was intact. Even in its weakest concentration, 509 had protected the cells against mouse and chicken retroviruses. The news quickly made the rounds of the building, releasing a wave of euphoria. "It was as if we'd suddenly discovered a miracle cure to heal all humanity's diseases," David Barry would remember.

For the nineteenth time, Marty St. Clair carefully made up a package addressed to Sam Broder and his team at Bethesda. To identify the substance, she wrote on it the letter *S*, the nineteenth letter of the alphabet. Thus did 509 became "Compound S."

Beyond that abstract code lay the hope that Marty St. Clair would express with typical modesty: "Perhaps we had taken a small step towards saving a few people."

* * *

The man flying from Washington to Raleigh that icy morning in February 1985 was carrying the concrete expression of that hope. In his test tubes the medical research scientist Sam Broder had confronted Compound S with concentrates of the living retrovirus that was killing one or two patients in his hospital every week. He had been able to establish at once that the product impeded the replication of the virus, by breaking its genetic sequence. Thus, the virus was unable to conquer the fresh cells. The result was so spectacular that in his mind's eye Sam Broder was already injecting all his condemned patients with "herring sperm." But the impulsive cancer specialist was well aware that months, possibly even years, separated him from the fulfillment of this dream.

First he would have to wrest the necessary authorization from the FDA. Sam Broder had often clashed with the bureaucratic encumbrances of this organization. Broder knew how diligent FDA officials were in ensuring that a remedy had no toxic effects before allowing it to be tried on humans. Still, as a responsible man of science conscious of the dangers of all experimentation, Broder had to admit these officials had their uses. Had they not rid his country's pharmaceutical industry of a tragic succession of deceptions, frauds, and criminal abuses?

America had taken its time, however, to put its house in order: it had taken the death, in 1937, of 107 children poisoned by a cough syrup before the U.S. Congress decided to vote in a law regulating the manufacture and sale of medicines. Since then the FDA had constantly been stepping up its surveillance as much over foodstuffs as over pharmaceutical products. Now it had some seven thousand inspectors, among them doctors, chemists, toxicologists, veterinarians, biologists, nutritionists, and statisticians. Its inspectors' range of competence extended to silicone breast implants, artificial hips, contact lenses, pacemakers, insulin syringes, and other biomedical matters. The FDA also monitored blood products and the radiological dangers presented by medical substances or equipment. Some of their problems were almost beyond belief. Ever since manufacturers had been obliged by law to guarantee that their products were both effective and not hazardous to humans, it had been necessary for numerous controllers to check that the 300,000 products sold without prescription satisfied these two conditions. In fact, they had already discovered that one-third of the seven hundred active ingredients contained in over-the-counter remedies were either harmful or had no curative effect whatsoever. It was thanks to the FDA's persistent effort that American children had been spared the tragic effects of thalidomide, the barbiturate responsible for the birth of hundreds of deformed babies in Europe.

Sam Broder knew that the FDA never gave its authorization for a medicine to be tested on humans unless a program of experiments had been carried out on animals that was so extensive and so complex it sometimes took several years. The FDA specifically demanded that the harmlessness of a product be established on at least two varieties of rodents—usually rats and mice—then on guinea pigs, rabbits, and dogs, and at last on monkeys. The trials must be conducted according to set procedures, with increasing doses over specified periods of time. The substance tested must first be injected intravenously, then administered by oral means. Each phase of the process must be controlled by a series of thorough biological and toxicological tests. Finally, it was imperative that the results obtained be detailed in reports, the most modest of which ran to several hundred pages.

It was to set up this titanic task with the directors of the Burroughs Wellcome laboratory that Sam Broder came rushing to Research Triangle Park that morning in February 1985. The greeting he received pleased him. David Barry was immediately disposed to invest the two or three million dollars needed for the first animal experiments. However, the young vice president in charge of research had several obstacles to overcome, starting with the opposition of the company's chairman, who, from his general headquarters in London, raised objection after objection against the venture. Not to mention the antivivisectionists and the societies for the protection of animals who went into action as soon as they heard about the proposed experiments. Opponents of animal testing had gone so far as to blow up the British cottage of Sir John Vane, one of the principal directors of Burroughs Wellcome, before launching a commando raid to free hundreds of animals from the laboratories in Beckenham, Kent, not far from London. Afraid they might suffer a similar attack, those in charge of the American branch had recently reinforced the defenses around their premises with barbed wire, alarm systems, and guard patrols. "But nothing and nobody was going to stop us," David Barry would say. "Even if it had only killed two or three thousand patients to date, AIDS was a major plague. We had a duty to do our bit to bar its way."

There remained one last obstacle, and no small one at that. Marty St. Clair's round containers had used up all of the tiny quantity of thymidine that Janet Rideout had found. The laboratory had to procure more of the precious and costly herring sperm needed to manufacture the molecule. Telexes and telephone calls were sent out to research centers aroung the world to try to round up all existing stocks. But the harvest was thin in the extreme, barely a few hundred grams. A breakdown in supply seemed likely before the Burroughs Wellcome chemists had even gotten started on synthesizing and manufacturing the rare molecule themselves. Still, what did that matter? At least, the ball was rolling.

How many animals—white mice, rabbits, dogs, monkeys—were put through agony that winter by the virologists in the North Carolina laboratory in order to work out the toxicity of Compound S? Such was the fear of violent action against the animal houses at Research Triangle Park that the figure was kept a fiercely guarded secret. As for Sam Broder and the FDA inspectors, they would have every reason to be satisfied. Not only did David Barry's team systematically carry out the program of requisite experiments, but they went much further. They tried to find out how thymidine circulated in the blood, what the duration of its effectiveness was at different doses, whether it could pass through the protective membranes of the brain. "It was fantastic," David Barry would recall. "The lights would be on all through the night. No one went home anymore. We knew we were the best people to rise to the challenge. And what we were after wasn't payment for overtime, but a constant and increased supply of herring sperm so we could conduct more experiments. Thymidine was our currency. It meant more to us than the dollars we were paid."

48

A Home for the Dying Overshadowed by Skyscrapers
New York, USA: Summer 1985

From his spacious office in downtown Manhattan, the mayor of New York contemplated his city with fondness and melancholy. In eight years of office, Edward I. Koch had achieved a feat of strength. He had checked the decline of municipal finances, slowed down the exodus of large corporations, restored the confidence of investors, and reduced serious crime. All the same, this audacious bald-headed bachelor had few illusions. This proud city of his still contained many areas of poverty and violence. Every day he was called upon to find the solution to some instance of pressing injustice. More than 400,000 unemployed and 850,000 needy depended on social services for their major support. In certain neighborhoods, hundreds of thousands of blacks and Puerto Ricans were crammed into nightmarish ghettos where the chances were slim of dying of natural causes. The hot spots of New York were a haven for half the United States' drug addicts. Police stations recorded an emergency call every second, a theft every minute, a holdup every quarter of an hour, two rapes and a murder every five hours, a suicide and a death by overdose every seven hours.

That summer of 1985 a new and terrible affliction had been added to this somber picture. The Atlanta CDC bulletin revealed that

New York was harboring a quarter of all American AIDS victims. The epidemic was affecting 2,140 people, twice as many as in the previous year. Despite its outstanding medical infrastructure encompassing nearly one hundred hospitals and five centers for medical research, the city was not managing to cope with the emergency. A fair number of establishments were still refusing to take patients. When they did resign themselves to doing so, it was only to isolate them like people with the plague or even worse, to scatter them between different departments in a way that exposed them to numerous additional infections. Only a few, such as the old St. Clare's Hospital, were equipped with special units where AIDS was not looked upon as some shameful evil. But these wards had too few beds and could not meet the growing need. The ostracism of the victims, the rapid spread of AIDS among black and Hispanic drug addicts without resources, gave rise to a predicament from which there appeared to be no escape. In the absence of any family or anywhere to take them in, numerous patients whose hospitalization the state could not justify found themselves condemned to the streets. Faced with the urgency of the situation, Ed Koch decided to set about finding a suitable place to house some of these unfortunates. In the borough of Queens he unearthed an unoccupied wing of a municipal old people's home, but his project met with such local resistance that he was forced to abandon it. Disheartened, he appealed to someone he thought was the very person to come to his aid. Perhaps a Catholic bishop could touch the hearts of his electorate better than a Jewish politician could.

*　　*　　*

The archbishop, John Cardinal O'Connor, reigned over two million parishioners in the archdiocese of New York. He was as sensitive as the mayor to the injustices and misfortunes of the Big Apple. Formerly chief chaplain in the American navy, it was he who had created the special AIDS treatment unit at St. Clare's Hospital. His motto was engraved on the entrance to his office on the top floor of his headquarters on First Avenue: "There can be no love without justice." True, the intransigent stance he had adopted on abortion and the civil rights of lesbians and gay men had at times lost him support for his crusade on behalf of the poor and homeless, but his dedication to charity was recognized by most

New Yorkers. The organization he had at his disposal made him
one of the city's most powerful leaders. He was head of numerous
hospitals, a college of medicine, day care centers, homes for young
people and the elderly, higher education establishments, dozens of
primary and secondary schools. Some of them were planted, like
St. Simon's School, right in the heart of the worst urban jungle. A
budget of several hundreds of millions of dollars furnished by the
donations of the faithful and municipal subsidies provided for the
needs of this formidable network of medical, social, and educational
assistance.

The mayor's SOS evoked an immediate response from the prelate.
It was not long before his staff discovered at the northern end of
Manhattan an old disused building belonging to the convent of the
Holy Name of Jesus. Its location within the confines of Harlem
seemed ideal. The archbishop ordered work to begin at once on
rehabilitating the building. Just as had happened in Queens, however, so here the project provoked an uproar among the residents
of the neighborhood. They organized meetings, threatened to use
force to prevent the patients' arrival, and flooded the prelate with
a deluge of petitions. The bishop's personal intervention could not
silence popular discontent. Bitterly disappointed, O'Connor was
forced to capitulate.

Far from making him lay down his arms, this defeat served rather
to spur him on. After weeks of searching, his staff found a five-
story presbytery in Greenwich Village near Saint Veronica's Church.
Only two priests lived in the building; the once flourishing parish
was now practically devoid of churchgoers. It would be easy to
move the priests elsewhere and turn their residence into a home for
some twenty AIDS patients. To celebrate this happy discovery, the
mayor invited the archbishop and his assistants to the Peking Duck,
one of his favorite restaurants in Chinatown. As usual on important
occasions, Ed Koch himself carved the duck for his guests. Then
they went on to the presbytery at 657 Washington Street to visit
the premises and give some thought to their arrangement.

Providence could not have chosen a more symbolic site. The gay
liberation movement had begun a few blocks away, on a stifling
night in June 1969, on the famous Christopher Street, which in-
tersected Washington Street. Saint Veronica's presbytery was right
in the heart of New York's gay ghetto. Despite vigorous campaigns

to try to change people's behavior, the neighborhood had remained a sexually active center. Several bathhouses had been closed but others survived, as did some of the haunts for sadomasochistic pleasure.

Contrary to the hopes of the mayor and the archbishop, the gay community greeted the project with distrust and outright hostility. The prelate's earlier pronouncements that homosexuality was a sin clearly had something to do with this attitude. Militant gay groups were afraid that behind the welcoming facade there lurked a "repentance factory." Richard Dunne, the energetic director of the Gay Men's Health Crisis, an organization active in support of AIDS victims, expressed his concern "at seeing occupants of the home subjected to religious indoctrination and attempted conversions to heterosexuality right up until their deaths."

The nongays in the neighborhood also made their reservations known. To allay their concerns, meetings were held in Saint Veronica's Church to educate the local residents. Doctors explained that the proximity of a hospice for this type of patient did not represent any kind of danger to the community. A committee of citizens was nominated and the issue put to an informal referendum. In the end, an overwhelming majority accepted the creation of the first New York center to take in destitute people with AIDS.

*   *   *

Nevertheless, Cardinal O'Connor's tribulations were not over yet. He had to find staff sufficiently motivated to make the home work. Over the past decade, attitudes had changed dramatically in the Catholic Church. Few religious workers accepted the idea of devoting their entire life solely to the relief of physical suffering. Sixty percent of sisters caring for the sick had left that kind of work, and the average age of those who remained was over sixty-five. Most nuns had given up their habit, preferring to shop for clothes like other women at Macy's or Bloomingdale's. They wanted comfortable accommodation and salaries proportionate to their work. In vain, the prelate sought an alternative by using lay people. But as soon as he uttered the word "AIDS," no one wanted to hear about the job anymore.

Only one person could help him resolve his problem: the indomitable nun who had wrested the dying from their hell on the sidewalks of Calcutta. Since the creation of her home for the dying, Mother Teresa had extended her work to the rest of the world, especially to those rich countries of whose countless difficulties and hidden poverty she was well aware. "Often the poor are more outcast and more neglected there than in India," she observed. To a Western world incapable of resolving the problem of those excluded from its prosperity, she had sent her dark-skinned Indian sisters, dressed in their simple cotton saris, their feet clad only in sandals. She had opened hospices, dispensaries, soup kitchens, night shelters in the poor suburbs of great capitalist cities. In Melbourne, Rome, London, Detroit, Marseilles, Rio, Chicago, Los Angeles, long lines of the unemployed, the homeless, the hungry, and the uprooted stood outside the doors of these refuges every day. And even in New York, right in the heart of the South Bronx, a nightmare section of the city burned out by fires and strewn with garbage, where the infant mortality rate was higher than in the Calcutta slums, Mother Teresa had opened in 1971 a center that dispensed food and clothing to thousands of unemployed blacks and Hispanics, to drug addicts, to all those the great American dream had somehow overlooked. To John O'Connor's predecessor, who wanted to know what salary package her Missionaries of Charity would want, Mother Teresa had replied: "Your Grace, serving Christ is our only paycheck."

The "saint of Calcutta" arrived in New York one stormy day in July 1985 for an inspection tour of her American houses. She had no idea that some people were looking to her as a messiah. With the same infallible instinct that had guided her throughout her life to where the need was greatest, Mother Teresa agreed to take charge of the first home for AIDS victims.

49

A Mink Coat for a Woman Resurrected from the Dead

Rockville–Bethesda, USA: Spring–Summer 1985

It would have been easier to imagine her striding across the links of some golf course or advertising fashion in the pages of *Harper's Bazaar*. This ravishing brunette, who looked so elegant and athletic, was not exactly anyone's idea of a government official. Yet at thirty-five, Dr. Ellen C. Cooper occupied one of the key positions in the steel-and-glass beehive located in the rural outskirts of Washington that harbored the general headquarters of the Food and Drug Administration. As medical inspector of the department of antiinfectious drugs, she was one of the authorities most courted by the American pharmaceutical industry. She was also one of the most feared because it would be her decision to authorize the testing of new antiviral substances on humans prior to consent for commercial use.

The daughter of a Philadelphia lawyer, nothing in her training had predestined her for an administrative career. She became a doctor of medicine at the age of twenty-six after studying at Yale, then specialized in infectious diseases in children. The reading of an FDA employment ad had one day made her take a closer interest in one of the principal viruses in child pathology, the virus that causes chicken pox. The mechanics of contagion were being studied in depth by the FDA laboratory. Ellen Cooper had joined one of the research teams. Two years later, the federal agency named her to the post of medical inspector she now occupied. However, in the medical world, she was more widely known as the mother of triplets. A photo of three endearing blond heads—Emmy, Benjamin, and Kimberley—presided in a place of honor on her desk, among the piles of scientific reports that filled her office. Ellen Cooper spent twelve to fourteen hours a day reviewing hundreds of pages of documents, analyzing their diagrams, dissecting their conclusions. There were so many she took them home with her to continue studying them in the evenings and even on Sundays, after a traditional stroll along the Potomac with her children and her husband, a well-known Washington lawyer. "An ordinary civil servant's life," she would recognize, "but one which gave me the satisfaction of going head-to-head with some of the most important public health problems."

Now the AIDS tragedy propelled Inspector Ellen Cooper right into the middle of a crucial drama. Could the herring-sperm-based medicine be tested on humans and if successful, be widely used as a treatment against the devastating disease? She and she alone would have to decide.

*　　*　　*

On Monday, April 22, 1985, the vice president for research at the Burroughs Wellcome laboratory came to submit to her the arguments in favor of such experiments. To support his application, David Barry brought with him a bulky report showing that AZT had a toxicity level acceptable to humans. Since that summer of 1953 when Dr. Jonas Salk had presented proof to the FDA inspectors that his vaccine against poliomyelitis could put an end to the tragedy, no other document of quite such importance had entered the prestigious womb of the FDA. No stenographer would record the discussion that took place around the oval table in the conference room on the third floor. Yet there was something historic about that meeting. Four years after a doctor from Los Angeles had diagnosed the first case of the epidemic, two years after biologists at the Pasteur Institute in Paris had discovered the fatal retrovirus, officials from the FDA and scientists from the pharmaceutical industry were getting together to develop the clinical protocol for testing the first possible weapon devised against AIDS.

"The task was enough to give us all nightmares," David Barry would say later. First, because of the lack of precedents. No product had yet successfully been tested against such a complex disease, one about which we knew so little. Then, there were numerous unknown factors relating to AZT itself. It hadn't been possible to fathom its overall pattern of action, and its toxic effects had only been assessed for a few short weeks on animals. What would happen in humans in the event of prolonged use? "We were steering blind," David Barry would say. One of the major questions concerned the choice of the first human guinea pigs. What would the criteria for that choice be? Should they, as the FDA representative wanted, give priority to patients whose condition suggested imminent death or to patients still in the early stages of the illness? Should they limit the clinical trials exclusively to victims of full-blown AIDS, and thus eliminate those who were only suffering from the preliminary mild form of the disease, which specialists called AIDS-related complex? Should they take all cases irrespective of whether they were suffering from pneumocystis pneumonia or Karposi's sarcoma or just one group and not the other?

The debate went on for several hours. In any case this was only the prelude to a long succession of discussions between representatives of Burroughs Wellcome, the oncologist Sam Broder, and Ellen Cooper. They all felt the same impatience. They were all particularly frantic because the effectiveness of AZT against the AIDS virus had been confirmed under test-tube conditions by Drs. Dani Bolognesi of Duke University and Robert Yarchoan of the National Cancer Institute. The diligent cooperation of Ellen Cooper pleased her partners, who were not used to an FDA official showing so much zeal. "She committed her triplets to the care of her husband and her mother-in-law and immersed herself in our endless stream of reports," David Barry marveled. The young FDA official provided the best explanation that summed up the sense of urgency they all felt: "We weren't looking at medicine designed to clear the nostrils of common-cold sufferers. We were trying to save the lives of patients who were dying daily while their doctors watched helplessly."

*   *   *

In spring 1985, the early studies performed on animals at Burroughs Wellcome showed that AZT had to be administered for prolonged periods in order for it to be effective. These studies also showed that AZT was better assimilated through intravenous therapy than by oral absorption. The drug's effect would last only for two hours. These three findings presented serious difficulties: it meant patients would be confined to hospital for several weeks, possibly months, simply for the purpose of receiving six to eight injections daily. The simplest solution would have been to develop a treatment to be taken orally at home, but experiments had revealed that in certain species, particularly rabbits, the body assimilated only 20 to 30 percent of the AZT taken in this fashion. What would the percentage be in humans? Only a test on patients could provide the answer. But American law was implacable here: such experiments could not be conducted until an official request had been made by the laboratory concerned and the approval of the FDA had been given. In spite of all Inspector Cooper's goodwill, the granting of FDA authorization to test would inevitably take a long time.

"We decided to risk a shortcut that was a tiny bit illegal," David Barry would confess. The tragic history of AIDS would show that the first milligrams of AZT administered to humans were taken by its three principal inventors, starting with the vice president himself. The experiment was carried out privately, away from indiscreet eyes. "What a revolting concoction!" the audacious doctor later said, referring to the bitterness of the orange juice he swallowed that day for breakfast. There were no tablets or capsules as yet, so he had been forced to dissolve the powdered herring sperm in fruit juice. Together with his two accomplices, he had already had a small quantity injected into his veins the previous day. A blood sample afterward confirmed the total assimilation of the substance. Similar blood checks after consumption by oral means were not as conclusive: only 70 percent of the AZT had passed into the blood. This percentage was confirmed over three consecutive days of experimentation.

David Barry was satisfied. He would be able to suggest an initial course of treatment to the FDA inspector. As he had anticipated,

Ellen Cooper did not fail to be surprised at the precision of the dosage of AZT advocated.

"How do you know you have to give exactly this additional quantity if taken by oral means as opposed to intravenous injection?" she wondered.

"Our computers have worked it out," responded David Barry imperturbably.

"My God!" exclaimed the young woman. "You've got some pretty extraordinary computers."

Another surprise lay in store for Ellen Cooper. "And why do you recommend mixing the product with a little sweet liquid?" she asked.

"Quite simply because that blasted herring sperm is horribly bitter, even more so than quinine," he replied.

"How do you know?"

David Barry felt the trap closing on him, but Ellen Cooper had the delicacy not to press the issue. She was too shrewd not to know that sometimes it was better to let the alchemists keep their secrets. One week later she confirmed the FDA's official consent. The demanding organization had granted its authorization in record time. The tests for the effectiveness and the toxicity of AZT in humans could begin.

* * *

The date of July 3, 1985, will remain firmly engraved upon the memory of the oncologist Sam Broder. That day, in his hospital at Bethesda, a young furniture salesman from Boston named Joseph Rafuse became a test pilot for science when he was given the first human dose of the first AZT treatment against AIDS. Obviously his dose was much stronger than those secretly given to the three colleagues at Burroughs Wellcome. "Sam and I linked our drip up to the infusion catheter," Dr. Robert Yarchoan recalled, "and held our breath as the drops fell one by one into his body. The first hour was critical. If the patient went into anaphylaxis, a violent reaction of biochemical intolerance could kill him." At the beginning of the night, his temperature shot up. The two doctors raced to his bedside and managed to cool down the fever. At dawn Sam Broder, exhausted, took off his white coat and uttered a few words to his assistants: "We're carrying on with the experiment."

There would be nineteen of them in all; nineteen men and women. They were selected by Sam Broder for his hospital on the Bethesda campus* because of the rarity and gravity of their symptoms. The experiment for which they were acting as guinea pigs was not designed primarily to cure them, but to establish that the drug was not likely to aggravate their condition or most importantly, kill them. Each patient was required to sign a document of eight typewritten pages certifying that he or she had volunteered, accepted the risks involved in the experiment, and in case of accident, absolved the center of all responsibility.

The protocol of clinical trials provided for the progressive increase of the doses of AZT, administered first intravenously for two weeks, then orally for the next four weeks. Studies on rats and dogs had shown tolerance levels up to forty milligrams of AZT per day per pound of weight. The doctors would start more modestly with doses of three, seven and a half, fifteen, then thirty milligrams. They would double the quantity for oral consumption. As the days went by, Sam Broder's hopes grew. The side effects were almost negligible: a decrease of barely 10 percent of red cells in three patients, headaches in ten others, some shivering in only one. On the other hand, the positive results were almost immediately apparent: a general weight gain of five pounds on average and a conspicuous increase in the number of T-4 lymphocytes, the sentinels of the immune system, revealed in fifteen out of the nineteen subjects. Two other patients showed complete elimination of a traumatic infection in their nails. Six patients eliminated their fever and nocturnal sweating. Several other subjects displayed a complete elimination of the retrovirus from their white cells. Two of the sick people were enjoying what amounted to a virtual resurrection.

*   *   *

The first dramatic case was the wife of a Washington doctor, an attractive nurse infected by a blood transfusion. Her name was Barbara. Her AIDS had been diagnosed in the course of her honeymoon to France. For the biologist Dannie King, director of the AZT project at Burroughs Wellcome, "Barbara epitomized every-

---

* Two patients were also treated at the Duke University Medical Center.

thing that was tragic about the disease. She did not belong to any of the risk groups, and what was more, she had chosen to make a profession out of caring for others." Neither Sam Broder nor his collaborator Robert Yarchoan had ever seen such lesions before. The young woman was suffering from a general infection of the mucous membranes of the mouth. Her tongue, her palate, her gums, the inner lining of her cheeks, her throat, her lips, were just one open wound, an inflamed expanse of bleeding ulcerations. "It was as if a punch in the face had knocked all her teeth out in one blow," David Barry explained. "She was really going through agony. Unable to eat for weeks, by now she was just a living skeleton. Apart from her husband and her doctor, no one dared to go into her room."

One day when he was helping her to slip on a dress that had become far too big for her fleshless body, her husband, knowing it was something she had dreamed about for a long time, said to her gently, "Darling, as soon as you've put on a few pounds, we'll go and buy you a mink coat."

Barbara's condition was so desperate that the promise seemed almost cruel. After two weeks of treatment with AZT, however, the young woman's disfigured face began once more to take on human form. She could speak normally again. Her oral lesions receded and ultimately disappeared. For three months she had been incapable of feeding herself; now she could eat normally. She managed to get up and dress herself. She started to take coquettish pride in her appearance again. Her strength returned and she had a burning desire to go back to active life. Barbara had not forgotten her profession. One day, Sam Broder was surprised to find her in a white lab coat busy nursing some of the other patients. Despite a few bouts of anemia promptly rectified with blood transfusions, her recovery was so sustained that, after four weeks, she was able to leave the hospital. On that memorable occasion she firmly filled out a turquoise silk dress bought in Paris that was a particular favorite—a dress she had not put on for months. Dr. Broder could not conceal his emotion. He and his whole team accompanied the woman and her husband to their taxi. As they disappeared into the vehicle, Barbara turned to her husband. "Darling," she said, "don't forget you owe me a mink coat!"

*   *   *

The second "resurrection" was also so spectacular that Sam Broder used this case to persuade Dr. Ellen Cooper to allow him not to interrupt treatment after the initial six weeks for the thirty days' rest interval prescribed by the protocol. This stoppage, customary in such experiments, is designed to give the patient some respite in order to eliminate eventual toxic effects. The FDA inspector considered an interval of this kind important.

This time the patient was an actor from Palm Beach, Florida. The particular virulence of his condition had made such an impact on his doctor, Margaret Fischl of the clinical center at Miami University, that she had sent him to Sam Broder without a moment's hesitation. In this case, the virus had attacked the brain. The man was paralyzed in his lower limbs. He had completely lost his ability to speak and was suffering from mental problems as well. "A man in his prime, fit, flamboyant, whom AIDS had reduced in the course of three months to the state of a cripple dragging himself about on two crutches," David Barry said. The impact AZT had in three weeks on this living corpse left both the Burroughs Wellcome laboratory authorities and those at the Bethesda hospital dumbfounded. Not only could the patient stand up unaided, but he even began to gambol about the corridors. Better still, he amused himself by scrambling at top speed down twelve flights of stairs to the ground floor and then, equally rapidly, clambering back up again in a race against the elevator, a feat he took great delight in repeating several times each day.

After six weeks of therapy, Sam Broder telephoned Ellen Cooper to ask her to agree that treatment of this exceptional subject not be interrupted with the fateful thirty days' cutoff.

"I've heard about the case," she grumbled. "He's a professional actor. Artistic people like that are capable of all sorts of hoaxes."

"Come and take a look for yourself," the doctor insisted.

Thirty minutes later, the incredulous young woman made her entrance into the room. She was astonished by the scene that awaited her. If it was an act, the former paralytic had perfected it to a fine art. He seized a crutch in either hand, jumped onto his bed, and brandishing them at the visitor, exclaimed, "Here are the instruments by which I was able to haul myself into this room three weeks ago!" He hurled the two crutches like javelins into the waste-paper basket at the other end of the room and added, "And here's what AZT has done for me." With all the suppleness of an acrobat, he leaped to the ground, threw himself down on his stomach, and began a series of push-ups with the cry, "My arms are as strong as my legs!"

Ellen Cooper was speechless. Eventually the former invalid got up and stood in front of her.

"Do you want me to show you how I go up and down the twelve floors of this blasted building?"

"No, that won't be necessary. I believe you." Ellen Cooper offered a smile of complicity. She left the room accompanied by Sam Broder. Laying a companionable hand on the cancer specialist's shoulder, she reassured him, "Okay, Sam. You got it. Don't interrupt his treatment."

50

Make Each One Feel That He Is Loved and Respected
New York, USA: Autumn 1985

"If I had the balls, Doc, I'd throw myself out of that window."

Dr. Jack Dehovitz looked with surprise at the luminous blue eyes burning with defiance and the thick ruffle of bristling auburn beard that made Josef Stein look like a Hebrew prophet. The ex-archaeologist was obviously having a bad day. It was the first time he had openly expressed the desire to die. This was common among some gays with AIDS. A few of them actually carried it out. Doctors attributed these suicidal tendencies to a self-destructive guilt complex exacerbated by the disease, sometimes combined with alcohol and drug abuse. That morning, Jack Dehovitz decided to treat his patient's morbid attitude with jocularity:

"Quit *kvetching!*" he responded briskly in a mixture of English and Yiddish that made them both burst out laughing.

For the doctor attached to the AIDS unit at St. Clare's Hospital, every working day began with a visit to his favorite patient. "Josef was so open, so intelligent, so full of humor and bursting with charm," the doctor would recall. "His Jewish culture and his long stays in Israel had drawn us together. I used to like going into his room with a few phrases of Yiddish or Hebrew that no one else could understand. With Josef I could at last laugh and talk about something other than the disease."

The same was true for the other members of the staff. They took every opportunity to go and see Josef Stein, smoke a cigarette, have a cup of tea, laugh at his jokes, listen while he related the adventures he had had, excavating among the ruins. Even when the chemotherapy had worn him to tatters, he never let visitors leave without having breathed into them a little of his dynamism and joie de vivre. "To those of us hammered day and night by disease striking people our age," the doctor said, "watching them in the throes of a death involving unbearable suffering, Josef brought fresh air and vitamins. In the sometimes unbearable situation that autumn, it took a Josef Stein to restore our morale."

For the patients, their physical nightmare was combined with a mental anguish that often aggravated their own ordeal and the task of those caring for them. "If you tell your family or friends you have cancer, no one will make an issue out of your morality," Terry Miles would explain. He was the "clinic coordinator" at St. Clare's, a thirty-year-old bachelor from Florida, in charge of the care and moral support of the nursing teams. "An AIDS patient has automatically to face disgrace," he added, "the consequence of a way of life considered reprehensible. His 'shameful' disease is regarded as a punishment. Hence the terror behind the heartrending question: 'Am I going to be treated as an ordinary patient or am I going to be excluded like a pariah?' "

Naturally, reactions varied from individual to individual. For the New York bus driver Frank Korda, a puny little fellow of twenty-eight with plastered-down hair, covered from head to toe with the hideous violet splashes of Kaposi's sarcoma, AIDS had been relieved by a small slip of a woman attentive to his every whim.

"I knew Frank was gay before he knew it himself," his mother, an operator at a Manhattan telephone exchange, would recount. "I took him to a doctor in the hope that he would be able to do something. My other son was quite the opposite, so macho. At sixteen, when he discovered his homosexual tendencies, Frank was totally confused. He confided in his brother, who said: 'Talk to Mom about it!' I knew he'd tried to go out with two or three girls. He said to me: 'Mom, I'm gay.' I told him: 'You're my son, that's all that matters to me.' All I asked was that he stayed a man. It was that time in the sexual revolution when a lot of gays were dressing up as girls. I said to him: 'Your sexual preferences are one thing, but I won't have you making yourself look ridiculous by disguising yourself as a woman. Whatever you do, do it with dignity and respect.' I got to know the boys he was mixing with. He brought them home. They were nice boys. Most of his friends adopted me as their mother.

"One day, Frank fell ill. It all began with his losing weight for no accountable reason. Although he'd never been exactly plump, I could tell he was losing maybe one pound a week. He didn't realize what was happening. Suddenly bruises appeared on his legs and he started to cough. At night I listened for his breathing. It made a very distressing sound like a piston. Last April, he said to me: 'Mom, I've got AIDS.' I'd heard the word before. One of our neighbors, who was a warden at Sing Sing penitentiary, had told us about a prisoner who'd died of AIDS. I'd paid very little attention at the time. When Frank told me about his illness, I broke down and sobbed. Then I went to look for my Bible. I have a firm faith and I thought there must be a reason for this ordeal. I said to Frank: 'There is a meaning for everything the Lord allows. Perhaps He wanted to use you.' I read him passages from the Scriptures. He started going to church. The church people in our parish were wonderful. To get them all to pray for him, I told them my son had cancer. In his case, it wasn't a lie.

"Twice Frank nearly died. The last time, the people looking after him gave up the struggle—all of them except the Lord and me. I stayed with him day and night. I fed him a spoonful at a time. I filled him full of vitamins, tonics, ice cream, all the things he liked. Above all, I never stopped encouraging him to fight, hope, and want to live. Every day, in the room next door, the nurses were closing some dead person's eyes. Frank is still there. No one else in the ward is as fiercely resolved to bear the disease. He has made me promise that if the worst happens to him, I will be a mother to the other patients. Many of them have been abandoned by their families. A lot of the parents will accept that their children have AIDS, but not that they are gay."

*   *   *

That autumn of 1985 there was no mother, no family, or companion in the life of twenty-seven-year-old Randy, a former drug-addict prisoner at Sing Sing. Years of isolation in a top-security wing there had transformed the New Jersey longshoreman into a wild animal, ever ready to pounce on anyone who ventured into his hospital room. His lungs were riddled with pneumonia, but there was no shortage of breath: he did not speak, he screamed. Whenever someone came running in response to his uproar, he would greet them with a barrage of insults and threats. He was a difficult patient who severely tried the nerves of Dehovitz and the staff. He confirmed their belief that looking after AIDS patients was as much a question of tender loving care as a purely medical issue.

"Going into a patient's room to spend a little time listening to him can be an act of therapy a hundred times more effective than giving him an intravenous," Jack Dehovitz would say. "Making him feel he is respected, considered, loved, that no one is judging him. What can be more life supporting than taking his hand, applying a little balm to a painful limb, and massaging it gently? Certain patients would tell you that no one dared to touch them for months. What is terrible is dealing with an illness where we have no cure, and all we can try to do is to give our patients the best possible quality of life for the time that remains to them."

The ethnic and social diversity among the patients required constant adaptation to each individual situation. Getting through to people, conquering their distrust, allaying their fear, took a wealth of patience and imagination that only a willing and highly motivated staff could provide.

The nurse Ron Peterson, a marine veteran of the Vietnam War who switched to modern dance prior to his nursing career, had the idea of providing gymnastic courses for St. Clare's patients. "It was a revelation," he would say. "All at once people found they could do something with their bodies, that they weren't just paralyzed wrecks confined to their beds. I even taught dance movements to poor guys stuck in wheelchairs." Ron had seen so many broken, despairing men in Vietnam that he took a keen interest in helping patients to put their affairs in order and come to terms with the idea of death in such a way that, "when the time came, they would not die hating themselves."

Strangely enough, the terror the disease inspired did not discourage the influx of candidates wanting to work in this special care unit. "AIDS is the tragedy of our generation," Terry Miles, the young clinic coordinator, would say. "I'm here because I believe it's my duty to take part in the struggle and do everything I can to help win it." Other applicants with similar commitments had personal reasons for their involvement. Usually they knew someone who had AIDS or had already died of it. Some were gay themselves and were conscious that because of their lifestyle they were at risk.

Still, it was difficult to teach at St. Clare's Hospital that they would first and foremost have to "help the dying to die." A number of nurses cracked up very quickly and disappeared after a few days. Others were under so much stress that their behavior changed to a point where they had to be sent away, like the nurse who, finding himself surrounded by drug addicts, began frantically to down pints of coffee. The addiction of his patients had contaminated him. Others discovered their own homosexual tendencies when brought into contact with gay patients and took flight. Yet others became so attached to their patients that they couldn't bear to see them die. "Day after day, they would go back to the room the patient had left, with a bunch of flowers in their hands and their eyes brimming with tears," one nurse would remember.

That autumn of 1985 was particularly murderous at St. Clare's. At one point the disease claimed three or four victims in less than a week. "An atmosphere of mourning, helplessness, depression, fell over the whole department at that time," Terry Miles would recount. "The whole thing seemed to be getting more difficult." The former Vietnam marine Ron Peterson felt he was losing his grip. Unable to confide in his friends, in the end he went to see a psychoanalyst. "Anyone confronted with that sort of situation needs to talk to someone about what they're going through. Otherwise you risk projecting your anxiety onto the patients." To ward off this danger, Terry Miles organized group therapy sessions for the staff. There they could all come and air their grievances, unload their frustrations, and share their anxieties with regard to a particular patient. "It was invaluable to be able to exchange impressions, express your misery, be comforted by your colleagues, feel that you were not alone, that others were facing the same crises," a black nurse named Gloria Taylor acknowledged.

*   *   *

A veteran of the intensive-care units for open-heart surgery at several major New York hospitals, Gloria was one of the mainstays of St. Clare's. With her generous bosom, her unaltering smile, and her Southern accent, she was like a black character from an antebellum plantation. No one could have taken on her work with more fervor and compassion. A woman from a humble background, she came in each morning from Queens to help patients on the point of death pass away with dignity. AIDS had robbed her of her dearest childhood friend. "He was my foster brother. My mother had adopted him as her son. He was gay, but that had never counted for much with us." When she knew he was about to die, she had him admitted to the hospital where she had been working. She fought like a tigress for him to be treated decently, "but because of this terrible disease that no one knew anything about, he was treated as if he had the plague." His death under such circumstances upset her so much, she had wanted to burn her nurse's uniform. It was then that she read an article in a newspaper announcing the opening of a special unit at St. Clare's. She rushed at once to the address given. "All I wanted," she would say, "was to give others the gentleness and kindness my little brother had been denied." Each patient entrusted to her became thereafter her "little brother." She had a gift for welcoming new patients and putting them instantly at their ease. "Hi, I'm Gloria and I'm pleased to meet you and be able to look after you; I'd like you to call me by my first name. You'll see, we're going to get along just fine." As she explained to her colleagues, "when people are dying there's no time for all that Mr.- or Mrs.-ing." This familiarity prompted an immediate complicity between her and her patients, even those who seemed most suspicious or hostile. That autumn, Gloria, with her overflowing tenderness and her innate gifts as a nurse, brought a little relief to the nightmare at St. Clare's.

The most difficult cases were kept for her, like that of Damien, a twenty-eight-year-old decorator whose brain was gradually being consumed by AIDS. "He was a marvelous man but as stubborn as a mule. He could shut himself off for whole days without speaking at all. He still knew how to hold a fork in his fingers, but he no longer knew that next he was supposed to raise it to his mouth to feed himself. Getting him to swallow a few mouthfuls became an obsession with me. Every spoonful of food, every swallow of liquid he took were my only pitiful victories over his illness. I would sit for hours on the edge of his bed playing with him, telling him stories, coaxing him into taking a little ice cream or yogurt." Everyone at St. Clare's performed the impossible to encourage people to take some nourishment. Dispensers of soup, salad, desserts, and other delicacies had even been installed in the corridors so that the least desire to nibble at something could be satisfied at any hour of the day or night.

One morning Gloria entered Damien's room and found him sitting on his bed eating his excrement. "I thought my heart was going to stop. I stood motionless, incapable of saying or doing anything. Finally, I asked: 'Is it good?' What else could I say? He threw me a mischievous look and replied: 'Very tasty.' When he finished, he took the end of his sheet and carefully wiped his lips. He then cleaned his fingers and wiped the rim of his plate like someone with good manners. Then he beamed with pleasure. I felt like screaming, but no sound could come out of my mouth. All that was left were my tears, to curse the virus which had destroyed the sanity of my little brother."

*   *   *

Gloria and her nursing teammates at St. Clare's had many other occasions, that autumn, to curse the diabolical virus, which Robert Gallo and Luc Montagnier were both claiming to have discovered. The growing number of drug-addict patients made the task at St. Clare's more difficult with each passing day. Like Randy, the ex-longshoreman, many patients had spent long periods in prison.

"Drug addicts were very different in character from homosexuals," Gloria would explain. "They denied their illness. To them, only one thing counted: getting their drug allowance. If you said to them 'That syringe will kill you,' they would answer: 'I couldn't give a damn. I'll take that risk.' First they had to be detoxified because keeping active, aggressive drug addicts in the ward was out of the question. AIDS, they couldn't give a damn. What they wanted was to take a trip. We had to part company with some sick people whose friends continued to supply them. Others we had to put in quarantine. It could take three or four weeks before we were able to reduce their dosage and therefore their drug addiction, depending on the level of intoxication. For those used to up to four hundred dollars' worth of powder a day, it took longer. You couldn't take it too fast for fear of killing them. Too abrupt a withdrawal could cause patients to sweat and hallucinate and trigger suicidal behavior. So we took it a step at a time with the help of substitute medicines.

"Junkies are extraordinary comic actors ready to resort to all kinds of subterfuge: pretending to be dying for lack of drugs, or claiming some upset had made them sick so they needed another dose. But with an old dog like me, they got nowhere. I won't forget our conversations.

" 'Just show me where you've vomited,' I asked one of them one day. He wore an expression of sincere regret. 'Impossible, Gloria, I've flushed it down.' 'You've flushed it,' I insisted. 'It's six weeks since you've gotten out of bed and now all of a sudden you've managed to get to the toilet?' He looked at me, unperturbed. 'Yeah, Gloria, today I managed to walk to the toilet all by myself.'

"The poor guy was covered with Kaposi's pustules. Herpes had eaten up half of his retina. He was almost blind. He had maybe three months to live. He laughed at our efforts to treat him for AIDS. What he wanted was his fix. He would have sold his father and mother for a capsule of powder."

If the slaves of hard drugs were a class apart in the confines of St. Clare's, survivors of the bathhouses did not always get away without similar urges for their fix. From simple poppers to injections of cocaine offering their bursts of adrenaline and twelve hours of guaranteed cheap nirvana, drugs were also a habit for numerous hypersexual gay men. Of all the drug addicts Gloria tried to win over that autumn, none gave her more trouble than Randy, the former inmate of Sing Sing. His yells and vulgarity brought a reign of ever greater terror to the corridors of St. Clare's.

Gloria Taylor's Story

By now Randy weighed no more than about a hundred pounds, but he still had the strength of Hercules. He used to try and scratch and bite me every time I picked him up like a child to carry him to the shower. In the space of six weeks, I succeeded in turning him into a lamb. I managed to make him discover something he had never felt in his life before: that someone loved him. I put him in a wheelchair and took him from room to room. Soon he had made a whole host of friends among the other patients and staff. He used to call me "baby." He had become the most affectionate of guys and I couldn't bring myself to accept the idea that he was going to die. He knew exactly what lay in store for him. He had already witnessed the horrible deaths of two of his friends. He used to say to me: "I don't want to go like that."

One morning, he took hold of my hand and said, "Baby, I'd like you to arrange a party in my room and invite all my buddies. I want to say good-bye to them."

He sent me out to buy toys for his little two-year-old daughter, whom he had only seen once through prison bars. He also wanted to see his parents again. He hadn't had the chance to give them a hug for fifteen years, since just before his first burglary. He also got me to invite one of the wardens from Sing Sing he had liked. As Christmas was drawing very close, I suggested he get his parents a present. "What might they like?" he asked me.

I'm not personally very religious, but I always encourage patients to seek support and comfort wherever they can, and especially in their faith. In the nurses' offices there's a sheet of paper posted with a list of all patients who want the presence of a minister of the church. A letter before each name identifies their religion: *C* for Catholic, *H* for Hebrew, *P* for Protestant. It's known as the pastoral list.

"You know what, I think the nicest gift for your parents would be for you to invite the chaplain to your party, too," I answered. "That way he'll be able to anoint you with the holy oils in their presence."

"Yeah," he exclaimed, delighted, "I think you're right. I couldn't give them anything better."

On the day of the party, there were about twenty people around his bed. Some had brought cakes, others flowers, and even balloons and garlands. Someone had come with a tape recorder. The room was filled with jazz. Randy was having more and more difficulty breathing, every gesture took an effort, but his face shone with a serene joy. The chaplain recited the last rites, then made the sign of the cross on Randy's forehead with cotton wool steeped in oil. In distress, his mother burst into tears. She left the room. Then Randy said a few words of farewell to each one as if he were going away on a journey. I had sat his daughter on his bed. He stroked her cheek with his thin, wrinkled hand. He seemed happy.

Suddenly, he was shaken with spasms. His breathing became irregular. I put the oxygen mask on him, but he tore it off. He smiled at us. His eyes sought out his mother. Not finding her, he made a sign to me to come nearer.

"Baby, give me your hand," he murmured.

He seemed content. I saw the lids close gently over his eyes like a theater curtain at the end of the last act. The virus had taken another of my "little brothers."

51

A Hundred Pounds of Herring Sperm to Avert a Tragedy

Research Triangle Park–Bethesda, USA: Autumn 1985

It really did look like a miracle. Since July 1985, when the on-cologist Sam Broder had begun to administer AZT to nineteen patients in his hospital at Bethesda, Barbara had been able to choose the mink coat her husband had promised her and take up nursing again. There was plenty of grounds for hope. But in medicine, nothing is more illusory than a miracle. "The legitimate euphoria those promising starts evoked mustn't be allowed to make us lose sight of the reality of the situation," David Barry of Burroughs Wellcome would say. "We had been picking our way through the unpredictable world of viral infections for too long to allow our-selves to be taken by that sort of success, spectacular though it might be." Dr. David Barry could remember the experience he had encountered while he was an intern at Yale with idoxuridine given to subjects suffering from fatal viral encephalitis. The biochemist who had developed this substance had tried it out on three patients. Two having survived, he concluded a little too quickly that the product was effective in 66 percent of the cases. As it happened, not only did it prove to be dangerous, but it even accelerated the deaths of several people. "The scientist who recommended this treatment had not studied the evolving effect of the disease, nor had he taken into account the fact that a certain percentage of sick people always survive their illness," David Barry explained. "An individual's immune reactions can vary from one day to the next without our understanding why. That could have been what had happened in Barbara's case. To claim that her apparent cure was due to our AZT was to confuse our wishes with facts. It might just be an instance of spontaneous recovery."

David Barry had good reason to be cautious. The history of therapeutics abounds with deceptive phenomena. First of all, there is the famous "placebo effect," the astonishing progress attributable to suggestion alone. Better morale often activates the appetite, which awakens the immune defenses that can check certain pathological manifestations. The fact of being involved in clinical trials in a highly specialized environment—where patients are more closely monitored—can also prove to be decisive. How were the researchers to know whether these various elements had had a role to play in the results achieved, and if so, what role? In any case, even if they had been able to prove the beneficial effects of AZT on the majority of the first patients treated, this initial experiment on humans was too limited, both in terms of duration and in the number of participants. The researchers were not in a position to predict whether this improvement would last. In the long term the virus could show itself to be resistant to the medicine as side effects would come to light after prolonged use. "In short, the benefits reaped initially could disappear at any moment," David Barry said. The false hopes vested in other substances, such as the HPA-23 that Rock Hudson had tried without avail, should serve as a lesson to the Burroughs Wellcome team to redouble their caution and discretion. But how could a similar discretion be expected of patients who found themselves apparently saved after taking AZT?

*   *   *

As soon as he got back to Florida, the comedian, who only a few weeks earlier had been unable to walk without crutches, proclaimed loudly and clearly in front of television cameras that a medicine had just cured him of AIDS. "Everyone who has the disease should have the right to AZT treatment," he declared in the course of paying homage to the laboratory that manufactured it. David Barry recalled, "Our switchboard was immediately jammed with requests." He himself did not hesitate to answer numerous callers. Sick people whose almost inaudible voices signaled their imminent end mustered what was left of their strength to beg for the remedy. Parents of drug addicts described the agony of their children with cerebral toxoplasmosis, which was making them blind or crazy. Activists rang to express their indignation that AZT was not already on sale at drugstores.

There were also people who telephoned to report "I've just had diarrhea and I sweat a lot at night. If I'm not given something, I know I'm going to die. Please send me some of your medicine at once." An anxious mother explained that her fifteen-year-old daughter had just lost her virginity to a man with a reputation for bisexuality and that she was convinced she had caught AIDS. As she had read in the press that by taking AZT there was a chance of arresting the effect of the virus, she wanted to know how to obtain the necessary doses. Lawyers and film agents intervened on behalf of their clients, who often included well-known politicians and actors. They offered the most extravagant sums and were at times highly unpleasant. Some of them had no qualms about threatening lawsuits "for failing to assist a person whose life was endangered," even making death threats if their appeals went unanswered.

There were also poignant requests from practitioners confronted with the horror of the disease. David Barry would remember the call from Dr. Durack of the clinical center at nearby Duke University. A jovial father of four children, he begged David Barry to send some AZT for a nineteen-year-old boy who was a hemophiliac. His name was Steve. Originally from a town in the far reaches of South Carolina, he had contracted AIDS as a result of a blood transfusion. Despite his weakness and his increasingly severe bouts of illness, he had been struggling to keep up his secondary studies. Two months before his exam, parents complained about the presence of an AIDS carrier in the institution their children attended. The headmaster asked him not to come back to school. Rising to the challenge, Steve completed his studies by correspondence and graduated with distinction. The graduation ceremony should have been one of the finest days of the few months that he had to live. But he was denied permission to take his place among his classmates or mount the platform to receive his award. Instead he was obliged to follow the celebrations, hidden behind a curtain, out of sight. And it was through this same curtain where, after everyone else was gone, he was stealthily presented with his certificate on the end of a pair of fire tongs. A few days later, an overwhelming attack of shingles covered his body with ulcerations so painful he had to be taken to the hospital and installed in a room apart so that his groans would not upset the other patients. The lack of any support from his family added to his pain.

"How was I to remain deaf to such injustice?" David Barry asked. The vice president of Burroughs Wellcome put a small bottle with capsules of AZT in his pocket, got in his car, and sped to the hospital. "The poor kid was in agony," Barry recalled. "There was no chance of his surviving six months, the minimum time stipulated for anyone to be able to take part in a clinical trial. In the face of so much suffering, a criterion of that kind seemed highly incongruous. I handed the AZT over to his doctor and I wished Steve all the luck in the world." Four weeks later his shingles had disappeared and he was able to join the other teenagers in his town as they ran from house to house collecting the traditional Halloween candies. As an act of defiance against the death he had just beaten, he chose to dress up as a skeleton.

*   *   *

People were not content just to telephone. Some of them turned up at Research Triangle Park to besiege the Burroughs Wellcome laboratory. The media had so highly praised the medicine that they were bent on getting some for a relative or someone close to them at any price. The employees in the reception area needed unlimited patience to make these visitors, the bearers of last hope of so many people condemned to death, understand that it was impossible to grant their requests. One day, David Barry received a call for help from one of the receptionists: a man was refusing to leave until he had spoken to the manager. He went down to the lobby accompanied by his colleague Tom Kennedy, an Irishman adept at untangling the most delicate situations. They found themselves face-to-face with an extremely thin man in his fifties who looked like a tramp. The unfortunate individual told them with heartbreaking sincerity that his companion was dying in Miami. "He's my whole life," he said. "Ever since he's been unable to eat, I've stopped eating myself. His suffering is my suffering. I won't leave here until you've given me the means to save him." David Barry explained that his company had plans for wide-scale experiments in which his friend would certainly be able to take part. The visitor remained unreceptive to this reasoning. "It was tragic and touching at the same time," the doctor said later. "That man was giving us a magnificent lesson about love, but our consciences as men of science were commanding us not to respond to his supplication."

Among the appeals that reached the pharmaceutical laboratory that autumn was one from a New York doctor. Dr. Jack Dehovitz represented an example of the growing frustration felt by hundreds of American doctors faced with this intolerable situation: a medicine did exist, it had already shown itself to be effective, but it was not available to patients. Haunted by the suffering of Josef Stein, and the numerous other patients who lay in agony at St. Clare's Hospital, Jack Dehovitz urged those in charge in North Carolina to "get a move on so we can at last have something to give those accusing us of letting them die without doing anything."

*   *   *

Certainly, they had to get a move on. But with what? The clinical trials carried out on Sam Broder's nineteen patients and the two patients from the medical center at Duke University had used up the very last grams of AZT accumulated the previous spring when they had bought up all the world's reserves of herring sperm. The chemists at Burroughs Wellcome, for their part, had not yet succeeded in reproducing in the laboratory the famous substance contained in the sea fish's sperm. There was good reason for this delay: the synthesizing of thymidine is highly complex. It requires a sequence of seventeen operations and a level of knowledge that very few laboratories in the world had mastered at that time. The production of AZT also presented certain dangers that necessitated the construction of special equipment, including enormous glass tanks to prevent the explosion of the thymidine molecules on contact with metal elements.

A solution to the lack of base material was found thanks to Sam Broder. He remembered that twenty years earlier, the National Cancer Institute had acquired all of the world's herring sperm in existence at the time—about a hundred pounds—for an experiment on patients with cancerous tumors. It had been very swiftly recognized that the product did not have the beneficial effect anticipated. The experiment was abandoned. Persuaded that the stock must still be there forgotten in the depths of some dusty storeroom, the cancer specialist appealed at once to the unit of Developmental Therapeutic Programs. He asked the employee there to "dig out the hundred pounds of herring sperm as a matter of urgency." A few minutes later, the unusual cargo had been located.

"Perfect!" exclaimed Sam Broder to the efficient official. "Send it immediately to the Burroughs Wellcome laboratory at Research Triangle Park. And don't, whatever you do, ask me to fill out a whole pile of forms. It's urgent. Just send the goods!"

His tone did not invite further discussion. The combatants against AIDS would receive their new supplies just in time.

52

A Celestial Welcome for the Commando Squadron in White Saris

Calcutta, India–New York, USA:
Autumn 1985–Winter 1986

It was one of the most beautiful scenes her nearly blind eyes could have witnessed. Through the milky veil of her double cataracts, Mother Teresa made out the contours of the procession as it made its way through the cathedral nave singing the *Magnificat*. That December morning, forty of her novices, with candles in their right hands, the scroll sealing the profession of their faith in their left, were about to take the vows of the Missionaries of Charity at the foot of the altar decorated with white lilies. At the head of the procession, the former little leper girl from the funeral pyres of Benares walked proudly and with obvious radiance. Ananda was dressed like her companions in the white silk sari of Bengali Christian brides, her forehead encircled with a coronet of flowers. Sister Ananda had overcome the obstacle of her karma. For her, that day was like a second birth. With a pounding heart, she came and knelt on the first step of the altar to receive the tokens of her new life from the hands of the archbishop of Calcutta. "Receive, my child, the symbol of your crucified spouse," declared Monseigneur Picachy, an Anglo-Indian originally from Bombay, as he handed her the olive-wood crucifix that the Missionaries of Charity wear on their chest. Then the prelate placed in her hands the humble white cotton sari bordered with blue that would be her only apparel from that day onward. "May this holy habit lead you ever in the steps of the Lord, may it give you access to the homes of the poor, there to be a bearer of His light and quench His thirst for souls."

When all the novices had received their crucifixes and saris, the procession made its way, singing, to the sacristy at the back of the church. The parents of the new sisters crowded after them to witness the act that symbolized the formal breaking of their children with the past. In the absence of her father and mother, whom she had not seen since they banished her, Ananda was thrilled to catch sight of Sister Bandona. The Nepalese sister had come from Benares to join in a day that was a coronation for so much effort, so many shared hopes. Behind her, Sister Ananda also recognized, under the thin veil of a red, festive sari, the reassuring smile of Domenica, her old Mauritian friend from the home for the dying. Next to her was her new husband, the German doctor Rudolf Benz, looking younger than ever with his perpetual diamond in his ear and his hair tied back in a ponytail.

Next, Mother Teresa made her entrance, a pair of scissors in her hand. In an emotional silence, she cut the long black braids of Sister Ananda and her companions to symbolize the severance with the past. Traditionally their parents carefully gathered up in cotton squares these relics of the world they had just left. The novices then had to change out of their bridal outfits into their religious habits. A sister handed them candles, which they lit from the one Mother Teresa was holding. Then the procession returned, singing, to the cathedral nave. The solemn moment had arrived. Heard against the creaking of old fans that stirred up the moist air, there rose the clear, firm voice of the former little ex-leper from Benares.

"I, Sister Mary Ananda, vow and promise to Almighty God and to the Blessed Virgin Mary, in your hands, Mother Mary Teresa, poverty, chastity, obedience, and wholehearted free service to the poorest of the poor."

With this pledge, on December 8, 1985, Ananda became the 2,458th sister to join the order Mother Teresa had founded.

*   *   *

A noisy and joyous celebration awaited the new "brides of Christ" on their return to the convent on Lower Circular Road. As on the occasion of real Indian weddings, families, friends, all the sisters, novices, and postulants from Calcutta and its surroundings, had gathered in the courtyard decorated with flowers, lanterns, and streamers.

Their foreheads marked in accordance with Indian tradition by a red dot of welcome, and garlands around their necks, Sister Ananda and her companions were embraced by Mother Teresa. Her face radiant with happiness, the elderly nun blessed them one after another.

"Let there always be a smile on your lips, Ananda," she whispered as she placed her hands on the young sister's head. "Never forget that it isn't just your work that the poor need, but especially a joyful heart."

Sister Ananda moved ahead to join the crowd in celebration. Arrayed before her all in white, the postulants were dancing energetically in a ring to the sound of a harmonium and *bhajans*. They were ancient rhythmic Bengali songs, half hymns, half poems celebrating the name of Jesus and his saints. Others were scattering a shower of rose, jasmine, and marigold petals from the stories above. Yet others were throwing confetti or waving the flames of multicolored candles as they danced.

Tradition had it that these celebrations were brought to a conclusion with the announcement of the sisters' postings. Unable this year to read the list herself because of her failing eyes, Mother Teresa asked Sister Paul to make the announcements for her. Sister Ananda knew this would be a major turning point in her life. "We all felt very strange as Sister Paul went through our names, and then read the names of towns and countries most of which we had never heard of. I had to wait almost to the end to learn that Mother Teresa had decided to send me to New York. The very next day I was to go and live in the United States with three other sisters, to work in a home for the sick." One comforting piece of news relieved Sister Ananda's apprehension at the prospect of this adventure into a foreign world. Sister Paul, the nun who had trained her at the home for the dying during her novitiate years, had been chosen by Mother Teresa to run the new Missionaries of Charity hospice in New York.

*   *   *

The American customs officials at John F. Kennedy Airport were amazed. They had rarely seen such a strange assortment of baggage come off an airplane before. It was as if immigrants from the previous century were landing on American soil with their few miserable possessions. There were buckets, secondhand cooking utensils, cardboard boxes tied up with pieces of string, patched jute sacks crammed full of linen and rags, mattresses rolled up in bits of cloth, old umbrellas, plastic sandals, brooms, aprons, and even Indian newspapers. On each pile of this unlikely bric-a-brac was scrawled a name and address inscribed in blue ink: MOTHER TERESA—NEW YORK—USA.

That was the rule. Every time the Missionaries of Charity went to start a home anywhere, even when it was in one of the richest capitals of the West, they took with them from Calcutta everything they needed. Mother Teresa had given strict instructions to the archbishop of New York with regard to the furnishing of the building on Washington Street. The spirit of poverty of all her institutions must be respected, especially when it came to the basement that was to serve as her community's convent. For beds there were to be no box springs and plump mattresses, but simple metal frames salvaged from other people's rejects, on which the sisters could lay out their straw mats. For furniture all they would need would be a bench and stools. Packing cases or cardboard boxes would serve as shelves on which to keep their prayer books. There would be no need for a refrigerator or a washing machine, much less air-conditioning or television. Not one penny was to be wasted, even on toilet paper.

The daughter of the Benares cremator would long remember the amazing reception New York had in store for her. "It was the first time in my life I had seen snowflakes falling out of the sky. Little by little the trees, houses, and cars hid themselves under a vast white sari. It was enchanting!" Wide-eyed with amazement, Sister Paul and the other sisters shared that enchantment. Soon the car belonging to the young volunteer coworker who had come to collect them was practically engulfed in a maelstrom of "white cotton." For superstitious Indian women sensitive to such manifestations of the forces of nature, this snowstorm could only be a sign from heaven, the welcoming greeting of their Creator. Dazzled, Ananda could not help thinking of the canticle of Daniel. The words of the prophet she had so frequently recited in the blazing heat of Calcutta were becoming a reality. Her clear voice intoned happily, "O ye frost and cold, O ye ice and snow, praise ye the Lord; praise Him and magnify Him forever." Taken up at once by the other sisters, repeated at the top of their voices, the psalm provided the joyous accompaniment for their journey through the squall to the door of their New York home.

Another surprise awaited Ananda. The two workmen busy installing the telephone for the future hospice had skin even darker than hers. It came as a great shock to someone who ever since she was a child had believed herself condemned to social abjection and who had always associated dark skin with ugliness. The ex-pariah from Benares was exultant. "The good Lord was showing me that He had created beautiful beings much darker than me!" she would say. "He wanted to convince me that I wasn't as ugly as I'd always thought I was."

There was no end to the astonishment America evoked that day in the travelers from Calcutta. Despite Mother Teresa's recommendations, well-wishers had too zealously equipped the house with all the household appliances an American home would normally have. Sister Ananda stood rooted for a long time in front of the battery of machines that occupied the far end of the living room. Apart from the refrigerators she had seen in Calcutta in the shop windows of Park Street, on the way to the home for the dying, all these devices were as strange to her as satellites orbiting in outer space. Sister Paul was quick to use her authority to ask for the immediate removal of this superfluous equipment. Only the large pipe fixed to one of the walls escaped unnoticed. Wanting to find out what it was for, Sister Ananda burnt her fingers. The young Indian girl had discovered one precious advantage of modern comfort in a city with arctic winters—central heating.

Her exploration of the basement brought other surprises. The workmen renovating the old presbytery had made one installation they regarded as so basic that they had not even informed the archbishop. To them it went without saying that a shower room would be indispensable to the visitors, even if they were holy women used to the poverty of Calcutta. Neither the funeral pyres of Benares nor the leper clinic on the banks of the Ganges nor the home for the dying had prepared Ananda for this extraordinary discovery. Mouth and eyes agog, she surveyed with a mixture of interest and fear the large shiny shower head attached to the ceiling. Timidly she touched one of the tap handles. Did you really only have to turn it for water to spurt from this metal spring? She could not believe it. Like so many Indians, Sister Ananda had an almost carnal relationship with water. Since earliest childhood her days had constantly been taken up with carrying water, sometimes to the point of exhaustion. She had never filled a bucket or a pitcher other than with the strength of her own arms. That grueling daily task had deformed her skeleton and imbued her with an almost religious respect for water, an acute sense of its value and scarcity, of the absolute necessity to conserve it. In India people could not afford to waste it. One used the same water first for washing oneself, then for washing the laundry, and finally for washing the floors.

Sister Ananda crossed herself, reached out a trembling hand, and turned the handle. At once a veritable deluge rained down from the ceiling. Hypnotized, she watched the flow of water. She was gripped not so much by the sight of the powerful jet as by the sound that it made, reviving memories of the monsoon's beating down upon the Ganges River, the sudden battering of tropical showers that turned the fields around Benares green again, a bombardment from heaven bringing a little coolness to the baking heat of summer. Ananda listened in ecstasy to the falling water. Caught up in the spell of her memories, she threw herself under the shower fully dressed. Arms outstretched, head bent back, she gave herself up to the marvelous stream. She felt the water, the heat, penetrate her as it had done in her childhood, when the clouds had dispensed their life-giving manna to humankind and its arid lands. Only an Indian could have savored that moment of communion, of unspeakable happiness. Once more she felt the urge to sing. "O ye showers and dew, praise ye the Lord, and O ye stars of heaven, praise Him and magnify Him forever . . ."

Drawn by the sound of Ananda's voice ringing out through the whole house, Sister Paul and the three other sisters came running. Seeing their companion enjoying herself like a child, they broke into howls of laughter. Mother Teresa could set her mind at rest. Her sisters were beginning their mission in New York with joy in their hearts.

53

Next Year in Jerusalem

New York, USA: Autumn 1985–Winter 1986

Life was not all tragedy at New York's St. Clare's Hospital. There were real celebrations, too. One evening in December, the whole nursing team, led by Dr. Jack Dehovitz, and all the patients on the floor who still had strength enough to walk a few steps, invaded Josef Stein's room to celebrate his departure with him. A new chemotherapy based on vinblastine, an herbal extract with anticancerous properties from the forests of the Amazon, had practically made the oral infection from his Kaposi's sarcoma disappear. The ex-archaeologist had started to eat again and had already put on several pounds. No one bumping into him in the street would have guessed he had AIDS and might not have long to live.

This victory had not been achieved without pain. Chemotherapy is an ordeal all patients dread because of its unpleasant effects— nausea, vomiting, migraine, diarrhea, sweating, shivering, skin eruptions, often in association with acute anemia. Some subjects react so badly to the toxicity of several medications that the functioning of their heart and breathing has to be monitored very carefully. Above all, people have to be prepared to break off treatment at any moment. There are, however, some odd exceptions. The nurse Gloria Taylor had a black transvestite in her care who "ate like a horse" after every chemotherapy session, whereas usually she had the greatest difficulty in getting him to swallow even a spoonful of soup.

Jack Dehovitz and his team were not laboring under any illusions: Josef Stein's apparent cure was only a temporary remission. In a few months, perhaps only a few weeks or even a few days, they would see him back again, hardly able to stand. All the drama of AIDS derived from these constant regressions. "We would stop one infection, control a tumor here or there, but it was no good. The disease would advance no less inexorably. For one thing, the virus is still there, and for another, the breakdown of the immune system favors the development of all kinds of opportunistic diseases. We have various forms of treatment we can use against the symptoms of infections and cancer, but alas, nothing against the virus itself. Complications crop up one after another, become worse, and eventually get the better of the patient's resistance." Dr. Sam Broder in his hospital at Bethesda, Michael Gottlieb in Los Angeles, Paul Volberding in San Francisco, and Willy Rozenbaum in Paris, like all the world's doctors having to deal with AIDS, shared Dehovitz's frustration that winter.

Always on the lookout for the sensational, the media, on the other hand, would periodically proclaim the discovery of some new panacea. That was how a television team from CBS happened to turn up one morning at St. Clare's Hospital to interview both a patient and a doctor about an experimental medicine based on interferon that purported to cure Kaposi's tumors. "The interviewer was bent on getting me to say come what may that I had enormous hopes vested in the substance and that I was very keen to use it," Dehovitz would recount. "Having experienced so many disappointments, I still had difficulty getting excited about any new treatment. Of course, I kept abreast of what was published about the product in question, and I knew that some of my colleagues had already used it. Without being particularly overenthusiastic, I simply expressed my intention of using it myself, on the same basis as other medications. The television team then descended on Josef Stein's room. After dramatically filming his lesions from every possible angle, the interviewer proceeded to inform him that a new remedy had just been found that could rapidly improve his condition. The film was shown that same evening during the news hour. My words had quite simply been cut to give more impact to the reaction of an AIDS victim discovering under the scrutiny of millions of television viewers that a new drug could save him. The result of this untimely reporting by the media was deplorable. The report shocked poor Josef so much that he caused a violent scene, accusing me of not trying to cure him because I wasn't making use of everything medical science was discovering."

Like most AIDS patients, Josef Stein took a very active interest in the development of his disease, in the treatment he received, and in the progress research was making. He read the *New York Times* attentively every day, combed through the news weeklies, and even medical journals. He kept a close eye on the television and radio news. By doing so he frequently left himself open to being taken in by the media, which often aroused false hopes in patients. This made the task of doctors even more complicated.

Some patients had no qualms about catching a plane for Mexico and the *farmacias* of Nuevo Laredo or Tijuana to buy remedies. These were prohibited by the FDA within U.S. territory. "In the name of what principles could I stop them when I had no alternative to offer them?" Jack Dehovitz would ask. "Had I the right to restrain men and women who knew they were threatened with imminent death from rushing off to the other side of the world in quest of some potential hope of prolonging their lives? Experience had unfortunately shown that none of the anti-AIDS drugs sold in Mexico or elsewhere were effective. I had looked after patients who had taken them, and unfortunately they had died just like the others. If I'd come across one single one who had been saved by those medicines, I would probably not have had any reservations about breaking the ethical rules of my profession to secretly get hold of these drugs to save some of the people who were dying daily before my very eyes."

*   *   *

That December morning, the spectacular improvement in Josef Stein's condition had brought an air of festivity to the whole floor at St. Clare's. The nursing staff's favorite patient was back on his feet, joyful, triumphant. Happy to have played some part in his friend's cure by going to appeal to the monks of the monastery at Latrun and the prophets of Israel, Sam Blum had brought with him a magnum of Dom Pérignon. "*L'chayim!* Let's toast to life," shouted the son of the Brooklyn rabbi as he poured champagne in the glasses.

"*L'chayim!*" they all repeated in chorus.

There was the sound of clinking glasses. Josef Stein hugged Jack Dehovitz. "You're the king of doctors, Doc!" The chronic infection of Josef's mucous membranes had given his voice a metallic tone.

The young doctor laughed. "Remember, no more *kvetching!*" he responded. "The ward is going to seem pretty empty when you've gone. We're all going to feel a bit lost. Don't forget to keep us in touch with your news."

"I'll send you a postcard from Jerusalem." Josef turned to Sam. "Isn't that right, old man? We're going to go there and provide a real surprise for our paralyzed friend and thank him for his prayers."

*   *   *

Two days before his anticipated departure for Tel Aviv, Josef Stein was awakened by an attack of vomiting that drained him so much he did not have the strength to get up. He could feel lesions once more swelling the lining of his mouth and throat right down into his trachea. Short but very painful fits of coughing began to shake him from head to toe. His high fever, accompanied by violent sweating and shivering, swiftly confirmed the symptoms of a crushing relapse.

Mustering all that was left of his strength, he telephoned Sam. Taking care not to alarm him, he suggested they postpone their journey to Israel to coincide with the following Passover.

"We'll use the opportunity to take our little monk to the Wailing Wall," he said. "What a fantastic act of thanksgiving that will be for him as well as for me!"

Relieved, Josef replaced the receiver. Before collapsing back into his bed, he allowed his hand to wander for a minute over the objects that cluttered his bedside table: the alarm clock he had used as a student; a small carved flint brought back from the dig in Israel, which was probably more than a hundred thousand years old; a silver photograph frame containing the picture taken at the archaeological site at Gezer with Sam and Philippe a few moments before the tragic accident; a copy of the Torah and an old leather-bound edition of the mitzvot, the Jewish commandments.

A ribbon marked one page. Josef had read and reread it many

times recently. He had analyzed every sentence, meditated on every word. It was the mitzvah relating to the prohibition of any attempt to take one's own life. This prohibition was based on a number of sacred texts. The work cited in particular was the rejoinder uttered by the famous rabbi Chanadiah ben Terodyan, who was burnt at the stake in the second century. When people cried out to him to cut short his suffering by inhaling the smoke from the flames deep into his lungs, he replied: "The Creator gave man his soul. He alone can withdraw it. No one has the right to hasten his own death." The chapter contained a reminder that Jewish law denies a person guilty of having terminated his life any religious service or show of mourning, including the keriah rite, the practice by which orthodox Jews show the deceased their sorrow by rending pieces of their clothes at his tomb. However, in the same work, Josef had discovered other commentators who had moderated the absolute intransigence of this commandment. Thus Rabbi Yore Deah had proclaimed that "any person whose existence has become wretched is authorized to abstain from doing anything to prolong it."

Having witnessed so many deaths around him at the St. Clare's Hospital, there was nothing Josef Stein did not know about the dreadful end that lay in store for him. Several times he had written letters on this subject, confiding in his monk friend in Israel. It wasn't the physical suffering in itself he dreaded, but the state of progressive degeneration that fatally destroyed everything that enabled a man to take pride in living. "I have no regrets," he had often reminded those around him. "I've loved everything I've done in life. If I had the chance to start again, I wouldn't change one bit of it." By signing the "do not resuscitate" form at the beginning of his first stay at St. Clare's, he had expressed his wish not to be kept alive by artificial means.

Feeling very sick that morning, he realized how much his condition had degenerated. He thought of the cruel plight of Philippe Malouf, condemned to live out his life in a wheelchair. He sensed that like him he would never again be able to stand on his own two feet as a man. Hadn't the time come for him to put an end to his futile struggle, while he still had the freedom of choice?

On the bedside table was the bottle of white capsules he had been given before he left St. Clare's. The hospital pharmacist had written their name on the label. Dilaudid was an analgesic much stronger than morphine. Josef surveyed with gratitude the small chemical capsules left in their container. They had eased his suffering and sustained his will to live on so many occasions. Usually, one was enough to ease even the most intolerable pain. How many would it take, he wondered, to put an end forever to the ultimate pain of an existence that was now so wretched?

Before seeking the answer, he wanted to speak to the friend who had so often exhorted him to accept his existence to the end, to listen to the voice of Isaiah proclaiming: "He was wounded for our transgressions and with his stripes we are healed." Josef Stein dialed the number of the Abbey of the Seven Agonies at Latrun. As he touched the phone digits, he could see again in his mind's eye the little cemetery behind the church, with its cypress hedge, its asphodel bushes, its rows of wooden crosses planted in the bare earth and marked simply with a series of Christian names.

Brother Philippe was not there. He had been driven into Jerusalem to undergo tests for a forthcoming operation that would give him back the complete use of his fingers.

"Can I give him a message?" asked the voice at the other end of the line.

"Just tell him that his friend Josef Stein wanted to say good-bye before leaving."

*   *   *

Next to the telephone there was always a small pad of paper. Josef Stein seized it and scrawled with difficulty: "Good-bye and mazel tov. I love you all." He tore off the sheet and placed it where it would be readily seen against his bedside lamp. He poured himself a glass of water, took the cap off the bottle of Dilaudid, poured the rest of the capsules into the palm of his hand, and swallowed them one by one.

54

"Life Is Life, Fight for It"
New York, USA: Christmas 1985–Winter 1986

Not since the great longshoremen's strike of the fifties and the demonstrations of the gay liberation movement in the seventies had the narrow street in Greenwich Village witnessed the arrival of so many journalists. Kept at a distance by a police cordon, the occupants of the neighborhood surveyed the most extraordinary of scenes. Scarcely recovered from a cataract operation, her lined face almost entirely obscured by thick, dark glasses, Mother Teresa was busy welcoming arriving dignitaries as they got out of their limousines amidst a maze of microphones and cameras. Mayor Ed Koch effusively shook the hand that the illustrious old lady extended to him under the delighted gaze of the archbishop of New York. John Cardinal O'Connor was triumphant. It was under the auspices of his archdiocese that, today, the first home for destitute AIDS patients was being opened.

On the wall to the right of the front door, the foundress of the Missionaries of Charity insisted a plaque be put up announcing the name of her congregation's new establishment. The cameramen jostled with one another to focus on the three words engraved on it. From now on, the former presbytery at 657 Washington Street would be known as the Gift of Love. Despite her tiredness, the nun had raised no objections to an official opening. "Every AIDS sufferer is the suffering Christ," she announced to the reporters clustering round her frail form. She had chosen Christmas Eve as the opening date because "Jesus was born on that night and I want to help each one to be born to joy, love, and peace."

She had personally chosen the first three residents. She had found them behind the bars of Sing Sing, a penitentiary with a sinister reputation, where she had been taken by an American nun who had dedicated her life to relieving the prisoners' mental and physical anguish. She had been horrified by what she had seen there. Drug abuse was rife in prisons and contaminated syringes spread the epidemic like wildfire. Sick people had no access either to appropriate care or to the slightest touch of psychological comfort. Mother Teresa considered their plight worse than that of the people dying on the sidewalks of Calcutta. She immediately asked for an initial group of three of the sickest to be entrusted to her care.

One of them, Daryl Morsette, aged twenty-seven, had been a dancer at the Electric Circus and the Gilded Grape, two discos in New York. One day when Daryl, an unshakable drug addict, lacked the money to buy his next fix, he had attacked a couple on a street in Manhattan. He found himself in Sing Sing, sentenced to six years' solitary confinement. He had six more months to serve before he could be eligible for parole. Mother Teresa moved heaven and earth to get two representatives from the New York State parole board to come to the convict's bedside and offer him early release.

The devout woman remembered the surprising exchange that took place on that occasion.

"Prisoner Daryl Morsette, you must appreciate that by virtue of this release, you cease to be in the charge of the State," one of the officials informed the prisoner. "That means that you forfeit the benefits of its social and medical support. From now on, you will have to cover all the expenses occasioned by your illness yourself."

The unfortunate man, who was in a very poor condition and covered with the bruises of Kaposi's sarcoma, nodded his head sadly.

"I don't know how many days I've got left to live," he muttered,

"but I'd rather spend them outside than behind these damn bars.
To hell with your medical protection. I prefer my freedom."

*   *   *

Mother Teresa was waiting, surrounded by a mob of journalists
and rubberneckers. Why had the ex-convict and his two sick fellow
prisoners, a couple of petty crooks by the name of Antonio Rivera
and Jimmy Matos, not arrived yet? When at last the flashing light
of an ambulance appeared at the end of the road, she rushed to
meet the vehicle. The pale, emaciated, bearded individual who was
about to get out recoiled for a moment when he saw all the cameras
and microphones thrust in his direction. Mother Teresa did not
recognize him as any of the three inmates of Sing Sing. She discovered then that their condition had seriously deteriorated and the
doctors at St. Clare's—where they had been admitted while they
waited for the Gift of Love home to be ready—had been forced to
place them all under intensive care. Another patient had been sent
in their place for the official inauguration of the home. Taken aback
by this unexpected welcome, Josef Stein allowed himself to be led
by Mother Teresa inside the building, which still smelled of wet
paint. He was even more surprised to be greeted there by the mayor,
the archbishop, and a representative of the governor.

*   *   *

Death had not been ready to take away the former archaeologist.
Suspecting the worst after his friend's telephone call, Sam Blum
had jumped into a taxi. He had arrived just in time. Josef was still
breathing. A stomach pump, intracardiac injections, infusions, oxygen: the St. Clare's mobile revival unit called to the spot had
managed to save the desperate man. The first thing he saw when
he opened his eyes was the fist that Dr. Jack Dehovitz was thrusting
into the air. A victory sign.

"Welcome back to the land of the living!" the doctor exclaimed
warmly.

"Why have you done this?" Josef reproached him in a whisper.

"I don't know, I had no part of it. The emergency rescue team
has done a good job. We're all very pleased."

"For more than three days, Josef didn't stop sobbing," the nurse

Gloria Taylor recalled. "Every time I went into his room, he would catch hold of my arm, squeeze it, and beg me to help him put an end to it all. He was forever pulling out his intravenous tubes so I had to tie his hands."

Once again the patient benefited from a spectacular remission. In under a week, thanks to specially adjusted chemotherapy, his oral infection disappeared, the coughing fits became less frequent. Soon Josef Stein was able to get up. "I felt like a NASA astronaut back from a moon walk," he would say. To force him to eat, every hour Gloria brought him a bowl of his favorite flavor of ice cream—strawberry. "I felt a bit confused. I was ashamed. I looked for the glint of reproach in people's eyes. All I found was kindness."

One morning, the hospital postman brought him a letter from Israel. His monk friend had heard from Sam about the suicide attempt. But Philippe Malouf made no reference to the incident. With his usual enthusiasm, he announced a piece of news that he saw as a marvelous sign. "I have just learned that my little Indian sister Ananda, whom I told you about, has been sent to New York to look after AIDS sufferers in a home Mother Teresa has opened. Providence has sent her to you, my brother. I beg you: go and see her at once."

Josef Stein was rereading his friend's letter when Gloria Taylor burst into his room. The black nurse was exultant.

"Get your clothes on, Josef, you're going on a short journey," she exclaimed. "Mother Teresa needs you."

*   *   *

Confusion reigned at the Gift of Love. Dressed in an embroidered white alb with a golden stole over his shoulders, Cardinal O'Connor flourished his aspergillum over the surrounding heads, sprinkling the freshly renovated building with holy water. As in all her centers throughout the world, Mother Teresa had decorated this home with the emblems of her faith. In the living room on the ground floor, adorned with a huge crucifix, she had herself chalked the words of the Hail Mary on a blackboard. She had been careful to write the last line—"Now and at the hour of our death"—in bold capital letters and underlined them twice. On a shelf on which the sisters had put a picture of her, she had placed two Bibles at the disposal of the sick, one in English and the other in Spanish for the benefit of the Hispanics. At the access to each landing, an inscription indicated the name she had chosen for the different floors. There was Christ the King floor, Saint Joseph, the Immaculate Heart of Mary, and the Sacred Heart of Jesus. The rooms had been christened in a similar way. Josef Stein's had been dedicated to Our Lady of Good Hope. It contained two iron bedsteads, a chest of drawers, a table, a chair, and an armchair covered in green simulated leather. A manifesto posted on the wall was the only decoration. Mother Teresa had composed its text one stormy night thirty years earlier in a leper colony set apart from an Indian village on the banks of the Ganges.

> *Life is an opportunity, benefit from it.*
> *Life is a beauty, admire it.*
> *Life is bliss, taste it.*
> *Life is a dream, realize it.*
> *Life is a challenge, meet it.*
> *Life is a duty, complete it.*
> *Life is a game, play it.*
> *Life is costly, care for it.*
> *Life is wealth, keep it.*
> *Life is love, enjoy it.*
> *Life is mystery, know it.*
> *Life is a promise, fulfill it.*
> *Life is sorrow, overcome it.*
> *Life is a song, sing it.*
> *Life is a struggle, accept it.*
> *Life is a tragedy, confront it.*
> *Life is an adventure, dare it.*
> *Life is luck, make it.*
> *Life is too precious, do not destroy it.*
> *Life is life, fight for it!*

—MOTHER TERESA

Stretched out on his bed, Josef Stein was meditating on these lines when a young sister in a sari came into his room.

"Her face was lit up by a big smile," he remembered. "She joined her hands together at chest height and bowed her head to greet me in her country's traditional way. Instinctively I knew that this was the spiritual fiancée of my monk friend from Latrun."

" 'I'm Sister Ananda,' she told me. 'I'm responsible for Christ the King floor.' "

55

AZT or Placebo: Russian Roulette
Pine Needle Lodge–Bethesda, USA:
Autumn 1985

Now the prime concern of the vice president of the Burroughs Wellcome laboratory and his main collaborators was the choice of strategy. Several options were open. They could start producing AZT right away, thanks to the providential gift of a hundred pounds of herring sperm that Sam Broder had managed to unearth. Above all, the imminent synthesis of thymidine by their chemists made massive production of AZT for wide distribution seem possible. It would cost millions of dollars, but it was workable. Because there was no other anti-AIDS medicine in existence, David Barry knew that such a decision would be welcomed with relief by the medical community, by patients, and by public opinion. It would also be approved by the compassionate woman inspector at the FDA, Ellen Cooper. "We were like the only available snowplow. Everyone was hoping we would clear a path through the storm," Barry would say. "Everyone was prepared to follow us blindly."

Yet the people in charge at Burroughs Wellcome chose a different course, one that would be more expensive and would not meet with public approval, but that was entirely consistent with the prestigious laboratory's rigorous scientific traditions. David Barry and his collaborators opted for more thorough testing of AZT. They wanted to submit it to the verdict of a "double-blind clinical trial." This would involve selecting several hundred patients, dividing them into two homogeneous groups, and administering the AZT to the members of one group while the others were given a neutral product known as the placebo. Neither the patients nor the doctors were to know whether they were taking the medicine or the placebo, hence its description as "double blind."

A comparison of the medical condition of the subjects in the two groups at the end of the experiment would make it possible to evaluate the real effect of the product tested. Most treatments for cardiac disease, urinary and pulmonary infections, and infectious pathologies had been subjected to this system of control. "It was our duty to comply with this method," David Barry would say. "It was the only way we wouldn't be acting as sorcerers with thymidine. We didn't know enough about its benefits and its disadvantages."

There was a chance that this decision would provoke violent objections in the context of a fatal epidemic like AIDS. Michael Gottlieb, the Los Angeles doctor who had diagnosed the first cases of the disease, asked, "Giving people who were likely to die some placebo pills for months on end when a medicine might perhaps save them—wasn't that a violation of the most basic principles of medical ethics?"

*   *   *

A superb eighteen-hole golf course and stables for fifty horses made Pine Needle Lodge a favorite resort for North Carolina's riding and golf enthusiasts. That first weekend of November 1985, some unexpected guests had arranged to meet at this peaceful inn surrounded by pine trees. Dr. David Barry had invited all the key members of his staff there. He was counting on the pastoral calm of the setting to help him respond to the various pressing questions the organization of the double-blind placebo test of AZT would entail.

How many weeks should it go on for? How many subjects were to take part in it? On what basis should they be selected? Should they be in the initial stages of the illness or in its terminal phases? Should they be suffering from pneumocystis pneumonia, Kaposi's sarcoma, or both at the same time? What other medical parameters should be taken into consideration? An abnormally low number of white T-4 cells? A weight loss of more than sixteen pounds in the previous three months? A high fever for more than three weeks for no apparent reason? Regular nocturnal sweating and inexplicable diarrhea? Should drug addicts, children, pregnant women, nursing mothers, be excluded? Should the taking of other medicines, including ordinary aspirin tablets, be prohibited for the duration of the test, even if the subject's condition was deteriorating? The area to be explored was so incredibly vast that "one of us was always having to go and consult some specialist over the telephone," the virologist Sandra Lehrman would recount.

Added to this were the choice of hospitals to conduct the experiment and the checking of the results by the experts at Burroughs Wellcome, the detailed gathering of information, the strict accountability for the pills distributed to patients to prevent theft or illicit traffic, the dosage of treatment, its frequency, the monitoring of patients' physical condition with clinical and biological tests, the action to be taken in the event of negative reaction, the assessment of incidental factors, and the kind of infringements committed by patients that would warrant their exclusion from the experiment. All these considerations were discussed methodically, one by one, analyzed and recorded. The statistical specialists could then store this mass of data on their computers to work out the directives and questionnaires that would form the basis for treatment procedures. One item in particular triggered a special concern of the guests at Pine Needle Lodge. It involved the overriding principle of the operation, the guarantee of secrecy, so that no one would know who was being given the medicine and who was being given the placebo. It was decided that a code number on each bottle would correspond with the code number of the patient for whom it was destined. The key to this code would be locked away in a safe. Only one scientist would know the combination. Built like a sheriff, Richard H. Clemons, aged sixty, was ideally suited for the job. The son of an Iowa farmer, at eighteen he had deserted his father's cornfields to satisfy his craving to be a scientist. His specialty was experiments on human guinea pigs. His colleagues could rest assured that the armor-plated safe in his office would be as inviolate as the gold reserves at Fort Knox.

Before bringing their weekend's work to a close, David Barry and his associates gave a name for the operation that they had just broadly outlined. This was the fifty-third offensive that the pharmaceutical laboratory was launching against viruses. It was called Operation 53.

*   *   *

Two months later, twelve doctors—ten men and two women—found themselves at the National Institutes of Health on the Bethesda campus. They shared the same commitment to caring for AIDS patients, the same frustration at the abortiveness of their efforts, and the same enthusiasm at the prospect of taking part in the experimental testing of a medicine that offered a glimmer of hope. Chosen by the Burroughs Wellcome staff, they all worked in cities where the epidemic had struck with particular intensity. Among them was Dr. Michael Gottlieb from Los Angeles. Despite his reluctance to give death-threatened patients a placebo, he had come to the conclusion that "the most compassionate and moral thing to do was to find an effective treatment as quickly as possible."

The twelve doctors had been called together by David Barry to put the final touches to the clinical procedures for Operation 53. Experts from the NIH and FDA and Atlanta-based CDC were also taking part in this meeting. The seminar at Pine Needle Lodge might have cleared the way, but there were still several major points to be resolved.

Based on the AZT supply, the Burroughs Wellcome researchers calculated that they were in a position to provide the necessary doses of AZT for 125 subjects over a period of six months. The number of participants admitted to the clinical trials was therefore fixed at 250 patients. Half would be given AZT, the other half the placebo. Drug addicts were eliminated because their addiction would force them to take drugs likely to falsify the results. Children under twelve were also excluded because of the dangers of toxicity. To guarantee that the experiment would be as homogeneous as possible, some health officials suggested that only men should be selected. David Barry considered such discrimination to be contrary to medical ethics, and it was decided that women would be included. Next they agreed on the principle criterion for eligibility: a life expectancy of at least six months. Contrary to usual practice in this type of experiment, however, the condition of candidates was required to be very serious. For the Burroughs Wellcome team this involved a risk: if AZT proved to be ineffective in severely affected subjects, there was a good chance of its being rejected altogether. The risk was no less considerable for the patients themselves, the likelihood of dangerous, possibly fatal, toxic reactions being inevitably higher in very weakened organisms. On the other hand, if the product was shown to be effective, the results would be all the more eloquent. Again out of the desire to guarantee maximum homogeneity among the subjects, a very rigorous clinical common denominator was chosen: the subjects must all have suffered their first attack of pneumocystis pneumonia within the last three months. This automatically excluded those patients in whom AIDS had only manifested itself in the form of Kaposi's sarcoma. David Barry would justify this decision by the fact that the life expectancy of patients with Kaposi's sarcoma varied considerably according to the location and extent of their lesions. In cases involving only cutaneous attacks, survival could extend to five years. Once the mucous membranes of the internal organs were affected, the expectancy could be reduced to a few weeks.

The outcome of this consultation was a monumental protocol, 262 pages long. The list of tests and analyses alone over the six-month period involved several hundred entries. Certain tests intended to disclose eventual attacks on the brain were so complicated that Burroughs Wellcome would hastily be obliged to make provision for the training of a special staff to take charge of them.

All they had to do then was fix D day. Wide-scale experimental testing of the first anti-AIDS medicine would begin on February 18, 1986.

56

"The Crucifix on Your Chest Isn't Going to Protect You"
New York, USA: Winter 1986

In the course of his nine-year reign over his capricious city, the major of New York had had many reasons to become blasé. He had probably heard more extravagant speeches, been subjected to more pressure, and been on the receiving end of more threats than any other municipal official. Yet, Ed Koch could not remember ever before being confronted by as tough an interlocutor as the visitor he received on that January 2, 1986. The most hard-nosed union leaders, the most demanding activists, even the outlandish troublemakers from among the racial, ethnic, and religious organizations in this melting pot, all seemed like choirboys to him by comparison with the wrinkled old woman who was fiercely and relentlessly subjecting him to blackmail in the cause of virtue. Her eyes still protected by dark glasses, Mother Teresa was admonishing the son of Polish Jewish immigrants who had become the custodian of the largest city in the United States.

"The three convicts that the authorities were kind enough to let me have before Christmas are only a tiny minority of AIDS sufferers among many. The New York State penitentiaries are bursting with them, Mr. Mayor. There are at least another two hundred and fifty.

I'm begging you to get the governor to release them so my sisters and I can look after them and help them to die with dignity."

"Mother, those prisoners are all criminals, some of them are dangerous killers," objected Ed Koch firmly. "They can't be allowed to go free just because they're in poor health."

"By inflicting AIDS on them, God has punished them more severely than human justice, Mr. Mayor. Don't you think they deserve our compassion?"

"All right, I'll speak to the governor about it," Ed Koch eventually promised. "While we're waiting for his decision, I'll try and find you another building in New York so you'll be ready to take them when the time comes."

"A building in New York?" protested the nun. "Out of the question! What we need is a house in the country. In India and elsewhere, governments and private individuals have given us land on which we've been able to provide homes for lepers. Today there are 178,000 of them on our farms and in our villages. They grow their own vegetables, rear chickens, and farm fish. They have even built their own houses. You should come and see for yourself, Mr. Mayor. You'd find it very interesting."

Ed Koch scratched the few small remaining curls on the back of his head. The prospect of going on a tour of Mother Teresa's leper colonies was not one he greeted with particular relish.

"People with AIDS are very sick, Mother," he observed. "Sometimes they haven't even got the strength to stand upright. What's more, most of them have no qualifications of any kind. How do you propose to transform them overnight into carpenters, plumbers, and electricians?"

Mother Teresa swept the air aside with her large callused hand. "If lepers who have lost their fingers, hands, feet, can manage to build their own houses, why shouldn't people with all four limbs succeed in doing the same? If they don't know how to go about it, we'll show them. Volunteer professionals will come and give us a hand."

"And what will you do about equipping and furnishing all these lodgings?"

A mischievous smile accompanied her favorite response. "God will provide, Mr. Mayor."

"In any case, what you're asking me can't be done in a day," replied Ed Koch, visibly exasperated. "It'll take time. Come back and see me in three months."

No argument could deter this fiery representative of the suffering people.

"I'll give you the necessary time," she conceded. Then, pointing a finger at her host, she added in a firm voice, "But you can be sure I won't give you any peace until it's done."

She stood up and placed a small slip of paper on the mayor's desk before taking her leave.

After seeing the nun out, Ed Koch read the message she had left for him: "The fruit of silence is prayer, the fruit of prayer is faith, the fruit of faith is love. And the fruit of love is service to others. Mother Teresa."

The devout woman's call for the release of all prisoners with AIDS and their installation in a rural community had the effect of a bombshell. The press devoted substantial front-page articles to it. Somewhat shaken, Mario Cuomo, governor of the state of New York, promised to consider releasing the most severe cases. Several owners of land and disused agricultural buildings offered them to the municipality of New York. Strangely, it was among the local Roman Catholic hierarchy that this audacious suggestion met with a degree of reticence. "That old woman and her farm are giving me nightmares!" announced Msgr. James Cassidy, who was responsible for social welfare and health care in the archdiocese. "She has no appreciation of the way things are in New York. She still thinks she's in the slums of her precious India!"

*　　*　　*

Of course New York was different from Calcutta. The young Indian sisters would soon realize this fact. In the course of the twenty years she had spent running the home for the dying in Calcutta, Sister Paul had tended more than fifty thousand dying people without being answerable to any authority apart from her conscience. Since she had assumed responsibility for the Gift of Love, home, fire, hygiene, health and building inspections, the obligation to have recourse to all kinds of safety measures, to wrap up every bit of garbage in an inviolable container (which much to her regret deprived the garbage pickers of some income), in short all the niggling regulations of an American city seemed to her to be clamping her mission of charity in an intolerable iron collar. When, one day, a zealous official wanted to check the electrical wiring, she chased him away crying, "It's not your business how we do things here!"

What was more, in a vast metropolis where there were as many opinions as there were citizens, the presence of Catholic nuns looking after the AIDS "unclean" could hardly fail to provoke all kinds of reactions. "There was always somebody ringing at the door," Sister Ananda would recount. "There were people who wanted to encourage and help us; people who came to curse us and run down the sick; people claiming to have some miraculous cure. There were wonderful people, but a lot of deranged people, too, such as I'd never encountered at the leprosy clinic in Benares or the home for the dying in Calcutta."

The fact that there were a high percentage of drug addicts among the first sick people welcomed into the Gift of Love did not sit well with the gay and lesbian residents of Greenwich Village. The Indian women's integration into the neighborhood suffered as a result, until the day came when Sister Paul decided not to limit the services of her small community exclusively to AIDS sufferers. The soup kitchen set up on the steps in front of Saint Veronica's Church and the visits to the poor and the elderly soon earned the sisters community support. "It was not long before the Gift of Love and its team came to represent a haven of compassion and hope for all the local inhabitants," Terry Miles, the clinic coordinator at St. Clare's, noted. St. Clare's Hospital had appointed him to supervise the medical care the sisters provided their residents. He found himself at once disconcerted. "Those Indian women arrived from their country with the idea that they were going to carry on helping the dying to die in peace," he would observe. He had to make them understand that this was quite a different situation. "Our sick people are not poor wretches picked up off the street. These are Americans in the prime of life, struck down by a fatal virus. Giving them a bed, a daily bath, a little food, and words of comfort are not enough. Like all citizens of this country, they are entitled to appropriate medical treatment. It's our duty as people caring for them to think in terms of biological tests, intravenous treatment, injections, oxygen, medicines." This pep talk left the sisters completely indiffer-

ent. "I might just as well have been talking Greek or Chinese," Terry
Miles would say. "My reasoning was totally alien to the thinking
of these women, who considered their prime mission to be that of
accompanying the dying on the road to paradise and not trying to
prolong their pitiful existence."

Terry Miles still shudders at the thought of the difficulties he
encountered in preparing the Gift of Love team for its real task.
"Talking about sperm, sex, libido, risk groups, to nuns brought up
in the strictest Catholic morality seemed an impossible aim to me,"
he would acknowledge. "They knew practically nothing about
AIDS as a disease or about the sexual habits of the majority of
victims it hit. The information sheet they had received on their
stopover in Rome wouldn't have enlightened a child of six. They
had to be taught everything." Terry Miles played devil's advocate.
"The crucifix on your chest isn't going to protect you," he told
them. "Quite the opposite, patients will take great delight in shocking you. Be prepared to hear the worst."

Support for him in this instructor's role came from an unexpected
quarter. Intrigued by the urgent recommendation of his friend at
the Abbey of Latrun, Josef Stein had asked to stay in the home for
a few days to get to know Sister Ananda better. It was not long
before the Indian girl and the American ex-archaeologist were
bound by a mutual compassion. He was immediately touched by
"the way she gave others her undivided attention." Whether it was
the gentleness of her gestures, her gift for discerning the least of
his pains or his lightest distress, the intensity of her looks or the
purity of her smiles, Josef Stein had never before felt the quality of
such love. "Her religious motivation might not coincide with my
convictions, but nevertheless this woman made every one of her
patients feel he was the center of the world." One day, while she
was massaging his legs, Sister Ananda ventured to ask Josef Stein
about the origins of the violet pustules scattered all over his body.
Josef told her. He even made it his duty not to leave anything out:
the discovery of his homosexuality in a train, the gay revolution,
the bathhouses of San Francisco, his escapades in Israel, the evening
at the opera when the terrible verdict had been pronounced. Attentive to what her fingers were doing to his ravaged flesh, Sister
Ananda listened to him in silence, her eyes averted. From then on,
for her AIDS would have a face and a name.

*   *   *

Sister Paul was not so lucky as to have such a courteous patient to deal with. A few days into the new year, two orderlies from St. Clare's brought her Orlando, a thirty-two-year-old transvestite with outrageously reddened lips, masquerading in false eyelashes, false breasts, and a wig of long blond locks. He was wearing a black sheath dress that forced him to take tiny steps when he walked. Sister Paul's Indian-style greeting and sari provoked amused chortles on his part. He rushed to clasp her in his arms. The nun pushed him bluntly away.

"Darling, don't be frightened," he protested in his falsetto voice. "Sugar won't hurt you."

Sister Paul learned later why Orlando liked to be called Sugar. It was the pet name Humphrey Bogart had given his wife, actress Lauren Bacall, whose identity the transvestite assumed each night in the burlesque cabarets of lower Manhattan. To earn his living, Sugar also went in for prostitution in a moving van parked on the banks of the Hudson. From the many needle marks on his arms, it was immediately apparent that he also went in for hard drugs. His makeup could not hide the fact: AIDS had hit him hard. His whole body, right down to the soles of his feet, was just one purplish-blue expanse of Kaposi's tumors. Sugar knew he had only a few months left to live, but the disease hadn't knocked him out of action yet.

"Come on," said Sister Paul, "I'm going to see you to your room."

The transvestite batted his eyelashes furiously. "Oh, tut, tut, darling! Sugar never takes orders from anyone!"

They got off to a bad start. The sick man might not have a home or family, but at least he had friends. A noisy horde soon began to sow disorder in the Gift of Love. It was not long before Sister Paul understood the interest these visitors had in her curious lodger. The transvestite was one of their best clients. Every day, he injected three hundred dollars' worth of heroin into his veins.

Poor Sister Paul! Terry Miles was right. The evils of New York were far worse than the poverty of Calcutta. Still the nun was not to be daunted by that kind of reality: she would find a way to bring these weird Americans into line. Three days after Sugar's arrival she posted a notice at the entrance to the home, setting down the measures she had decided upon: the immediate and definitive expulsion of any patient found in possession of alcoholic beverages or drugs, the restriction of visiting hours to certain times, the discontinuance of the use of the telephone during the hours of religious functions, lights out at 8:30 P.M.

Such strictness raised an immediate outcry in the city's gay community. Staff members at St. Clare's also protested. Newspapers pilloried the "religious watch guards of Washington Street." Even when confronted with a fatal plague, Americans valued respect for individual liberties above the caring for its citizens whose lives were in danger. Sister Paul stood her ground, especially with regard to visiting times. In her eyes any visitor who was not a relative was a shameful relation: a partner in drinking, gambling, drugs, or sex. This intransigence posed a few problems with "buddies," who were none of these things, but just good friends. The extreme physical and psychological distress that AIDS occasioned had induced the gay community to create certain organizations for mutual aid and support, of which these well-intentioned visitors were often the dedicated representatives.

The most remarkable of these organizations, the Gay Men's Health Crisis, had been created as early as 1981, almost five years before Mother Teresa and her sisters opened their home in Manhattan. The founders were the scriptwriter and novelist Larry Kramer and five of his New York friends. The six men wanted to make up for the government's slowness to take action with regard to the epidemic. The organization was soon to become a model of its kind. As Sisters Paul and Ananda were only beginning to take care of their first patients, GMHC already had some 1,600 volunteers and 70 permanent staff supporting more than 2,000 patients. Its help included legal assistance and clerical work on behalf of patients, and group sessions for their families and the people close to them. It conducted important education and prevention programs, and responded day and night to distress calls via a hot line. For the year 1985, the switchboard volunteers of GMHC answered some 52,000 calls. If the primary object of GMHC had been to bring assistance to gay men hit by AIDS, the scope of its action had soon widened to all categories of AIDS victims, as well as women, heterosexuals, hemophiliacs, IV drug users, and even children. Without GMHC, the plight of New York's AIDS sufferers would undoubtedly have been even more tragic.

Each volunteer "buddy" had charge of a patient who had found himself particularly isolated. He would help him to put his personal affairs in order, spend long hours with him every day making him eat and keeping him from being bored. He would run errands for him, comfort him, help him in his last hours, look after the formalities after his death. The nursing team at St. Clare's, who had long ago come to appreciate that these "buddies" were indispensable, gave Terry Miles the task of getting Sister Paul to relax the regulations at the Gift of Love. "I could tell the problem was a question of language. In the nun's mind the word 'buddy' conjured up every possible depravity. I suggested she substitute the term 'concerned visitor' and the matter was resolved." With another of his interventions, on the other hand, Terry Miles failed dismally. In vain he pleaded that television would help sick people to forget their predicament and alleviate their boredom. Sister Paul objected that, on the contrary, it would prevent friendships from developing between the residents of the home. It would be better to provide them with parlor games, books, records, and cassettes than to "let them coop themselves up all day in solitary degradation in front of a screen." The television set, brought by a generous donor, was never removed from its carton.

*   *   *

Gradually, the iron discipline imposed by Sister Paul was accepted. Terry Miles ended up recognizing the benefits of it himself. Each time he visited he was amazed at the amount of work that had been done. "Those Indian sisters had made that ramshackle old building really sparkle. Everything was so clean you could have eaten off the floor." What amazed this American agnostic most was "the way the sisters had of surrendering everything to the will of the God they served. Whenever a difficulty arose, whenever they needed something, they would raise their arms to heaven and say in the most natural way in the world: 'The Lord will provide.'" Terry Miles was astonished when one day Sister Ananda obliged the cook to make the dessert they had planned for lunch despite the fact that there was only one egg left in the house. "I can't make a cake without eggs," protested the cook apprehensively. The nun told her calmly to trust in Providence. She was right. Soon afterward there was a ring at the door. It was a neighbor bringing them a dozen eggs.

The fourteen first beds at the Gift of Love were always filled. Gay men and drug addicts—the two risk groups primarily affected by AIDS at the time—were about equal in number, the latter being principally blacks and Hispanics. Terry Miles frequently visited the home to help the sisters by sharing his experience acquired at St. Clare's. However, he had a hard time convincing them of the importance of a specially tailored diet for each case. The vegetarian nuns, accustomed to offering their dying Indian patients only a spoonful of rice or lentils, found no benefit in the idea of nutrition. Their meals were primarily composed of a thick soup, whereas patients also needed more proteins and calories from meat, fish, and cereals. The capricious appetites of AIDS patients ran counter to the rigid mealtime schedule at the home.

Terry Miles patiently resolved each problem as it arose. Soon he was so proud of his nurses in their saris that he would claim: "The only bit of luck an AIDS sufferer can have is that of falling into their hands."

The clinic coordinator never suspected what torments sometimes beset those women, as ever smiling, they went about their ministry. One morning, during prayers in the chapel, one of the sisters broke into sobs.

"I can't take it anymore," she moaned through her tears. "We're not being asked to look after lepers or people who are dying, but real monsters, pariahs that God has cursed, outcasts that he has punished for their sins. It's beyond me to respect and love them."

Sister Paul took her in her arms, wiped away her tears, and tried to calm her. "It's because God has punished them that we must offer Him their suffering and ours."

That was when Sister Ananda intervened. "These men are neither monsters nor sinners. They're just victims. I have lived through some of their moral and physical degradation. I've been abused as many of them have been. No, little sister, their illness isn't a punishment, but the proof that God loves them, as He loves me, as He loves you, too, in your anguish."

57

Japanese Mushrooms and Chinese Cucumbers for the Desperate

New York, USA: February 1986

Indian women only show their emotions with extreme reserve. That morning, however, Sister Ananda's utter amazement could be read all over her face. One of her inmates had disappeared. No one had seen Josef Stein leave the Gift of Love home. He had gone without leaving any message. There had been no prior intimation of this flight. Quite the opposite. Despite the fact that he was neither indigent nor homeless, the former archaeologist had taken it upon himself to ask to be allowed to prolong his unexpected stay with Mother Teresa's sisters.

His condition had grown steadily worse since his arrival for the inauguration of the home. Having receded somewhat, his Kaposi's lesions had subsequently returned in full force. He had new ones all over his body, including his mouth and his tongue. The absorption of solid food was so painful for him that he had gradually stopped eating. For years in Calcutta, Sister Ananda had dealt with people racked with hunger who could not manage to swallow any food. In New York, she had to tackle this same problem. Here she followed the dietetic advice of Terry Miles. "There is no one quite like her for providing some chocolate ice cream balls or a little honey that would glide down your throat and make you want to climb the Himalayas," Josef Stein would say. All the same, it had not been enough to keep him there.

It would take the sisters in the home and Dr. Jack Dehovitz several weeks to find out the motive for his escape. Yet the newspaper clipping found by his bedside table should have told them. It was an article from the *New York Post* about an AIDS medicine that had just produced "almost miraculous results on the first human guinea pigs treated in the cancer hospital at Bethesda." The text announced the forthcoming wide-scale clinical trials of AZT. As soon as he read this news, Josef Stein had latched onto the idea of being able to take part in the experiment. Waiting until the sisters were confined to the chapel, he had dragged himself to the telephone on the ground floor to call one of the three New York centers designated to conduct the experiment.

"Even if I only had a one-in-two chance of being given the medicine, it was my last hope of pulling through," he would later explain. "It was absolutely vital I took part in the operation." The voice at the other end of the line asked him various questions. When Josef mentioned the word "Kaposi," the conversation stopped short. That form of AIDS officially eliminated him from selection.

"Don't lose heart," the speaker recommended. "If it's successful, AZT will be distributed to all patients without distinction."

"How soon?" ventured Josef Stein.

"In about a year."

A year! For a man who sensed a little of his life slipping away from him each day like "a continuous hemorrhage," they might just as well speak of a century or a millennium! And yet instead of making him give up, this clearly defined deadline jolted him like a shock wave. "It was astonishing," he would recount. "Two months earlier, I'd swallowed I don't know how many pills to have done with it once and for all, and there I was suddenly consumed with a frantic desire to keep this appointment in one year with AZT. Back in my room, I reread all the information I had accumulated prior to my suicide attempt about the palliatives available from underground channels."

*   *   *

There was nothing unusual about Josef Stein's reaction. In their desperation at feeling themselves condemned to die before a medicine had been found to cure them, a growing number of American patients were pouncing on alternative treatments that winter in early 1986. Thus hundreds of victims—in the final stages of the illness or simply seropositive—were crossing the Mexican border to purchase antiviral medicines at extortionate prices. These were treatments not yet authorized by the FDA. Following Rock Hudson's example, other patients went to France or Israel to take advantage of treatments used in those countries. Yet others preferred to seek a cure in the U.S. itself from a network of dispensaries that were more or less clandestine.

They were known as "guerrilla clinics." Every week, they dealt with some two thousand patients. There, AIDS was treated with a pharmacopoeia that was at the very least original, including as it did an acid used to develop photographs, a soya derivative, an extract from a Japanese mushroom, and the bark of a tree found in the Brazilian Amazon. One of the most sought after of these fortuitous remedies was manufactured in his apartment in San Francisco by an employee in a factory for orthopedic equipment. It was a mixture of dinitrochlorobenzine, ethanol, and a capillary lotion sold in the trade. The mixture had been reported by several medical reviews. Applied daily to the lesions of Kaposi's sarcoma, it had, so it was said, the power to stimulate the activity of the immune system.

In New York, AIDS sufferers had access to a telephone answering machine that gave an address on West Twenty-third Street where, for two hundred dollars, they could buy a medicine based on egg yolk imported from Germany under the label AL-721. In San Francisco, the hotline to Project Inform, a voluntary organization to support sufferers, provided callers with information about various experimental treatments available on the West Coast. One of them involved a preparation based on the roots of a Chinese cucumber. Known as Compound Q, this product had apparently shown itself under test-tube conditions to be endowed with the remarkable capacity to kill selectively the cells infected by the virus and spare the healthy ones. A number of patients would have themselves injected with this providential panacea. For want of preliminary tests for its toxicity, the Chinese cucumber would be the cause of many tragedies. Some of its imprudent consumers found themselves paralyzed, blind, suffering from dementia, or in a coma.

Even real doctors sometimes turned to strange remedies in their
desperation. In Miami, some physicians offered capsules of fresh
calves' embryos capable, so they assured people, of obliging the
thymus to stimulate the reproduction of T-4 lymphocytes. Again
in Miami, travel agents organized excursions to a Caribbean island
where a laboratory produced a certain substance that had been
christened "reticulose" and whose inventors extolled its curative
powers in the press. In nine days, it was supposed to cure Kaposi's
sarcoma and infectious pneumocystis pneumonia. It could also be
found in Mexico and Central America at the astronomical price of
$6,000 for twenty-one days' treatment.

*   *   *

"When orthodox medicine and its great professors abandon you
to the most horrible death, when all the scientific pundits with their
Nobel Prizes let themselves be flouted by a miserable virus despite
their phenomenal research budgets, how can you fail to go after a
last glimmer of hope no matter where, in hell if necessary?" Josef
Stein asked. That winter, it was among the banana trees and the
clusters of Caribbean jacarandas on St. Martin island that the former
archaeologist's last hope was glimmering. A French doctor who for
the last thirty years had made his home in this Caribbean paradise
was administering a vaccine obtained from mice he had infected
with the AIDS virus. Apparently the man was not a charlatan. He
even enjoyed a reputation for being an authentic researcher. Unlike
most owners of "guerrilla clinics," he sought no publicity and in
many instances, offered his vaccine free of charge. Some journalists
had not hesitated to present him as a kind of Dr. Schweitzer.

"St. Martin island was only a four-hour flight from New York,"
Josef Stein would say later. "I was sure I could be back within three
days. My little escapade would pass almost unnoticed."

58

281 Guinea Pigs for a Handful of Bitter Capsules

New York–Los Angeles–Miami–San Francisco, USA: Spring–Summer 1986

Dr. Paul Volberding was one of the twelve practitioners appointed by the Burroughs Wellcome pharmaceutical laboratory to take part in the double-blind placebo testing of AZT. Ever since the day he had discovered the lesions of one of the West Coast's first cases of Kaposi's sarcoma on a gay male sauna attendant, Paul Volberding had never stopped caring for AIDS victims. His consulting room on the fifth floor of San Francisco's old General Hospital was one of the busiest treatment centers in the gay capital of America.

That spring of 1986, he had among his patients the companion of a newspaper vendor who had died of AIDS four years previously. At the time, he had desperately fought to save the unfortunate man. In the absence of suitable medicines, he had lost the battle. Now Paul Volberding hoped to avenge his failure with the companion of the deceased. The fact that his patient was suffering from pneumocystis pneumonia, diagnosed less than ninety days earlier, qualified him to take part in the AZT trials. Before announcing the good news to the patient, however, the doctor had to perform the tests prescribed by the organizers. One of them, to test cutaneous sensitivity, caused the appearance of nodules two millimeters larger in diameter than permitted by the selection criteria. The difference was so minimal that Paul Volberding at first considered disregarding it. Was not his primary duty as a doctor to assist a person whose life was endangered by every possible means? On the other hand, did he have the right to deceive, even in such a negligible way, those who had put their trust in him in the higher interests of science? The friendship he had with this patient further complicated his unbearable dilemma. "How do you explain to someone dear to you who is expecting you to work miracles that you have to deprive him of a chance of survival because of a detail like that?" After two days and two nights of being torn by the dilemma, with death in his heart, Paul Volberding gave up the idea of having his friend benefit from the only chance of finally receiving treatment. "My honor as a servant of science required that I respect the rules of the game to the letter."

*   *   *

The rush was on. Everywhere the number of patients meeting the criteria for eligibility exceeded the quota allocated to each of the twelve centers. Violent incidents sometimes occurred. At the University of California hospital in Los Angeles, rejected patients threatened Dr. Michael Gottlieb with cries of "Genocide! We all want AZT!" As might have been expected, the selection gave rise to disturbing questions of conscience. Why choose one particular candidate as opposed to another? Dr. Oscar Larry Laskin of Cornell University medical center in New York and several of his colleagues resolved to overcome the "emotional difficulty" by adopting the old commercial practice of "first come, first served." Elsewhere fortune smiled on those who just happened to be there at the right time. As for Paul Volberding, he decided to entrust the selection of his contingent of patients to chance. He directed his assistant Roby Wong to "draw their names out of a hat."

The great majority of the 281 subjects finally accepted—144 were given AZT and 137 the placebo—came to the experiment with a positive attitude. They had all read and duly signed the five-page document that spelled out in no uncertain terms the dangers they were risking. "One of the side effects of AZT is a decline in the number of red cells significant enough for several transfusions to be necessary," the text declared before going on to enumerate other possible side effects, such as migraine, slight mental confusion, states of anxiety, nausea, painful cutaneous eruptions, together with an eventual decline in the number of white cells, which could give rise to a variety of infections.

Hardly anyone was put off by these warnings. "Such was the desperation that most people would have taken cyanide if they'd been told it might check the ravages of the virus," one doctor would explain. Above all else, patients felt reassured to know that their state of health was going to be kept under close surveillance. What was more, they had been told that in the event AZT proved successful, they would be the first to be given it on a permanent basis. This was a vital advantage because the remedy made no claims to curing AIDS, only to stopping the proliferation of the virus. According to Roby Wong, Dr. Volberding's assistant, "a good many of them also felt proud to be able to take part in a scientific venture which could further medical research."

For all this, Operation 53 was not launched to unmitigated praise. Some patients suffered from being treated like guinea pigs. "By throwing us this life preserver, they had us at their mercy," one of them would say of the organizers. "They would give you your ration of capsules for a week and direct you to take two every four hours including at night," another would complain. The restriction of being forbidden to eat anything for an hour before or after each dose was "a particular hardship as AIDS makes your appetite very temperamental," another would explain. The real agony for each patient was putting up with these torments in the knowledge that, as one said, "we might just be swallowing a load of quack powder."

A number of patients would speak of how, in the early weeks, they were haunted by the idea of being brutally rejected from the experiment. "No one really knew whether certain symptoms caused by the evolution of our AIDS were likely to disqualify us," one of them would confide. "One day, I had the panic of my life after telling the doctor in charge that I had taken an aspirin tablet. I thought he was going to tear out my tongue. I learned my lesson and never mentioned the medicines I went on taking to alleviate my petty aches and pains. Nor would I mention any unusual symptoms. It was a question of life and death." Some subjects would complain about their doctors keeping them in the dark about the progress of their condition. "They took my blood at every opportunity, but no one wanted to tell me whether or not I was better," a Los Angeles architect protested. Others tried to break through this information blackout by having tests carried out in private laboratories, "to find out the truth." Yet others were worried about the delay involved in analyzing the results when time had become, as a sick Broadway actor would confide, "a key factor in this damned disease."

These recriminations were not the only discordant notes that marked the beginnings of Operation 53. A number of doctors were quick to criticize certain aspects of the protocol that, in their view, posed a serious moral problem in the light of this tragic epidemic. Of the 22,000 cases of AIDS identified in the United States since 1981, death had already claimed more than half. The average life expectancy, once the disease had been diagnosed, was rarely more than two years. Those afflicted with opportunistic illnesses such as pneumocystis pneumonia had little chance of surviving more than six months. More and more researchers were even convinced that the virus caused irreversible brain damage prior to the appearance of the first symptoms. For Barbara Starrett, a New York doctor who had dedicated herself to AIDS sufferers, "frankly it's inhuman just to give patients a little lactose and then expect them not to take any remedy to prevent or treat secondary infections resulting from their AIDS." Such arguments could not be taken lightly.

*   *   *

AZT or placebo? The rule of secrecy produced an obsessional neurosis in certain patients. Some were overjoyed at the slightest nausea or the most ordinary headache, persuaded that it meant they were absorbing the real medicine. Others sought to double their chances by sharing with another patient their combined rations of capsules. To put himself out of his misery, a Miami patient used a ruse the Burroughs Wellcome researchers had not anticipated. He sliced open the gelatine casing of the capsule to taste the powder. The sweet taste of the substance sent a shiver down his spine; he had just found out that he was being given straightforward "sugar pills." Another patient, on the other hand, discovered that his product tasted bitter, proof that it was AZT. In Miami, where the gay community maintained a very effective network of underground information, the implications of the bitterness of the medicine spread like wildfire. "Patients came to collect their ration of capsules as usual, but as soon as they got home, they would open one up to taste the contents," one doctor observed. "If it was bitter, they carried on with the treatment. Otherwise, they threw the bottle in the garbage can and rushed to catch a plane to try their chances elsewhere by getting themselves admitted at another center."

Dr. David Barry was devastated. "In the course of the one hundred and sixty double-blind clinical trials we had already conducted, never before had anyone opened up a single one of our capsules." He asked his chemists to make the placebo as bitter as the AZT. Then he sent his inspectors out to the twelve centers to substitute new coded bottles for the old ones. But the unfortunate doctor's troubles were not yet over. In their frustration at not being able to identify what they were being given, several patients in San Francisco and Miami had the composition analyzed by specialist laboratories. It was a few days before the Burroughs Wellcome technicians found an answer to this latest stratagem. They added a particular molecule to the AZT and the placebo that made it impossible to distinguish between the two.

The doctors conducting the clinical trials also tried to deduce the secret by observing the patients closely. Since they had no right of access to the results of the patients' tests, they tried to guess from their general progress which were being given the benefit of AZT. Favorable signs such as increase in weight could sometimes prove deceptive because this might actually be due to the effect of earlier antibiotics given to subjects when their pneumocystis pneumonia had first been diagnosed. "Remissions at the beginning of treatment are common," Paul Volberding explained. "They're called the honeymoon. They can last seven or eight months, until the inevitable and often fatal relapse. The improvement in a number of our patients' conditions could not automatically be attributed to AZT."

By the second month, it became apparent in each test center that subjects were falling into two very distinct categories: those who were better to a point where they could resume an almost normal life, and those whose condition was growing consistently worse. The distinction was so flagrant that several doctors asked the Burroughs Wellcome authorities to put an end to the secrecy and allow the distribution of AZT to those who had been given the placebo.

One of the principal American authorities in the field of AIDS treatment, Dr. Margaret Fischl, in charge of the Miami center, provided David Barry with observations that left no room for doubt: AZT was effective. "It was a heartrending dilemma," David Barry would say, "but it was my duty to see the experiment through to its conclusion."

*   *   *

Two events helped to expedite matters. On March 15, 1986, the celebrated British review *Lancet* published an article that was immediately taken up by the national press. In it, Dr. Sam Broder gave notice of the encouraging results registered in the first tests of AZT on humans carried out at his Bethesda hospital the previous autumn. Coming from such an authority, the news gave rise to an enormous wave of hope. Patients, doctors, newspapers, gay organizations, and numerous well-known personalities demanded that the medicine be distributed to all AIDS sufferers immediately.

It was then that the death of the subjects identified by the numbers 102, 412, 452, and 808 occurred in May and June. These deaths led the inspectors from the FDA and Burroughs Wellcome to consider the premature curtailment of Operation 53. No one at the pharmaceutical laboratory knew any more than the doctors at the experimental centers what substance the deceased patients had been receiving. It had been planned that this information would only be divulged at the end of the clinical trials, that is to say at the end of the prescribed six months. That was the rule of the game. At least in theory. In practice, this particular type of experiment was actually reviewed by a group of independent experts known as the Data Safety and Monitoring Board. Every eight weeks, they were supposed to examine the reports submitted by the twelve centers in order to determine whether, from the point of view of scientific research and medical ethics, it was appropriate to continue the operation. They alone knew what each patient was receiving.

On August 1, the death of a sixth subject, killed by a crushing attack of pneumocystis pneumonia, marked the beginning of an onslaught. Six deaths would follow in the course of the same month. Worried, David Barry telephoned the president of the data monitoring committee to ask him if it was still ethically right to continue the experiment. He was surprised by the answer. The committee wanted to wait and examine the next results.

The ten thousand living American victims of the epidemic were not of the same opinion. A campaign to stop Operation 53 and trigger the immediate distribution of AZT to all patients was already in full swing in the media. It even had its passionate advocate: a warmhearted woman, a doctor of biology, member of the St. Luke's–Roosevelt Hospital's laboratory in New York, and also, incidentally, the wife of one of Hollywood's most celebrated film producers. An eminent expert on interferon, Mathilde Krim was passionately caught up in the AIDS cause. Indignant at the federal authorities' slowness to release funds to combat the disease, in the previous year she had joined forces with Dr. Michael Gottlieb of Los Angeles to create the American Foundation for AIDS Research. In the year 1986 alone, this private organization would distribute $1.6 million in research grants and aid to scientists working on AIDS.

Mathilde Krim was conducting her implacable fight that summer primarily on behalf of patients. "The double-blind clinical trial on AZT is an insult to morality," she did not hesitate to announce publicly during the course of a large demonstration held in New York. She proceeded to denounce altogether the small number of subjects selected, the restrictive criteria for eligibility, the use of the placebo, and the six-month deprivation of any other treatment, which gave "those who weren't being given the medicine plenty of time to die." She considered that AZT should at least be given "for compassionate use" to all patients who had only a little time left to live. "If the Burroughs Wellcome laboratories are not in a position to or do not want to manufacture enough AZT, then the federal government must sign contracts with other laboratories and distribute the medicine free of charge," she declared at every possible opportunity. And should anyone complain to her about a shortage of herring sperm, she would retort, "With warships in all four corners of the globe, the American government has the means to catch all the herring in all the world's seas." To those who raised objections about the high toxicity of AZT, she would respond, "Surely a man who has no more than six months to live has the right to take a risk and have one last chance to hope."

Mathilde Krim conducted her crusade on all fronts at once. She even managed to go to Washington to defend her cause in front of the U.S. Congress. Powerfully orchestrated by the gay organizations, supported by numerous political and scientific figures of all parties, encouraged by the media, the campaign to put a stop to the clinical trials and promote the general distribution of AZT did eventually move certain elected representatives of the American people. Democratic congressman Ted Weiss invited the principal protagonists in the debate to appear before the Committee for Human Resources over which he presided.

"Don't we have a duty to provide people who are dying with the means to fight to the last?" Mathilde Krim was quick to ask. The presence at her side of two dramatic supporters gave her question a poignant reality. One of them, who was thin in the extreme with a greenish complexion and face studded with Kaposi's tumors, gave testimony that overwhelmed the committee members. It made the ensuing discussion between experts relative to the advantages and disadvantages of double-blind clinical trials seem somewhat incongruous. "What I would like to hear straight from my doctor's mouth is that several remedies are being experimented on and that at least one of them is probably going to help me," he announced. "Instead, every time I see him, he has to admit that there is still no medicine available and there are as yet no plans for experimental trials in the area where I live. I'm sorry I have to vent all my anger on him when he's doing his best to keep me alive until the day they come up with something to cure me."

*   *   *

The Washington hearings gave rise to considerable emotion, but it was a cold statistic that actually clinched the decision. At the beginning of September, the twentieth death was registered. The experts on the Data Safety and Monitoring Board had only to glance at their lists to know which group the deceased belonged to. Of the twenty victims, nineteen had been given the placebo, only one AZT. Who would dare persist in such circumstances? The committee's decision was made public on the afternoon of September 11, 1986: the clinical trials were stopped. At last all patients were to benefit from the first AIDS medicine.

While a throng of cameramen, photographers, and journalists

pressed around David Barry and his collaborators, one man slipped quietly away from the room at the National Institute for Allergy and Infectious Diseases where the press conference announcing the forthcoming commercial distribution of AZT was to be held. Dr. Paul Volberding shut himself in a telephone booth and dialed a number in San Francisco. He wanted to be the first to tell his patient, the companion of his newspaper-vendor friend, the good news. Later, as he looked back on those moments of intense optimism, he would say, "For the first time, we were going to be able to do something other than stand by and watch our patients die."

59

"There Can Be No Greater Love Than Yours"
New York, USA: Autumn 1986

With a wail of sirens, the St. Clare's Hospital ambulance came to a halt outside the door to the Gift of Love home. With Sister Paul leading the way, all the nuns rushed out onto the sidewalk of Washington Street. Seeing the gleaming station wagon reminded Sister Ananda of the ramshackle old heap that used to bring the dying from the streets to Mother Teresa's hospice in Calcutta. That September morning, the two vehicles had one thing in common. Whether because of poverty or AIDS, their passengers were reduced to the same state of physical degradation. In the Indian woman's eyes, the man that the two orderlies were taking carefully out of the vehicle was a striking replica of the destitute taken to the place next to the Kali temple. He was a living skeleton with eyes bright with fever and breathing that came in gasps. She started as she recognized the thick ruffle of beard on the emaciated face.

"What a wonderful surprise to have you back, dear little brother," she exclaimed cheerfully to Josef Stein. "Be welcome."

Too full of emotion to answer, the American could only squeeze the nurse's hand with what little strength he had left.

A short time later Sister Ananda would hear from his own mouth the story of his escapade in the Caribbean in quest of a miracle cure. He had no sooner landed on St. Martin island where the doctor with the promising vaccine lived than he had felt the early signs of a devastating attack of herpes on his hands, stomach, and legs. Soon his whole body was one open wound. Transported to the local hospital, for thirteen days and thirteen nights he had endured pain enough to drive him crazy, to a point where the nurses had to strap him into his bed.

The attack had subsided on the morning of the fourteenth day. He had been able to call New York and make contact with Sam Blum, who had been looking for him everywhere. Fearing he might have gone off to Israel to put an end to his life there, Sam had alerted the monk at Latrun. No one had seen the fugitive or heard any news of him. Sam caught the first plane for St. Martin and arranged for Josef's return to New York. Twenty days of intensive care and chemotherapy at St. Clare's had brought about a spectacular regression of the infection and the partial restoration of his immunological defenses. Despite his extreme weakness, Josef had been authorized to leave the hospital. But Jack Dehovitz did not want him to go home. The doctor knew that one of the characteristics of the virus was the gradual destruction of the will to live. Two of his patients had committed suicide toward the end of that summer when they found themselves alone in their apartments.

Josef Stein obtained permission to go and spend a few days convalescing at the Gift of Love home. Welcomed back like the prodigal son of the Gospels, he returned to his room dedicated to Our Lady of Good Hope. "At that time our people were nearly all drug addicts whose behavor was usually violent," Sister Ananda would recount. "They were giving us a hard time, so Josef's return was like a Providential gift." A pretty paltry gift. The chemotherapy had literally poisoned his body. He was suffering from repeated bouts of nausea that at times prevented him from eating for several days in succession. He had to be fed with infusions of glucose serum.

One evening, as she passed along the corridor checking that all was well for the night, Sister Ananda heard him weeping. She went into his room, sat down on the edge of his bed, and took his hand.

"I'm frightened, little sister," he moaned.

The nun did not offer reassuring words. Her years spent with the dying of Calcutta had taught her that the touch of a hand could calm the worst anguish better than any comforting speech. At one point she felt Josef's fingers tighten on hers. His expression shone with an unexpected brightness. Such changes of mood were not always a good sign. In Calcutta, she had come across dying people who, just before surrendering their souls, had suddenly emerged from their state of exhaustion to grasp her hand and press it to their sex to express their gratitude.

"I love you, little sister," Josef Stein murmured simply. "I love you so much."

Sister Ananda remained with him until, calm at last, he fell asleep. Then she gently disengaged her hand, looking with tenderness at the gaunt face pitted with violet patches. Before tiptoeing away, she bent over him and in a gesture very alien to Indian tradition, kissed him on the forehead.

One morning, when he was feeling better, Josef Stein produced a large photograph album from an attaché case and invited his nurse to look through it with him. Thirty-four years of his life passed before Sister Ananda's wondering eyes like a film in slow motion. In the three years she had spent in the home for the dying in Calcutta, she had only seen its occupants stretched out in a state of absolute degradation. And yet how often had she imagined them proudly laboring in their fields, running between the long poles of a rickshaw, dressing themselves up in their festive clothes to be married, bathing with their children in the village pond. Today, she was discovering a dying man's past, a whole life made up of happy childhood scenes, family affection, mischievous adolescence, a young man's wanderings. Josef commented on the photographs for her one by one, trying in each case to make the context come alive again. When he came to the last one, the American said to her, "I'd like you to choose one of me you'd like to keep."

The Indian girl went back through the album and picked out a black-and-white snapshot that she felt best conveyed the spirit of life in the individual now prostrate before her. The picture showed a laughing young man standing on top of railings of the Golden Gate Bridge, defying the abyss below. It was a reminder of the time when, to pay for his archaeology studies, he had worked at night as a tollbooth attendant on San Francisco's famous bridge.

*   *   *

Jack Dehovitz could not believe his ears. Sure enough, it was Sugar calling him from the depths of Brooklyn.

"Doc! Doc," the drug-addict transvestite shouted at the top of his battered lungs, "we've hit the jackpot! I read in the paper they've found a medicine that works at last! I want you to shoot my veins full of it. I'm going to jump in a taxi and I'll be there."

The attentive care of Sister Ananda and her companions had enabled this colorful character to overcome his illness and clamber back onto the stages of the burlesque nightclubs where every night he gloried in playing the part of his lifelong idol, the actress Lauren Bacall. Jack Dehovitz knew that this recovery was only an illusion, that the Kaposi's sarcoma had not disappeared, that it was only lying dormant for a few weeks or a few months. His violet pustules would resurge and break through his makeup and spread to other parts of his body and possibly creep into his lungs, his liver, his heart, and his brain.

"It was pathetic," the doctor would say as he remembered that telephone call. "Sugar couldn't have learned of the existence of AZT by reading the newspaper. He was completely illiterate. It must have been via the underground telegraph that was already operating between patients."

*   *   *

The giant postcard showed the ancient city of Jerusalem sprawling in the shelter of its antique ramparts, its abundance of bell towers, cupolas, terraces, its interlacing flights of steps, its labyrinth of alleyways. "I am writing these lines myself," announced Philippe Malouf, the monk at Latrun. "An operation has given me back the total use of my fingers. This is to let you know that our community gathered together this morning for the official opening of the monastery museum. A plaque denotes the name by which it will be known from now on: the Josef Stein Museum of Palestinian Antiquities. I've been put in charge of welcoming visitors. Alleluia, Josef! Join with me in singing *Leshannah haba'ah beyerushalayim*— 'Next year in Jerusalem!' "

The Josef Stein Museum of Palestinian Antiquities! Josef was in ecstasy. His heart was pounding, his eyes brimming with tears. All at once he remembered his years as an archaeologist, his excitement at discovering the vestiges of ancient times unearthed by the monks' plough from beneath their vineyards.

The arrival of Sister Ananda cut short his reverie.

"Come and look, little sister, at what I've just been sent by your 'spiritual fiancé' " he cried, brandishing the postcard. "That's Jerusalem!"

Jerusalem, the celestial city of the Bible! The Indian nun was fascinated by the marvelous confusion depicted in the panoramic view. Josef tried to help her imagine the noise, the shouting, the voices, the clamor of the markets, the muezzins' call to prayer, the chime of the churchbells, the sound of the shofars, all the racket that rose constantly from this entanglement of humanity, beliefs, and holy places. He choked in the process. At times his voice was so weak that she guessed at rather than heard the words: Golgotha, Via Dolorosa, Ecce Homo, names she had come to know as she knelt in the chapel in Calcutta during her years as a novice.

Jack Dehovitz interrupted their pilgrimage. The doctor was wearing a triumphant expression unusual for him. "I want to be the first to bring you the glad tidings!"

Josef raised his arm to interrupt him. "First take a look at this photo," he said, handing him Philippe Malouf's card. "Don't those stones remind you of anything?"

Dehovitz flashed a melancholy smile. "Jerusalem! Israel! The most unforgettable moments of my life. I wanted so much to do my *aliya*, stay there forever. But it was the Yom Kippur War. My parents made me come straight back to America. I didn't have the courage to resist them. Afterwards, it was too late."

Josef closed his eyes to get a better grip on his own memories. As if to defy his physical annihilation, his memory conjured up virile, shocking scenes. "Doc, if you only knew what I got up to there! It's the only time in my life when I really let myself go. Those boys could be so beautiful, affectionate, and available; the least intimation and any one of them was yours. On the beach, in a public park, in the toilets of some restaurant, in your bed. If there had been such a thing as AIDS at that time, I think I could have infected the whole of the Middle East single-handed."

The honesty of this recollection took Jack Dehovitz aback. Never before had his friend alluded to his homosexuality in such an open way. On the contrary, his modesty and discretion had been remarked upon by all those who looked after him. The doctor wondered whether this letting go was a sign his condition was worsening, evidence that the virus had attacked his brain.

Josef let out a cynical laugh and changed the subject. "So what's this great news then, Doc?"

Jack Dehovitz took a bottle of AZT out of his pocket and put it in his patient's hand. "They've finally come up with something!"

Josef inspected the white capsules. They looked like the ones he had swallowed when he had wanted to put an end to his life.

"When do I start?"

"In a week or two. As soon as I have obtained authorization to get the first doses of your treatment."

"Authorization?"

Jack Dehovitz explained that, for the moment, only cases judged to be desperate could have the benefit of the medicine. Their doctors had to submit a formal request "for compassionate use."

"And do you think I'll still be here in a week's time to swallow the little pills so 'compassionately' provided?"

*   *   *

Three days later, a surprising spectacle was to greet Sister Ananda outside the door to Our Lady of Good Hope room. Josef Stein was stretched out as naked as a baby. He seemed delighted to be making such an exhibition of himself. "Naked I came into this world, naked I want to leave it," he announced.

The nun had no need of explanations. She understood that the virus had reached her protégé's brain and that he was giving up the fight. The effect of this surrender was immediate: in the hours that followed Josef Stein was struck by a fresh attack of pneumocystis pneumonia. Each fit of coughing seemed likely to deliver the last blow. The lesions of Kaposi's sarcoma had reached his salivary glands, burning his tongue and throat with a burst of fire no liquid could quench. Alerted by the sisters, Jack Dehovitz had come at once. The doctor still wanted to hope that such grave symptoms did not necessarily mean the worst. An infusion of vinblastine made it possible provisionally to fend off final defeat. A few days later,

Sister Ananda was surprised to discover her patient calmly sitting up in his armchair, savoring with delight a whole cup of strawberry ice cream.

The former archaeologist's immunological defenses were too exhausted, however, for this respite to last for long. Soon his body would no longer respond to the medicines. The cough reappeared, drier and more painful. Eventually the proliferation of pustules in his mouth blocked the entrance to the esophagus altogether, preventing the passage of the tiniest morsel of food. Even the relentless dedication of his Indian nurse proved futile against the bottling of his throat.

The situation very quickly grew worse. His lungs ceased to play their part properly. Short of oxygen, his heart had more and more difficulty in circulating the necessary blood to his vital organs. Gradually the machinery began to break down. One evening, the American signaled Sister Ananda to come to his bedside. He took hold of her hand.

"This time I know it's really the end," he said softly as his eyes sought her confirmation.

She gave it with a slight movement of her head.

Josef began to suffocate. The "hunger for air" that accompanied the last agony of so many AIDS sufferers was horrifying. The nun tried to place an oxygen mask up to his face. Josef pushed it away.

During his visit that evening, Dr. Dehovitz did the only thing that was still medically available to him. He put his stethoscope to the dying man's chest. He was not surprised to "hear" nothing really abnormal. He knew that like deep-sea sharks, AIDS parasites destroyed their prey silently. "In any case, I wasn't there to treat him," the doctor would say. "I was just there." He had felt his friend's gaze follow every one of his movements. "His expression burned into me. It seemed to be saying: 'Don't waste your time. It's no use anymore.' "

"Is there anything you'd like me to do for you?" inquired the doctor, concealing his emotion.

The bearded man's face slowly turned toward the window where Sister Ananda had hung up the picture of Jerusalem.

"Yes," murmured Josef, "I would like you to take my little sister Ananda to the monastery at Latrun, one day, to meet her 'spiritual fiancé.' And then I'd like you to take her on a visit to Jerusalem."

"Done, old buddy," the doctor assured him as he sought his friend's hand under the sheet to shake on their agreement. He noticed that Josef had pulled out the intravenous tube that was still there to infuse a bit of life. The doctor tried to connect it to the catheter again, but Josef stopped him.

At that point several people came into the room and formed a half-circle around the patient. His eyes lit up with such joy at the sight of his visitors that Jack Dehovitz was surprised. He had noticed that the look in AIDS sufferers' eyes gradually dimmed like a rheostat turning down a lamp. News of the imminent end of one who had brought a little humanity to the corridors of St. Clare's had reached the nearby hospital. Those who had liked and looked after him came to say good-bye. There with Sister Paul, Sister Ananda, and Dr. Dehovitz were Gloria Taylor, Palma, Ron, Terry Miles, Jack Lekko, all his companions through a long ordeal that their generosity, devotion, and skill had helped to alleviate a little.

Josef surveyed them at length, one after the other, trying silently to convey his gratitude to each one. He was smiling. With difficulty he breathed in a little air and said in a gasp, "There can be no greater love than yours."

With these words he took a final gulp of air and died.

EPILOGUE

Three hundred thousand people have already shared Josef Stein's cruel fate. Today between six and ten million individuals are infected with the AIDS retrovirus. The statistics are terrifying. Two million women and some two hundred thousand children have been infected. In several parts of the world the disease has reached staggering proportions. In certain areas in Africa, 10 percent of the population is affected. In the orphanages of Haiti, more than one in two babies is a carrier. Out of 2,200 Romanian children examined in February 1990 in the hospitals of Bucharest and Constanz by the Organization of World Doctors, more than a third were found to be infected as a result of blood transfusions and repeated use of polluted syringes, a finding so tragic that experts had no reservations about referring to an "epidemic of pediatric AIDS." In New York City alone, it is estimated that before the year 2000, fifty to a hundred thousand children will lose a father or mother or both to AIDS. If a vaccine is not very quickly discovered, experts of the World Health Organization anticipate that in that same year 2000 about fifteen million people will be carriers of the virus. There will then be six million people with the full-blown disease.

*　　*　　*

Sugar, the transvestite drug addict, was the first resident of the Gift of Love to benefit from the discovery of AZT. Despite episodic relapses that oblige him to spend short spells in Mother Teresa's New York home, he still parodies his idol, the actress Lauren Bacall, every night in the burlesque shows of lower Manhattan. Every four hours, the ringing of his wristwatch's alarm reminds him to swallow two capsules. Sugar is one of thirty to forty thousand AIDS sufferers whose prolonged survival can now be attributed to this medicine.

The substance tested by Marty St. Clair in her laboratory in North Carolina is to date the only commercially available remedy effective against AIDS. New experiments periodically enlarge its range of effectiveness. Two double-blind clinical tests carried out in August 1989 on several hundred subjects who were seropositive but showed no symptoms of the disease revealed that AZT retarded or prevented the outbreak of AIDS.

The medicine was nevertheless to become the subject of criticism, starting with what was considered to be its exorbitant, even scandalous, price. In the United States, where more than 30 million citizens do not benefit from any health insurance, half the AIDS victims do not have the means to pay for treatment, the annual cost of which amounts to over $6,500. During the summer of 1989, activists from the gay movement chained themselves to the balconies of the New York Stock Exchange to protest against the spectacular profits of the Burroughs Wellcome Co., whose shares were showing a rise considered to be immoral in the dreadful context of the epidemic. In New York and San Francisco, protestors invaded pharmacies and stuck red labels on all the firm's products with the accusation "AIDS exploiters." One of the fathers of AZT, Dr. David Barry, had to appear before a Congressional committee to face hostile questioners and explain how the price of the medication was justified by the size of investment involved in further testing and research. The announcement that the laboratory would distribute AZT free of charge for children with AIDS did not silence the debate.

Medical circles were further upset by the fact that serious side effects forced numerous patients to break off treatment after only a few months. Normally they would have expected to continue medication for life. A clinical trial of treatment with constantly decreasing AZT doses fortunately showed that the product remained fully effective with reduced side effects due to toxicity. Early in 1990, the Food and Drug Administration approved a regimen of six hundred milligrams a day, half the dose previously administered. The annual cost of treatment would therefore be reduced by half. As for the worries occasioned by certain signs of the virus's resistance to AZT, the Burroughs Wellcome biologists seemed to have found an answer by combining their medicine with other antiviral products under development. "Within a year, patients will be given a combination of AZT and several other substances," David Barry announced in December 1989. "With this synergy of different remedies we might even make AIDS a disease that can be controlled as easily as hypertension."

A report published in mid-August 1990 in the American *Annals of Internal Medicine*, however, was to alarm the medical community. According to this report, a study had just produced evidence that nearly half of the people with AIDS who have been taking AZT for a period of three years can be expected to develop an aggressive cancer called non-Hodgkin's lymphoma. Researchers admitted there was no absolute evidence that AZT directly causes lymphoma. Rather, they said, AZT was probably contributing to the cancer's increasing frequency by allowing more AIDS patients to live longer with weakened immune systems, so that there is more time for the tumors to appear. But, they cautioned, further study could show that long-term use of AZT may predispose patients to develop cancer.

*   *   *

After a year of furious controversy between retrovirologists, an international committee decided, in May 1986, to put an end to the battle of abbreviations that was pitting the French and the Americans against each other. The LAV and the HTLV-III finally became the HIV, an abbreviated version of "human immuno-deficiency virus," or VIH in French, for *virus de l'immunodéficience humaine*.

Ten months later, on Tuesday, March 31, 1987, President Ronald Reagan of the U.S. and Prime Minister Jacques Chirac of France signed an agreement in Washington burying the hatchet between Luc Montagnier's and Robert Gallo's teams. This agreement recognized the contribution of both groups without attributing the initial discovery of the virus responsible for AIDS to either one of them. It established the validity of both of the separate patent applications for the commercialization of kits to diagnose seropositivity and made provision for the division of the considerable commercial profits that would arise from them.

This Franco-American battle had seemed somewhat sordid in the light of the tragedy patients were undergoing and the urgent need to discover a curative treatment and a vaccine. Its conclusion was greeted with relief, even if some French scientists, such as Prof. Jean-Claude Chermann, codiscoverer of the virus, felt their compatriots had "capitulated to Robert Gallo's steamroller."

A remarkable investigation conducted by a Pulitzer Prize–winning journalist from the *Chicago Tribune*, Mr. John Crewdson, was to shed new light on the conflict that opposed the National Cancer Institute of Bethesda and the Pasteur Institute of Paris. In two lengthy articles published in November 1989 and in March 1990, Crewdson revealed a number of facts that seriously questioned the role played by Robert Gallo and his team at the National Cancer Institute in the codiscovery of the AIDS virus. The journalist's meticulous investigation concluded that Gallo's AIDS virus, the HTLV-III, was probably a contaminant from a specimen of the French LAV virus that the Pasteur Institute had sent to the American laboratory. More disturbing still was the revelation that the NIH had commissioned a number of inquiries on the activities at Gallo's laboratory during these crucial events. These inquiries had all been classified "confidential."

The very existence of these reports raises serious questions as to the attitude of the U.S. administration at the time. It seems obvious that it violated the law that obligated it to inform the Pasteur Institute lawyers fully about what exactly took place in Gallo's laboratory between 1983 and 1985. Various elements included in these inquiries could put in question the modus vivendi reached in 1987 and push the French, in view of the enormous sums of money involved, to reopen the case and ask for considerable indemnities. Congress has appointed an investigative commission to dig into the matter.

As for Robert Gallo, in a personal letter to the author of this book dated March 26, 1990, he has repeated his position: "The so-called new information 'found' by Crewdson was published in 1984–1985! This was known to all. The worst that can be said is that *one* of our isolates might be a mix-up with LAV. But, we reported 48 detections of HIV, not *one*, in our first papers. Of these, seven—*not one*—were successfully put into laboratory tissue culture. We had the choice of more than the one for the blood test. These contributions in early 1984 were what convinced the scientific world and established the blood test. The noise now is P.R. hype."

*   *   *

The growing rumors of scandal have not deterred Gallo and his team from an active presence on the AIDS scene. At the end of 1986, the controversial virologist's laboratory discovered a new family of the herpes virus, another disease born of sexual liberation. Research work established that this virus attacked the same T-4 lymphocytes as the AIDS agent, which made it a possible cofactor in the incidence of AIDS in individuals who were seropositive.

Over the last few years, Robert Gallo and his laboratory have also been applying themselves diligently to better understanding the process of cellular infection in order to be able to impede it more effectively. Among their most original work is a technique designed to neutralize the AIDS virus by means of molecular lures. It is known that in order to penetrate the nucleus of a cell, the virus has to attach itself to a particular protein from its coat. The idea of injecting large quantities of this protein into patients' blood to attract the virus and thus divert it away from healthy cells is an attractive strategy, which Gallo and his team are now endeavoring to perfect.

Parallel with this research, the Bethesda team is collaborating with an eminent French scientist, Prof. Daniel Zagury, to develop a means of stimulating the immunological defenses of subjects infected with the AIDS virus. Combined with the taking of antiviral medicines such as AZT, this immunotherapy could offer someone who was seropositive a good chance of not developing AIDS.

Robert Gallo and his research scientists also managed to grow cells of Kaposi's tumors in their test tubes. This enabled them to understand the development process of cancer of the skin. They discovered that the AIDS virus generates a protein that makes cells from surface blood-vessel tissue increase abruptly in size. This stimulation in turn gives birth to other proteins, which set about manufacturing a parallel network of small arteries. These arteries proliferate in the lining of the normal arteries, thereby causing lesions on the mucous membranes and the skin. "This work may not be particularly spectacular," Robert Gallo would acknowledge, "but I don't believe that from now on we shall need any major discoveries to get to the bottom of AIDS. We have adequate technology and the essentials of the requisite knowledge. Victory is only a matter of time, experimentation, and dedication to pursuing the numerous research options open to us."

The development of a vaccine is obviously one of those options. Assigned in 1988 by the American Cancer Institute to direct a task force to develop a vaccine, Robert Gallo initiated several research programs both within the confines of his own laboratory and abroad. His retort to the defeatists who predict that no vaccine will be available before the year 2000 is that there is a good chance of seeing one developed within five years.

In recent years, the conspicuous increase in manpower and finances devoted to the struggle against AIDS has multiplied the number of teams and research centers everywhere. The result has been a disruption of staff in some laboratories. In 1989, two of Robert Gallo's principal biologists, Flossie Wong-Staal and Mikulas Popovic, both left to go and head new research projects, one in southern California, the other in New Mexico.

* * *

The Bru room team at the Pasteur Institute in Paris would experience similar disruptions. Jean-Claude Chermann and Françoise Barré-Sinoussi flew Luc Montagnier's nest. After receiving the Louis Pasteur medal in 1987, Prof. Jean-Claude Chermann left for Marseilles to assume the directorship of a team attached to IN-SERM, the national institute for health and medical research, specializing in studying the role of the HIV in AIDS-related diseases. Françoise Barré-Sinoussi, for her part, set up a new work group at the Pasteur Institute in Paris. The laboratory of retroviral biology she directs will devote itself to, among other research subjects, the detailed comparison of AIDS viruses of African origin with those deriving from elsewhere. Her work is also geared to developing a vaccine. The Parisian biologist is more than ever convinced that to achieve this end greater knowledge is needed of the relationship between the virus and the cells that harbor it. Direct experimentation with a vaccine on man is not possible. The number of monkeys available precludes wide-scale testing. Thus, her team is working steadily on finding a model animal that is capable of being infected, yet is both prolific and cheap, such as a mouse or some other small mammal. Only with a guinea pig of this kind will it be possible to progress toward the ultimate goal of their research: the complete immunization of people against the AIDS virus.

As for Prof. Luc Montagnier, his worldwide fame now obliges him, like Robert Gallo, to devote a large part of his time to various associated activities outside his laboratory. Traveling to conventions, scientific conferences, meetings with clinicians and patients, his involvement in all kinds of committees, the demands of the media, all compete for his time. In a letter addressed at the end of 1989 to the author of this book, Luc Montagnier wrote: "AIDS is still my prime concern . . . research is making rapid progress and my collaborators and I still contribute actively to it, but I am finding fresh motivation in my contact with patients doomed to slow and inevitable extinction. Every death is a failure of our science, a failure I experience personally. That is why the essential aim of my research is currently to understand the illness and the role of the virus by means of three approaches: *in vitro* in the culture flask, *in vivo* with animals, and finally, at the patient's bedside. From this understanding will come rational therapeutic strategies and vaccines. Although we appear currently to be marking time, I am optimistic as far as the reasonably near future is concerned. I hope to see the post-AIDS era."

*   *   *

No one shared this hope as fervently as the American who, during the first years of the epidemic, had so incessantly goaded the scientific world into investing in research for a medicine. Promoted in 1989 by President Bush to the post of director of the American National Cancer Institute, today Prof. Sam Broder coordinates the largest world undertaking to prevent and cure "the dread disease." This responsibility has not divorced him from his oncology laboratory where, in 1985, he and his two collaborators, Hiroaki Mitsuya and Bob Yarchoan, had made the critical discovery of the effectiveness of AZT in vitro, before carrying out the first tests of it on humans. Since then, Sam Broder and his team have submitted dozens of other substances to the verdict of their test tubes and come up with a whole arsenal of therapeutic strategies. Eight anti-AIDS protocols are the current subject of their experiments. In the last six years Sam Broder has published more than a hundred scientific papers and articles in the most prestigious international journals. All of this work reflects the obsession that, now more than ever, haunts the Polish survivor from the Nazi holocaust: that of saving lives.

Dr. Michael Gottlieb, the Los Angeles immunologist who, in 1980, identified the first AIDS case, left the University of California hospital in Los Angeles at the end of 1986 to open private practices in two of the city's suburbs where, because of the density of the gay male population, AIDS was striking with particular virulence. His experience in the field of clinical trials earned Michael Gottlieb nomination to head the AIDS treatment unit at the Sherman Oaks hospital, where he actively pursues his own research into the effectiveness of new substances.

Having struggled for three years to relieve the suffering of patients he could not save, Dr. Jack Dehovitz chose to withdraw provisionally from the battlefield to devote himself to the prevention of the disease. He left St. Clare's Hospital in Manhattan for the New York State university health center, where he is in charge of several prevention programs directed at the numerous ethnic minority groups that make up the population of Brooklyn. Substantial federal grants also enable the doctor to launch extensive epidemiological inquiries aimed at a better grasp of the public health problems posed by the spread of the epidemic.

* * *

In France, the doctor of the fashion designer whose lymph node made it possible to identify the AIDS virus has remained at his post. Today Prof. Willy Rozenbaum's department at the Rothschild Hospital in Paris is one of the French centers specializing in the treatment of the disease. Two of Willy Rozenbaum's patients with opportunistic infections, in one case Kaposi's sarcoma and in the other pneumocystis pneumonia, have survived to lead normal lives, one for seven years and the other for three and a half. The doctor attributes these results to the constant advances in therapeutic skills. While he waits for a panacea or a vaccine, he is convinced that the ever more judicious and precise combination of antiviral medicines will make it possible to prolong the lives of an ever increasing number of victims.

* * *

Eight years after launching his medical detectives from the Atlanta CDC on the trail of the killer virus, Dr. Jim Curran is also still involved. He and his collaborators have established a direct link between AIDS and the resurgence of infections that had previously almost disappeared, primarily tuberculosis and syphilis. They have identified most of the disease's possible means of transmission and provided in a hundred or so issues of their weekly bulletin an impressive list of recommendations on how people should protect themselves against the epidemic. This titanic effort bore tangible fruit in educational programs in all the United States' schools, in national media campaigns, and in preventive action conducted in collaboration with numerous organizations. Jim Curran is more than ever resolved to fight. "We're only at the beginning of the AIDS venture," he declares. "We've only written the first chapter. With a little bit of luck, I shall live long enough to tell my children about our victory over the plague."

*   *   *

After four years of serving the destitute victims of the cruel disease, Sister Ananda and Sister Paul left the New York home to go and continue their mission of charity in China. Today they are working in a suburb of Shanghai where, in 1988, Mother Teresa successfully managed to open an orphanage for spastic and mentally handicapped children. Twice a year, an envelope bearing stamps with red flags brings Philippe Malouf news of his Indian spiritual "fiancée" to whom he is still linked through prayer and whom he still hopes one day to meet. At the end of 1986, the monk left the Monastery of the Seven Agonies in Latrun to join another religious community in the country of his birth, Lebanon.

His spiritual bond with Sister Ananda is one of countless links in the chain of solidarity created by Mother Teresa between those who suffer and those who do active work. As she had wanted, this chain "forms a rosary of compassion around the world." The card indexes of Jacqueline de Decker, whom illness prevented from fulfilling her vocation in India and whom Mother Teresa placed at the head of the association for sick and suffering coworkers, contain the names of 4,500 ill and incurable people who offer their suffering for the daily work of about 3,000 Missionaries of Charity scattered over some eighty countries. About forty letters arrive each morning at Jacqueline de Decker's Antwerp home from sick and incurable people hoping to become additional beads on the rosary. The requests are so numerous that she has been obliged to "marry" several correspondents collectively to one single sister working in the field. Thus, for example, she has linked the residents of a Belgian psychiatric hospital with a nun who cares for lepers in the slums of Tanzania.

Mother Teresa's relentless crusade in the service of the poor was crowned with some spectacular victories during the year 1989. The indomitable nun and her little Sisters opened no less than five homes for the destitute, the old, and the needy in the USSR. Two of these institutions are located in distant Siberia.

On April 11, 1990, a brief announcement from the Vatican informed the world that the Pope had accepted the resignation of Mother Teresa from her duties as superior of the congregation of the Missionaries of Charity she had founded in 1950. On September 8, 1990, she called the heads of her various institutions to Calcutta to elect her successor. Unable to reach a unanimous decision on one of the three candidates to succeed her, the Electoral College opted to re-elect Mother Teresa. She accepted the challenge as "the expression of God's will" and announced she would soon leave for Romania and Czechoslovakia to open homes for destitute children stricken with AIDS. But her failing health had prevented her from carrying out this project. In September 1989, a serious heart attack had stopped her from embarking on another venture that was to be the crowning achievement of her exhausting crusade, the opening of an orphanage in the country of her birth, Albania, the last bastion of communism in Europe. She nearly died.

When she came out of the hospital, she was informed that the author of this book had just learned he had cancer with several chapters still left to write. She was determined to send him a message of comfort immediately. On the very day of the surgery that would restore him to health, he received a letter from her in her own handwriting: "Dear Dominique, at the same time Jesus' gift of sharing His Passion comes to both of us. My prayer and that of our Sisters and our Poor will be with you. Let us thank God for His great love for us."

ACKNOWLEDGMENTS

First and foremost I would like to express my enormous gratitude to my wife, Dominique, who shared every moment of my long and difficult research and whose assistance was indispensable in the preparation of this book.

My deepest thanks to Colette Modiano and Paul and Manuela Andreota, who spent long hours correcting my manuscript and gave me the support of their encouragement. My grateful thanks, too, to my friend Dr. Claudine Escoffier-Lambiotte, author of so many remarkable medical writings, for the care with which she so generously checked the accuracy of the scientific passages; to my friend Jean Mariaud de Serres, and to Dr. Madeline Farbrother, who checked the medical terminology of the English translation.

This book is the fruit of patient investigation with the help of numerous scientists, doctors, nurses, and patients. Without their active and generous collaboration, it would never have seen the light. In the United States, I would firstly like to thank Sam Broder, now director of the American National Cancer Institute, for having offered me so much of his valuable time in this department at the Bethesda hospital as well as at his charming Rossmore Drive home with his wife, Gail, and their two daughters.

Similarly, I would like to express my appreciation to Prof. Robert Gallo for the innumerable meetings we had in his research laboratory in building 37 on the Bethesda campus, in his car along the roads of Maryland, in his favorite trattorias of Washington with his scientist friends visiting from abroad, and in his Thornden Terrace home with his wife, Mary-Jane, their two sons, and the piles of Italian pastries of which he is so fond. I am particularly grateful to him for organizing one of his "high masses" specially for my benefit so that I could meet all the associates in his team, particularly the biologist Flossie Wong-Staal, Bill Blatner, Mikulas Popovic, Zaki Salahuddin, and the many others I am unable to mention here.

The Atlanta CDC was one of the central pivots of my research, and I would like to extend my very special gratitude to the head of its task force, Dr. James Curran, and his medical detectives Drs. Harold Jaffe, Martha Rogers, and all their colleagues, who helped me reconstruct in detail the fantastic hunt they embarked on for the virus suspected of being the AIDS agent.

Among the American doctors who had to confront the first cases of the terrible epidemic out in the field, I would like to address my particular thanks to Dr. Michael Gottlieb for the many days we spent together reconstructing down to the smallest detail the discovery of the five first cases that would alert the attention of the world's scientific community. Similarly, my heartfelt thanks to Drs. Alvin Friedman-Kien and Joseph Sonnabend of New York, Marcus Conant and Paul Volberding of San Francisco, and Peng Thim Fan and Joel Weisman of Los Angeles for their valuable contribution to that part of my research. Finally, my special gratitude goes to Dr. Jack Dehovitz for the detailed account he was kind enough to give of the traumatic experience he went through in New York's St. Clare's Hospital in the daily exercise of his care for the victims of the scourge.

Without the kind cooperation of Dr. David Barry and his collaborators Richard Clemons, Sandy Lehrman, Dannie King, Marty St. Clair, and several others, I would not have been able to re-create the moments of anguish and hope that marked the momentous development of the first effective medicine against AIDS. I would like to thank them all for their contribution to my research in the workrooms of the Burroughs Wellcome laboratories on the Research Triangle Park campus. I would also like to thank Dr. Ellen

Cooper, representative of the Food and Drug Administration, for all the time she gave me in her glass beehive headquarters in Rockville, Maryland, helping me relive the peripeties that led up to the authorization of the trials of AZT on humans. My gratitude also goes to Dr. Mathilde Krim for the patience with which, in her private mansion in New York, she told me of how her campaign for the distribution of AZT to all patients had given those under sentence of death from AIDS a first glimmer of hope.

Among those condemned people, it goes without saying that, first and foremost, I would like to thank with much emotion and sadness Josef Stein. I shall never forget the long conversations we had at his bedside in the spring of 1986 when he was fighting the fatal virus with so much flair. I shall not forget how on the eve of his death, he had the postcard I sent him of my village, Ramatuelle—where he was never able to come and convalesce—put up on the window of his room next to the view of Jerusalem he had been sent by his monk friend in Latrun. I would like to include in this tribute all the other patients and all those who are so dedicated to their service, especially the archbishop of New York, Cardinal John O'Connor, and Msgr. James Cassidy, thanks to whom it was possible to set up the Gift of Love home for destitute AIDS sufferers; the director of St. Clare's Hospital, Richard Yezzo; Dr. Deborah Spicehandler; nurses Ron Peterson and Gloria Taylor, social workers George Lafontane and John Wright, the clinic coordinator Terry Miles.

A large proportion of my research was conducted at the Pasteur Institute in Paris and in several Paris hospitals, and so my sincere thanks go to Prof. Luc Montagnier for agreeing to spend some of his precious time reconstructing those memorable days of winter 1983 when he and his team were trying to rise to the greatest medical challenge of this end of a millennium. Among the members of that team I would especially like to thank Prof. Jean-Claude Chermann and Dr. Françoise Barré-Sinoussi, codiscoverers of the AIDS virus. In the very place where they had experienced their victory, they reenacted for me the many steps involved in their research into the famous reverse transcriptase enzyme that would turn out to be the "signature" by which the virus was identified. I include in this tribute Prof. André Lwoff, winner of the Nobel Prize for medicine, who was kind enough to give me the benefit of his advice; Prof. Daniel Zagury, who answered my questions at a time when he was trying out on himself the vaccine he is engaged in developing; Dr. Françoise Brun-Vézinet, who took the samples of the tumor cells that served to isolate the virus; Prof. Willy Rozenbaum, who agreed, in the course of several interviews in cafés near Claude-Bernard Hospital, to speak of the drama of his confrontations with the first AIDS patients. Similarly I would like to thank Dr. Christine Rouzioux, who told me the story of the development of the first seropositivity test; Dr. Jacques Leibowitch, who was kind enough to recount his memorable journey to Bethesda to try to persuade Robert Gallo to "give it everything he'd got." This list of acknowledgments would be seriously incomplete without the inclusion of Charles and Claudine Dauguet. The hours spent in their company in the very place where "Charlie" took the world's first photograph of the AIDS virus will remain among the most compelling memories of my life as a researcher and writer.

I would also like to convey my heartfelt gratitude to all those who gave unfailingly of their encouragement and affection during the long process of the researching and writing this book, particularly my daughter Alexandra, Rina and Takis Anoussis, Chuck and Red Barris, Julia Bizieau, Larry and Nadia Collins, Laura Fry, Françoise and Pierre Gautier, Alain and Clémentine Gomez, Marie de Hennezel, André Lewin and Catherine Clément, Anna and Jean-Bernard Mérimée, Heidi Wurzer.

I would never have been able to write this book without the enthusiasm and faith of my friend and literary agent Morton L. Janklow, together with Anne Sibbald and Cynthia Cannell, and the longstanding, loyal trust of my publishers: Robert Laffont in Paris; Mario Lacruz in Barcelona; Larry Kirshbaum in New York; Giancarlo Bonacina in Milan. I wish to extend my very special gratitude to my friend and translator Kathryn Spink, author herself of remarkable books on Mother Teresa, Brother Roger of Taizé, and Jean Vanier, founder of a chain of institutions for mentally handicapped children and adults. To Larry Kirshbaum goes also my special gratitude for his many valuable contributions to the American edition of this book.

I would like to express my very special gratitude, admiration, and affection to Mother Teresa and the sisters who contributed so much to my research, together with Jacqueline de Decker, Fr. Céleste Van

Exem, François Laborde, James Stevens, Brother Gaston, Brother Philippe, and Dr. Kumar Chanemougame.

Finally, it is thanks to the skills and talent of Drs. Pierre Leandri and Georges Rossignol, who operated on me, to the competence and dedicated care of their team at Saint-Jean-du-Languedoc's clinic in Toulouse that I am cured of cancer. They can be assured of my warmest gratitude.

INDEX